Essential Obstetrics and Gynaecology

E. Malcolm Symonds
MD FRCOG FFPHM FACOG (Hon)

Foundation Professor of Obstetrics and Gynaecology
University of Nottingham, Nottingham, UK

Ian M. Symonds
DM BMedSci BM BS MRCOG

Lecturer, Department of Obstetrics and Gynaecology, University of
Nottingham, Nottingham, UK

*Illustrated by Geoffrey Lyth BA and
Patrick Elliot BA(Hons) ATC MMAA AIMI RMIP*

THIRD EDITION

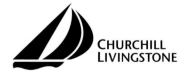

CHURCHILL
LIVINGSTONE

EDINBURGH LONDON NEW YORK PHILADELPHIA SYDNEY TORONTO 1998

CHURCHILL LIVINGSTONE
An imprint of Harcourt Brace and Company Limited

© Longman Group UK Limited 1987, 1992
Assigned to Pearson Professional Ltd 1995
© Pearson Professional Limited 1998
© Harcourt Brace and Company Limited 1999

◪ is a registered trademark of Harcourt Brace and
Company Limited

First edition 1987
Second edition 1992
Third edition 1998
  Reprinted 1999

Standard edition ISBN 0 443 05453 3

International Student Edition of 3rd edition published 1998

International Student Edition ISBN 0 4430 5551 3

British Library of Cataloguing in Publication Data
A catalogue record for this book is available from the British
Library.

Library of Congress Cataloging in Publication Data
A catalog record for this book is available from the Library of
Congress.

Medical knowledge is constantly changing. As new
information becomes available, changes in treatment,
procedures, equipment and the use of drugs become
necessary. The authors and the publishers have, as far as it is
possible, taken care to ensure that the information given in
this text is accurate and up to date. However, readers are
strongly advised to confirm that the information, especially
with regard to drug usage, complies with current legislation
and standards of practice.

Printed in China
NPCC/03

Preface to the third edition

The first edition of this book was published in 1987 and the second edition in 1992 and has been translated into Spanish and Mandarin. Dr Ian Symonds has joined me as joint author and has been a collaborator in revising and updating the text and in the addition of new sections. Textbooks tend to assume a life of their own by the third edition and I have received many suggestions as to how the book can be improved and expanded. Given the rapidly changing profile of the discipline, I started with the presumption that it will be impossible to satisfy everyone and that I must adhere to the principle of simple, direct and, at times, dogmatic statements. The book continues to expand, despite my best efforts to keep the text as focused as possible.

I am once again indebted to my secretary, Mrs Sue Kirk, for retyping the manuscript and to Mrs Jo Swallow for updating the section on imaging. Dr Simon Fishel revised some aspects of the chapter on reproductive biology and Dr Malcolm Anderson provided helpful advice on updating the chapter on the cervix. Finally, Margaret Oates, the only other author in this book, has contributed an additional chapter on the psychological aspects of gynaecology and I am greatly in her debt for the two chapters she has now contributed.

I have added an additional chapter on medicolegal issues which now form important determinants in the practice of obstetrics and gynaecology. Whilst these are matters that have a parochial aspect to them, the legal principles on which much of British legislation is based are reflected in the legal systems of many other countries.

It was a source of considerable regret to me that Mr Geoffrey Lyth retired shortly after the first edition was published. This year, I have been delighted to be joined by Mr Patrick Elliott who has created new illustrations and modified some of the earlier drawings.

Finally, I would like to acknowledge the forbearance of my publishers in accepting the delays caused by the exigencies of decanal life in revising this third edition.

Nottingham 1997   E. Malcolm Symonds

Preface to the first edition

This combined textbook of obstetrics and gynaecology presents the *essential* information required by medical students in their clinical course. At most medical schools obstetrics and gynaecology is given only 8 weeks of the clinical curriculum since there is a long-held belief that it is a postgraduate subject. Nothing, of course, could be further from the truth. Although obstetrics has become more hospital based, gynaecology has become increasingly important in general practice, with all the problems related to fertility regulation and the increasing awareness by women of the many functional disorders of the menstrual cycle. However, the fact remains that 8 weeks is the usual allocation for undergraduate clinical training in obstetrics and gynaecology.

Therefore, this textbook has been written to provide the core of knowledge which medical students need to supplement their clinical experience and help them to master the essentials of obstetrics and gynaecology in that short 8 week period. It has been planned to bridge the gap between the vast postgraduate tomes and the very brief list of facts in the 'pocket' books, providing students with one combined course book. I hope that it will also be of interest as an introduction to the subject for other health professionals.

As I have written each chapter, I have constantly reminded myself of a review written by an experienced paediatrician of an undergraduate textbook in which he counted 200 named syndromes. He had seen only four of these syndromes in a busy lifetime of clinical practice! I have tried to focus throughout on the common conditions encountered in clinical practice and not the small print required in an encyclopaedia text. Particular emphasis has been placed on certain chapters that form the physiological basis of obstetrical and gynaecological practice. For example, the chapters on physiological changes in pregnancy and on conception and nidation are essential platforms on which to build a knowledge of abnormal states of fertility and reproduction and therefore receive greater emphasis than many other sections.

Of course, some of the sections such as those related to the mechanisms of normal and abnormal labour remain essentially unchanged since these mechanisms were described by William Smellie and yet are still fundamental to an understanding of the management of parturition and its complications.

I owe a considerable debt to many people in compiling this textbook – first and foremost to Mr Geoffrey Lyth, who has thoughtfully designed and drawn the numerous diagrams and tables which have been planned to complement and enhance the text, and act as a series of 'aides memoire'. The line drawings have been kept as simple as possible with a limited use of colour to emphasize particular points that are central to the narrative.

I also owe a great deal to my staff over the years who have helped in the formulation of the text. In particular, Mr G. M. Filshie and Mr R. R. Sanders played an important role in the evolution of the notes that formed the basis of many sections of this text. Dr Margaret Oates in the Department of Psychiatry, University of Nottingham, wrote the chapter on mental disorders in pregnancy. Dr Alexandra Tobert made a major contribution to the chapter on sexual disorders. I am particularly grateful for their contributions. Mr Martin Powell, Professor Brian Worthington and Mrs Josephine Swallow all provided invaluable assistance with the chapter on imaging. The book has been read and helpfully criticized by Dr Keith Louden, Dr Martin Walker and Mr Michael Martin. Dr Malcolm Lewis provided helpful information on serology and microbiology, and Dr Richard Madeley on perinatal and maternal mortality.

The text has been typed by Miss Catherine Greasley, Mrs Ann-Marie Kay, Mrs Gillian Bradshaw and Mrs Kathleen Nicholson, but the real problems of organizing and completing the text have rested in the capable hands of Mrs Sue Alvey.

Finally, I owe a great debt to Mrs Sue Symonds for patiently reading and correcting the text, and to my son, Matthew, for correcting the spelling errors!

Nottingham, 1987   E. M. S.

Contents

1 History and examination in obstetrics

INTRODUCTION

There are many features that are common to history-taking in any section of medical practice. However, there are also special areas that are central to the history in obstetrics and gynaecology, and knowledge of these factors is essential to good practice in these disciplines.

The term 'obstetrics' relates to the study and management of normal and abnormal pregnancy. The term 'gynaecology' describes the study of diseases of the female genital tract. There is a continuum between both subjects so that the division is sometimes arbitrary. Complications of early pregnancy, such as abortion, are often considered under the title of gynaecology, but more properly lie within the definition of obstetrics.

OBSTETRIC HISTORY

The relevant history in obstetrics can be considered under the present pregnancy, previous obstetric history, and previous medical and family history.

Present pregnancy

The commonest presenting symptom of pregnancy is the cessation of periods, i.e. secondary amenorrhoea, in a woman having regular menstruation. Therefore, it is important to ascertain the date of the first day of the last menstrual period. It must be remembered that this information is often inaccurate, simply because many women do not record the days on which they menstruate and, unless the date of the period is associated with some particular event, precise dates are not remembered.

The length of the menstrual cycle is also important. Ovulation usually occurs on the 14th day before menstruation, but the time interval between menstruation and ovulation – the proliferative phase of the menstrual cycle – may vary substantially. The length of the cycle always describes the time interval between the first day of the period and the first day of the subsequent period. This may vary from 21 to 42 days in normal women, but menstruation usually occurs every 28 days.

It is important to ascertain the method of contraception employed prior to conception. The date of onset of the periods – the **menarche** – is recorded, although it is not particularly relevant to the obstetric history.

The **estimated date of delivery** can be calculated if one knows the date of the first day of the last menstrual period and the usual length of the menstrual cycle (Fig. 1.1). The average duration is 269 days from the date of conception. In a 28 day cycle, the estimated date of confinement can be calculated by subtracting 3 months from the date of the first day of the last menstrual period and adding on 10 days. About 40% of women will deliver within 5 days of the estimated date of confinement and about two-thirds within 10 days.

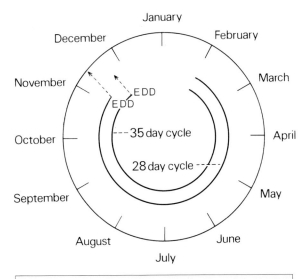

Fig. 1.1 Calculation of the estimated date of delivery (EDD).

If the normal menstrual cycle is less than 28 days or greater than 28 days, an appropriate number of days should be subtracted from or added to the estimated date of confinement. For example, if the normal cycle is 35 days, 7 days should be added to the estimated date of confinement. A history of taking oral contraceptive steroids may result in a delay in ovulation, particularly in the first cycle after discontinuation of the pill.

Obstetric history

- Period of amenorrhoea
- Previous obstetric history
- Condition of previous infants at birth
- Previous medical history
- Family history

Symptoms of pregnancy

In addition to the symptom of amenorrhoea, various other symptoms are common in early pregnancy.

Nausea and vomiting commonly occur within 2 weeks of missing the first period. Although described as morning sickness, vomiting may occur at any time of the day, particularly during the first 3 months of pregnancy. Thereafter, this symptom tends to disappear although it may sometimes persist throughout pregnancy.

Frequency of micturition occurs in early pregnancy and cannot be explained on the basis of pressure from the pregnant uterus as it tends to diminish after 12 weeks gestation.

Plasma osmolality falls soon after conception, and the ability to excrete a water load is altered in early pregnancy. There is an increased diuretic response after water loading when the woman is sitting upright and this response declines by the third trimester. However, it may be sufficient to cause urinary frequency in early pregnancy.

Excessive lassitude is a common symptom of pregnancy and may be apparent even before the first period is missed. Again, it tends to disappear after 12 weeks gestation but is often the most noticeable symptom experienced by many women.

Breast tenderness and '*heaviness*', symptoms which are really an extension of those experienced by many women in the premenstrual phase of the cycle, are common, and are particularly apparent in the month after the first period is missed.

Fetal movements or '*quickening*' are not usually noticed until 20 weeks gestation in the woman having her first pregnancy and 18 weeks in the second or subsequent pregnancies. However, many women experience fetal movements earlier than these times and others may succeed in reaching full term without ever being aware of movements.

Occasionally, an abnormal desire for a particular food may occur and this is known as **pica**.

Symptoms of pregnancy

- Secondary amenorrhoea
- Nausea and vomiting
- Frequency of micturition
- Breast tenderness
- Lassitude

Pseudocyesis

All of these symptoms and many of the signs may develop in the absence of pregnancy, giving rise to a condition known as **pseudocyesis**.

An intense desire for or fear of pregnancy may cause stimulation of the hypothalamus and release of gonadotrophic hormones. The condition may be particularly difficult to diagnose because the physical signs of early pregnancy will often be apparent.

Biochemical confirmation that pregnancy has not occurred will usually convince the patient, but subsequent sympathetic support will be necessary to resolve the anxieties associated with the condition.

Previous obstetric history

The term **gravidity** is the same as pregnancy, and a gravida is a woman who is pregnant. A primigravida is a woman who is pregnant for the first time, and a multigravida is a woman who has been pregnant several times (Fig. 1.2A).

This term must be distinguished from **parity**, which is a description of having given birth to an infant, alive or dead, with a birth weight of 500 g or more and a gestational age in excess of 24 weeks (Fig. 1.2B). Thus, a primipara is a woman who has given birth to one or more infants as a result of one pregnancy. Multiple pregnancies are counted as singleton as far as the term 'parity' is concerned. A multipara is a woman who has given birth on two or more occasions to infants weighing 500 g or more (Fig. 1.2C).

A nulliparous woman has not given birth to a viable infant (Fig. 1.2D). A grand multipara has given birth to viable infants on five or more occasions. Thus, a pregnant woman who has given birth to three viable singleton pregnancies and has had two miscarriages would be described as a gravida 6, para 3 – a multigravid multiparous woman.

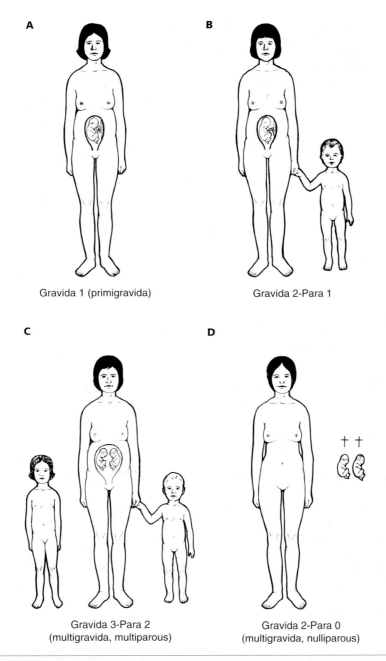

A Gravida 1 (primigravida)

B Gravida 2-Para 1

C Gravida 3-Para 2
(multigravida, multiparous)

D Gravida 2-Para 0
(multigravida, nulliparous)

Fig. 1.2 **A** Gravidity refers to the number of times a woman has been pregnant; **B** parity refers to the number of times she has delivered potentially viable children; **C** an example of multigravidity and multiparity; **D** a multigravid but nulliparous woman who has miscarried twice.

A parturient is a woman in labour, and a puerpera has given birth to a child during the preceding 42 days.

A record should be made of all previous pregnancies, including details of previous miscarriages and the length of gestation. In particular, it is important to note any previous antenatal complications, details of induction of labour, the length of labour, and the method of delivery. Complications of the puerperium, such as postpartum haemorrhage, infections of the genital tract and urinary system, a history of deep vein thrombosis and perineal complications may all have relevance to future pregnancies. The condition of each infant at birth and the birth weight, presentation at delivery and sex should be noted.

Previous medical history

Various medical conditions will have a significant bearing on pregnancy. Thus, it is important to note a history of diabetes, renal disease, hypertension, cardiac disease and thyrotoxicosis. Tuberculosis, syphilis and liver disease may all affect pregnancy, as may the drugs employed in the treatment of any of these conditions.

Family history

A wide variety of conditions which are genetically transmitted may have importance in the family history. In practical terms, most women will be aware of the family history of any major disorders and it is not necessary to list a catalogue of these diseases. An enquiry as to whether there are any known inherited conditions in the family will usually be sufficient, except where one or both partners are adopted and are not aware of their family histories.

Meticulous attention to the family history and past obstetric history, maternal age and medical condition may allow the precise risk of fetal abnormality to be estimated, and the appropriate prenatal screening tests to be implemented.

OBSTETRIC EXAMINATION

At the initial visit a complete physical examination should be undertaken.

Height is recorded, as it may provide the first indication of a small pelvis. Weight is recorded at the first and all subsequent visits.

Blood pressure is recorded with the patient supine and in the lateral supine position in late pregnancy to avoid compression of the inferior vena cava (Fig. 1.3). Apart from the effect this has on the blood pressure, the direct supine position may produce syncope and nausea in the mother, a condition which is known as the **supine hypotensive syndrome**. Blood pressure should always be recorded in the same way to give comparable measurements. Diastolic blood pressure should be taken on the fourth Korotkov sound as the point at

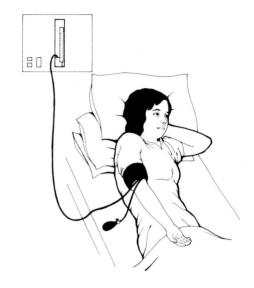

Fig. 1.3 Blood pressure recording standardized in the left lateral supine position.

which the sound disappears is often difficult to determine in pregnancy.

Head and neck

Many women develop pigmentation over the forehead and cheeks, particularly when the complexion is dark and there is frequent exposure to sunlight. This is known as **chloasma** (Fig. 1.4).

The colour of mucosal surfaces such as those of the mouth and conjunctivae should be examined for pallor, and the general state of dentition should be noted. Pregnancy is often associated with hypertrophic gingivitis. Dental caries should be treated and appropriate advice given in dental hygiene. Some degree of thyroid enlargement is normal in pregnancy, but abnormal thyroid enlargement associated with tachycardia should arouse suspicion of hyperthyroidism.

Heart and lungs

A careful examination of the heart should be made to exclude organic murmurs. Flow murmurs are common in pregnancy and are of no significance (Fig. 1.5). Occasionally a mammary souffle may be heard arising from the internal mammary arteries, which can be confused with a systolic murmur. The sound is audible in the second intercostal space, and will disappear with pressure from the stethoscope.

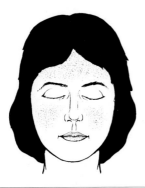

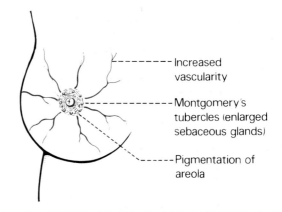

Fig. 1.6   Physiological changes in the breast in early pregnancy.

Fig. 1.4   'Chloasma' – facial pigmentation over the forehead and cheeks.

Breasts

The breasts show characteristic changes in pregnancy, which are apparent within the first 8 weeks (Fig. 1.6). The breasts should be examined to exclude the presence of any lumps and to note the condition of the nipples. Inverted nipples may give rise to difficulties with breast feeding and may be helped by the use of breast shields.

Abdomen

Examination of the abdomen commonly shows the presence of stretch marks or **striae gravidarum**. Marks from previous pregnancies have a silvery white appearance, whereas recent striae are a purplish red. The striae follow the lines of stress in the skin of the abdominal wall and may also occur on the lateral aspect of the thighs and the breasts. Hepatosplenomegaly should be excluded as well as any renal enlargement. The uterus does not become palpable as an abdominal organ until after 12 weeks gestation. The linea alba often becomes pigmented, and is known as the **linea nigra**. This pigmentation persists after the first pregnancy.

Limbs

The legs should be examined for evidence of varicose veins. Also, note should be made of any shortening

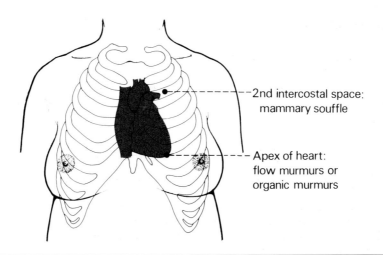

Fig. 1.5   Flow murmurs in normal pregnancy.

5

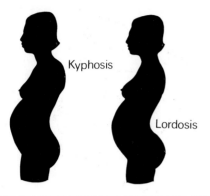

Fig. 1.7 Postural changes in pregnancy: with enlargement of the gravid uterus there is an increased lumbar lordosis and a tendency to some degree of kyphosis.

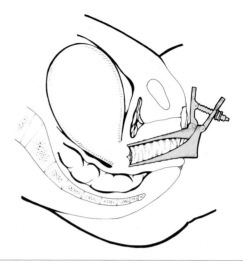

Fig. 1.8 Insertion of a bivalve speculum enables examination of the cervix and vaginal walls.

and of any skeletal abnormalities and, in particular, of evidence of any kyphosis or lordosis (Fig. 1.7). Normal pregnancy is associated with an increase in lumbar lordosis, which frequently causes lumbar backache.

Pelvic examination

Three functions are served by pelvic examination in early pregnancy at the first attendance. The examination should confirm the presence of a pregnancy, exclude any pelvic tumours and enable a preliminary assessment of the size and shape of the bony pelvis.

Signs of pregnancy

The mother should be examined resting comfortably in the supine position with her knees drawn up and heels resting together on the examination couch.

The vulva should be examined to exclude any abnormal lesions and to asses the state of the perineum in relation to any damage sustained during previous pregnancies. Varicosities of the vulva are common and may become worse during pregnancy.

Having completed the external examination, the next important stage is the internal examination. The essential point to remember about pelvic examination is that it should be performed with the greatest gentleness. Rough and painful examination reduces the amount of information obtained, as the pelvic floor and abdominal wall musculature will be tensed and the mother will lose confidence in the examiner.

Speculum examination is performed with the mother supine or in the left lateral position. If the left lateral position is employed, a Sims' speculum is used, but if the patient is examined in the supine position, a bivalve duckbill speculum is employed (Fig. 1.8). It is important to remember that the vagina runs posteriorly towards the sacrum and that the canal is widest transversely with an H-shaped cavity.

The blades of the speculum should be carefully smeared on the external surfaces with a thin layer of lubricant. The inferior blade of the speculum should be gently applied to the introitus and pressure applied towards the anus. The blades are then introduced in the line of the vagina, and when the blades are fully inserted they should be opened to expose the cervix. Remember also that the largest part of the vagina is the vaginal vault so that the speculum should not be withdrawn until the blades are closed.

The vaginal walls become more rugous as the stratified epithelium thickens with an increase in the glycogen content of the epithelial cells. There is a marked increase in vascularity of the paravaginal tissues so that the appearance of the vaginal walls becomes purplish red. There is an increase in vaginal secretions associated with vaginal transudation, increased shedding of epithelial cells and some contribution from the cervical mucus.

The cervix becomes softened and shows signs of increased vascularity. Enlargement of the cervix is associated with an increase in vascularity and

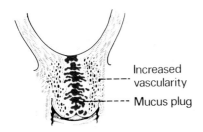

Increased
vascularity

Mucus plug

Fig. 1.9 Cervical changes in pregnancy include increased glandular content and a thick mucus plug.

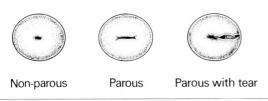

Non-parous   Parous   Parous with tear

Fig. 1.10 Appearances of the cervical os in relation to parity.

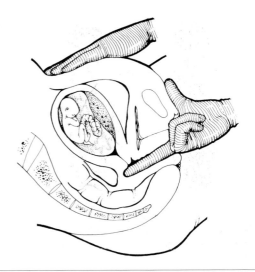

Fig. 1.11 Bimanual examination of the pregnant uterus.

oedema of the connective tissues, and cellular hyperplasia and hypertrophy. The glandular content of the endocervix increases to occupy half the substance of the cervix and produces a thick plug of viscoid mucus, occluding the cervical os (Fig. 1.9).

The cervix should be examined to exclude any evidence of pathology and of previous evidence of cervical damage. The nulliparous external cervical os is circular, while the parous os is a transverse slit, and this sometimes extends into the lateral vaginal fornix where cervical damage is sustained during childbirth (Fig. 1.10). A cervical smear is taken as a routine procedure in all women, and the speculum is then removed.

A digital examination is now performed. The middle finger of the examining hand should be introduced into the vaginal introitus and pressure applied towards the rectum (Fig. 1.11). As the introitus opens, the index finger is introduced as well. The cervix is palpated and feels softened.

The size and shape of the uterus is palpated bimanually. The abdominal hand compresses the uterus onto the vaginal hand. In early pregnancy the uterus feels soft and becomes globular in shape. It is palpable abdominally by 12 weeks gestation. Care is also taken to exclude uterine and ovarian tumours.

Assessment of the bony pelvis

The shape and size of the bony pelvis are critical determinants in the outcome of labour. The bony pelvis consists of the sacrum, the coccyx and two innominate bones. The pelvic area above the iliopectineal line is known as the **false pelvis**, and the area below the pelvic brim is known as the **true pelvis**. The latter is the important section in relation to childbearing and parturition. Thus, the wall of the true pelvis is formed from the sacrum posteriorly, the ischial bones, the sacro-sciatic notches and ligaments laterally, and anteriorly by the pubic rami, the obturator fossae and membranes, the ascending rami of the ischial bones and the pubic bones (Fig. 1.12). The shape and the dimensions of the true pelvis are best understood by consideration of the four planes of the pelvis.

The **plane of the pelvic inlet** or **pelvic brim** is bounded posteriorly by the sacral promontory, laterally by the ilio-pectineal line and anteriorly by the superior pubic rami and upper margin of the pubic symphysis. The plane is almost circular in the normal female or gynaecoid pelvis but is slightly larger transversely than antero-posteriorly.

The true conjugate or antero-posterior diameter of the pelvic inlet is the distance between the mid-point of the sacral promontory and the superior margin of the pubic symphysis anteriorly (Fig. 1.13B). The diameter measures approximately 11 cm. The shortest diameter, the one of greatest clinical significance, is the obstetric conjugate diameter. This is the distance between the midpoint of the sacral promontory and the nearest point on the posterior surface of the pubic symphysis. It is not possible to measure either of these diameters by

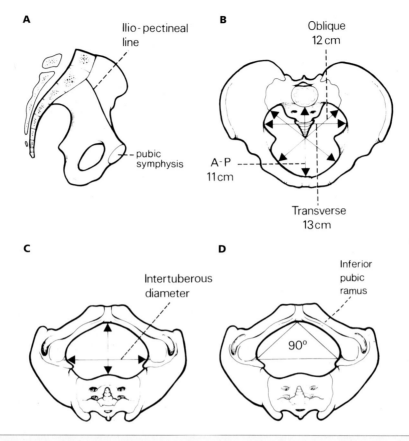

Fig. 1.12   **A,B** Inlet of the true pelvis bounded by the sacral promontory, ilio-pectineal line, pubic rami and pubic symphysis; **C,D** pelvis outlet bounded by the inferior pubic rami, the ischial tuberosities and the sacro-sciatic ligament; the inferior pubic rami should form an angle of 90°.

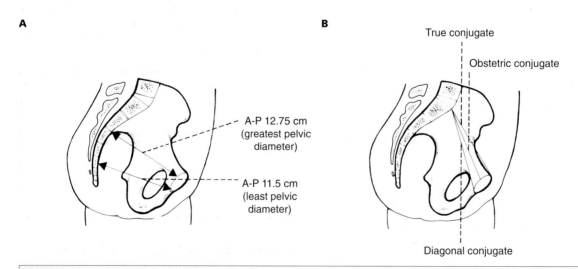

Fig. 1.13   **A** Antero-posterior diameters of the mid-cavity and pelvic outlet; **B** conjugate diameters of the pelvic inlet.

A   B

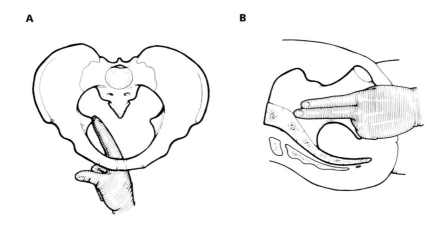

Fig. 1.14 **A** Clinical assessment of the ischial spines and the plane of least pelvic dimensions; **B** assessment of the pelvic inlet.

clinical examination, and the only diameter at the pelvic inlet that is amenable to clinical assessment is the distance from the inferior margin of the pubic symphysis to the midpoint of the sacral promontory. This is known as the diagonal conjugate diameter, and is approximately 1.5 cm greater than the obstetric conjugate diameter. In practical terms, it is not usually possible to reach the sacral promontory on clinical examination, and the highest point that can be palpated is the second or third piece of the sacrum. If the sacral promontory is easily palpable, the pelvic inlet is contracted (Fig. 1.14).

The **plane of greatest pelvic dimensions** has little clinical significance and has an anteroposterior and transverse diameter of approximately 12.7 cm. The antero-posterior diameter extends from the midpoint of the posterior aspect of the pubic symphysis to the junction of the second and third pieces of the sacrum. The transverse diameter passes laterally through the middle of the acetabuli. The only indication of the shape of the pelvis at this level is the curvature of the sacrum and the shape of the sacro-sciatic notch, which should subtend an angle of 90°.

The **plane of least pelvic dimensions** represents the level at which impaction of the fetal head is most likely to occur. The antero-posterior diameter extends from the inferior margin of the pubic symphysis and transects the line drawn between the ischial spines or the transverse diameter of the mid pelvis. Both the transverse (interspinous) and the antero-posterior diameter can be assessed clinically, and the interspinous diameter is the narrowest space in the pelvis (10 cm). The ischial spines should be palpated

to see if they are prominent and also to estimate the distance between them (Fig. 1.14A).

The **outlet of the pelvis** consists of two triangular planes. Anteriorly, the triangle is bounded by the area under the pubic arch, which should normally subtend an angle of 90°, and the transverse diameter, which is the distance between the ischial tuberosities, or intertuberous diameter (11 cm). The posterior triangle is formed anteriorly by the intertuberous diameter and postero-laterally by the tip of the sacrum and the sacro-sciatic ligaments. Clinically, the intertuberous diameter can be assessed by placing the knuckles of the clenched fist between the ischial tuberosities. The subpubic angle can be assessed by placing the index fingers of both hands along the inferior pubic rami, or by inserting two fingers of the examining hand under the pubic arch.

Obstetric examination at booking

- Height and weight
- Blood pressure
- Dentition
- Heart sounds
- Breasts/nipples
- Abdominal palpation
- Pelvic examination (smear)
- Legs
- Urinalysis

Obstetric examination at routine visits

At all antenatal visits, the blood pressure should be recorded and urine tested for glucose, protein and ketone bodies. Maternal weight should increase by an average of 0.5 kg per week from 16 weeks gestation, and the weight gain results from both fetal and maternal contributions. Maternal factors include contributions from breast enlargement, myometrial hypertrophy, an expansion of blood volume, retention of tissue water and deposition of fat and protein. The fetal contribution arises from the placenta and membranes, the weight of amniotic fluid and the weight of the fetus.

Rapid and excessive weight gain nearly always indicates abnormal fluid retention, and is often associated with pitting oedema of the legs, abdominal wall and fingers. Static weight or weight loss may indicate intra-uterine fetal growth retardation.

ABDOMINAL EXAMINATION

Palpation of the uterine fundus

The estimation of gestational age is the first step in examination of the abdomen in the pregnant woman; there are several methods employed to assess the size of the fetus. The ulnar border of the left hand is placed on the uterine fundus (Fig. 1.15). The uterus first becomes palpable suprapubically at 12 weeks gestation, and by 20 weeks gestation it has reached the level of the umbilicus. At 36 weeks gestation the uterine fundus is palpable at the level of the xiphisternum and then tends to remain at this height until term, or to fall as the head enters the pelvic brim. All methods of clinical assessment of

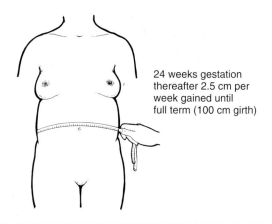

24 weeks gestation thereafter 2.5 cm per week gained until full term (100 cm girth)

Fig. 1.16 Estimation of girth circumference at the level of the umbilicus.

gestational age and fetal size are subject to considerable inaccuracies. The fundal height may also be described in relation to the xiphisternum.

Measurement of girth provides an alternative method of assessment (Fig. 1.16). Assuming that the average girth measurement in the non-pregnant state is 60 cm, no significant increase will occur until 24 weeks gestation. Thereafter, the girth should increase by 2.5 cm with each week of gestation, so that at full term the girth will be 100 cm. If the non-pregnant girth is greater or less than 60 cm, appropriate allowance must be made. Thus, a woman with a normal 65 cm girth would have a girth measurement of 95 cm at 36 weeks.

Measurement of symphysial–fundal height

A further method of assessing gestational age is based on the measurement of symphysial–fundal height. The distance between the uterine fundus and the top of the symphysis pubis is measured in centimetres. The mean fundal height measures approximately 20 cm at 20 weeks gestation and increases to approximately 36 cm by 36 weeks gestation. Thereafter the distance tends to plateau until full term. Using two standard deviations from the mean, it is possible to describe the 10th and 90th centile values. Using this technique on a serial basis, approximately 75% of all small-for-dates infants can be detected, and the maximum accuracy of detection occurs at 32–33 weeks gestation. It will be appreciated that accuracy is considerably less if the measurement is made after 36 weeks gestation.

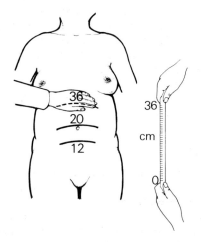

Fig. 1.15 Palpation of the uterine fundus: measurement of the fundus – symphysis height is a useful method of assessing gestational age.

The predictive value is lower for large-for-dates infants, and is stated to be lowest in approximately 65% of these infants. The technique is simple and easily applicable in routine antenatal care. It is particularly useful where other more precise measurements such as those from ultrasound cephalometry are not available routinely.

Palpation of fetal parts

Fetal parts are not usually palpable before 24 weeks gestation. When palpating the fetus, it must be remembered that the presence of amniotic fluid necessitates the use of 'dipping' movements with flexion of the fingers at the metacarpo-phalangeal joints. The purpose of palpation is to describe the relationship of the fetus to the maternal trunk and pelvis (Fig. 1.17).

Lie

The term **lie** describes the relationship of the long axis of the fetus to the long axis of the uterus (Fig. 1.18). Facing the feet of the mother, the examiner's left hand is placed along the left side of the abdomen, and the right hand is placed along the right lateral aspect of the uterus. Systematic palpation towards the midline will reveal either the firm resistance of the fetal back or fetal limbs.

If the lie is **longitudinal**, the head or breech will be palpable over the pelvic inlet. If the lie is **oblique**, the long axis lies at an angle of 45° to the long axis of the uterus, and the presenting part will be palpable in the iliac fossa. In a **transverse** lie,

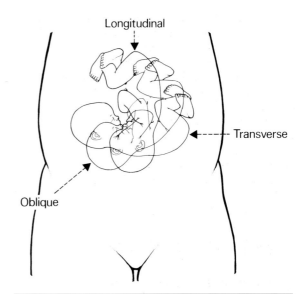

Fig. 1.18 Fetal lie describes the relationship of the long axis of the fetus to the long axis of the uterus.

the fetus lies at right angles to the mother, and the poles of the fetus are palpable in the flanks.

Having ascertained the lie and the position of the fetal back, it is important now to feel for the head and breech by firm pressure with alternate hands. The head is hard, round and discreet. It can be 'bounced' between the examining hands, and is described as being ballotable. The buttocks are softer and more diffuse, and the breech is not ballotable. The head should be sought in the lower abdomen or in the uterine fundus. Facing the mother's feet, firm pressure is applied over the presenting part. If the head is presenting, note is made of whether it is easily palpable or whether it is necessary to apply deep pressure.

The normal attitude of the fetus is one of flexion (Fig. 1.19) but, on occasions, it may exhibit an attitude of extension.

Presentation

In a longitudinal lie, the presenting part may be the head (cephalic) or the breech (podalic). In a transverse lie, the presenting part is a shoulder.

Depending on the degree of flexion or deflexion, various parts of the head will present to the pelvic inlet. Where the head is well flexed, the presentation is the **vertex** – the area which lies between the anterior and posterior fontanelles. If the head is completely extended, the **face** presents to the pelvic

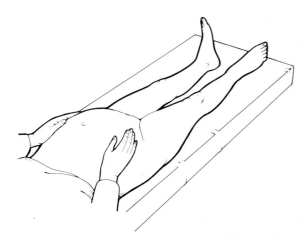

Fig. 1.17 Palpation of fetal parts necessitates bimanual palpation of the uterus.

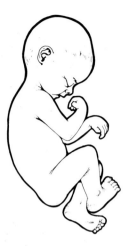

Fig. 1.19 The normal attitude of the fetus is one of flexion.

inlet (face presentation), and if it lies between these two attitudes the **brow** area presents (brow presentation). The brow is defined as the area between the base of the nose and the anterior fontanelle. The diameter of presentation for the vertex is the sub-occipito-bregmatic diameter (Table 1.1, Fig. 1.20). If the head is deflexed, the occipito-frontal diameter presents. With a brow presentation, the vertico-mental diameter presents

Table 1.1   Diameter of presentation

Presenting part	Diameter	Size (cm)
Vertex	Sub-occipito-bregmatic	9.5
Brow	Vertico-mental	13.5
Face	Sub-mento-bregmatic	9.5
Deflexed vertex	Occipito-frontal	11.7

to the pelvic inlet. Presentation and position can be accurately determined only by vaginal examination when the cervix has dilated and the suture lines and fontanelles can be palpated, and this situation pertains only in labour.

Position

Position must be differentiated from presentation, as the term describes the relationship of a denominator of the presenting part to the right or left side of the maternal pelvis:

Presentation	Denominator
Vertex	Occiput
Face	Chin (mentum)
Breech	Sacrum

Thus, in a vertex presentation, six different positions are described (Fig. 1.21). Viewed from below the pelvis these include right and left occipito-lateral, anterior and posterior positions. Except in advanced labour, it is very rare for a direct anterior or posterior position to be adopted. With a face presentation, the prefix **mento-** is included (Fig. 1.21), and with a breech presentation the prefix is **sacro-**. No such description is given to a brow presentation, as it has no mechanism of labour and cannot be delivered vaginally.

The position can be determined from abdominal palpation by palpating the anterior shoulder of the fetus. If this is near the midline and easily palpable, the position is anterior. If it is not easily palpable and the limbs are prominent, it is probably posterior. The position of the presenting part can be accurately determined only by direct palpation of the suture line or the buttocks through the dilated cervix.

The degree of flexion of the head can also be determined. A deflexed head tends to feel large and

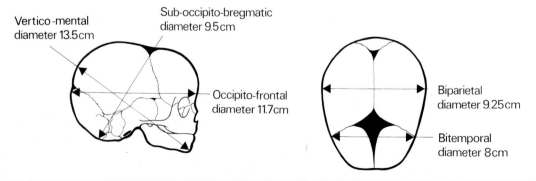

Fig. 1.20 Diameters of presentation of the mature fetal skull.

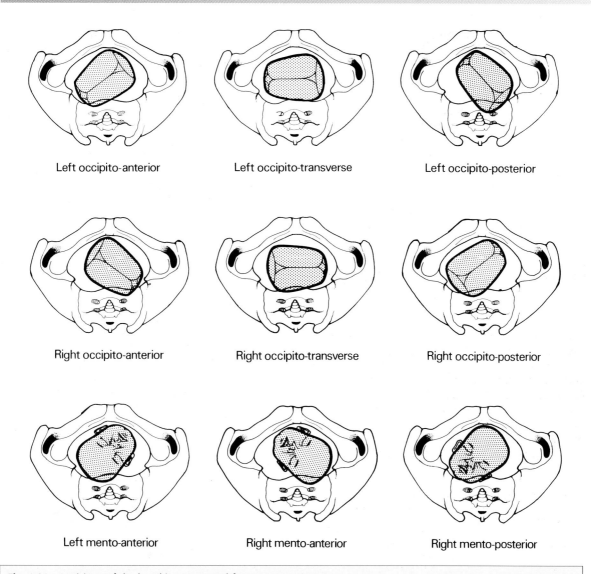

Left occipito-anterior   Left occipito-transverse   Left occipito-posterior

Right occipito-anterior   Right occipito-transverse   Right occipito-posterior

Left mento-anterior   Right mento-anterior   Right mento-posterior

Fig. 1.21 Positions of the head in vertex and face presentation.

the nuchal groove between the occiput and back is deep.

Station and engagement

The station of the head is also described in fifths above the pelvic brim (Fig. 1.22). Thus, a head that is only two-fifths palpable is engaged and is usually fixed in the pelvis. This is not invariably the case, as a small head may be mobile when it is engaged and a large head may be fixed but not engaged.

At the simplest level, a head that is easily palpable abdominally is not engaged, whereas a head that is presenting and is deeply engaged is difficult to palpate. This can be checked by vaginal examination, as the leading part of the engaged head is palpable at the level of the ischial spines.

Auscultation

Auscultation of the fetal heart is usually performed with a Pinard fetal stethoscope (Fig. 1.23). The instrument is placed over the anterior shoulder or in the midline in a posterior position and counter pressure is exerted with one hand on the opposite side of the abdomen.

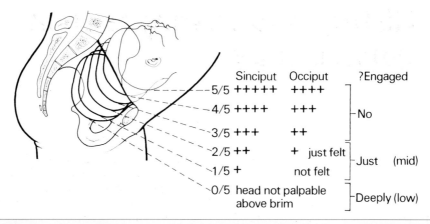

	Sinciput	Occiput	?Engaged
5/5	+++++	++++	
4/5	++++	+++	No
3/5	+++	++	
2/5	++	+ just felt	Just (mid)
1/5	+	not felt	
0/5	head not palpable above brim		Deeply (low)

Fig. 1.22 Stations of the fetal head.

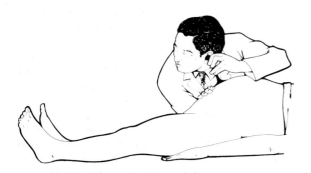

Fig. 1.23 Auscultation of the fetal heart.

With a cephalic presentation, the low frequency sound is best heard about 8 cm above the pubic symphysis, but with a breech presentation it is best heard at the level of the umbilicus. The rate and rhythm of the heart beat should be noted.

Abdominal examination of gravid uterus

- Fundal height in centimetres approximates to gestation in weeks after 20 weeks
- Lie
- Position
- Relation of presenting part to pelvic brim
- Auscultation of fetal heart

History and examination in gynaecology

Gynaecology is the study of diseases and disorders of the genital tract in women. In practice, the specialty now covers problems of reproduction in general, many of which do not fall within the realm of disease or disorder but have a social content such as therapeutic abortion, sterilization and contraception.

HISTORY

Details of the patient's name, age, marital status and occupation should always be recorded at the beginning of a consultation.

The history should be comprehensive, but not intrusive in a manner that is not relevant to the patient's problem. For example, whilst it is essential to obtain a detailed sexual history from a young couple presenting with subfertility, it would be both irrelevant and distressing to ask the same questions of an 80-year-old widow with a prolapse. The history must, therefore, be geared to the presenting symptom. It should be remembered that the presenting symptom may not always be related to the main anxiety of the patient and that some time and patience may be required to uncover the various problems that bring the patient to seek medical advice.

The patient's complaint

The patient should be asked to describe the nature of her problem, and a simple statement of the presenting symptoms should be made in the case notes. A great deal can be learnt by using the actual words employed by the patient. It is important to ascertain the time-scale of the problem and, where appropriate, the circumstances surrounding the onset of symptoms and their relationship to the menstrual cycle. It is also important to discover the degree of disability experienced for any given symptom. In many situations, reassurance that there is no serious underlying pathology will provide sufficient 'treatment' because the actual disability may be minimal.

A social history is important with all problems but is particularly relevant where the presenting difficulties relate to abortion or sterilization. For example, a 15-year-old female requesting a termination of pregnancy may be put under substantial pressure by her parents to have an abortion and yet may not really be happy about following this course of action.

Previous medical history

A detailed history of previous serious illnesses and operations – either general or gynaecological procedures – must be recorded. This description should take particular account of any endocrine disorders and any previous episodes of pelvic inflammatory disease. Chronic lung disease and disorders of the cardiovascular system are highly relevant where any surgical procedure is likely to be necessary. It is also important, where possible, to obtain any records of previous gynaecological surgery. Many women are uncertain of the precise nature of their operations. A family history of diabetes, tuberculosis and carcinoma of the genital tract should be noted.

Menstrual history

The first question that should be asked in relation to the menstrual history is the date of the last menstrual period. Omission of this one question may lead to serious errors in subsequent management.

The time of onset of the first period, the **menarche**, commonly occurs at 12 years of age and can be considered to be abnormally delayed over 16 years or abnormally early at 9 years. The term should be distinguished from the **pubarche**, which is the onset of the first signs of sexual maturation. Characteristically, the development of breasts and nipple enlargement predates the onset of menstruation by approximately 2 years.

The length of the menstrual cycle is the time between the first day of one period and the first day of the following period. Whilst there is usually an interval of 28 days, the cycle length may vary between 21 and 42 days in normal women and may only be significant where there is a change in menstrual pattern. It is important to be sure that the patient does not describe the time between the last day of one period and the first day of the next period, as this may give a false impression of the frequency of menstruation. Absence of menstruation is known as **amenorrhoea**, and frequent periods are known as **polymenorrhoea** or **epimenorrhoea** (Fig. 2.1). **Oligomenorrhoea** is the term used to describe infrequent menstruation.

The amount and duration of the period may change with age but may also provide a useful indication of a disease process. Normal menstruation lasts from 4 to 7 days, and normal blood loss varies between 30 and 120 ml. A change in pattern is often more noticeable and significant than the actual time and volume of loss. In practical terms, excessive menstrual loss is best assessed on the history of the number of pads or tampons used during a period and the presence or absence of clots. Excessive regular periods are described by the term **menorrhagia**, and irregular acyclic heavy bleeding is known as **metrorrhagia**. Periods that are both frequent and excessive are known as **epimenorrhagia** or **polymenorrhagia**.

The cessation of periods at the end of menstrual life is known as the **menopause**.

A history of irregular vaginal bleeding or blood loss that occurs after coitus should be noted, as should bleeding after the menopause.

Vaginal discharge is a common presenting symptom, and the colour, odour and relationship to the periods should be noted. It may also be associated with vulval pruritus, particularly in the presence of specific infections.

Another common presenting symptom is abdominal pain, and the history must include details of the time of onset, the distribution and radiation of the pain, and the relationship to the periods.

The presence of an abdominal mass may be noted by the patient or may be detected during the course of a routine examination. Symptoms may also result from pressure of the mass on adjacent pelvic organs, such as the bladder and bowel.

Vaginal and uterine prolapse are associated with symptoms of a mass protruding through the vaginal introitus or difficulties with micturition and defaecation.

Urinary symptoms

Common presenting urinary symptoms include frequency of micturition, pain or dysuria, incontinence and the passage of blood in the urine, or haematuria.

The sexual history

The history should include reference to the coital frequency, the occurrence of pain during intercourse – **dyspareunia** – and functional details relating to libido, sexual satisfaction and sexual problems.

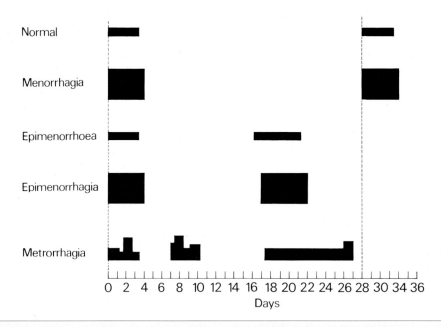

Fig. 2.1 Normal and abnormal patterns of menstruation: the large blocks represent excessive menstrual loss.

Gynaecological history

- Presenting complaint
- Previous gynaecological history and pregnancies
- Urinary symptoms
- Menstrual history
- Sexual/contraceptive history
- Medical history
- Social history
- Date of last cervical smear

A detailed obstetric history and a history of the patient's contraceptive practice, as previously described, should always be included.

THE GYNAECOLOGICAL EXAMINATION

A general examination should always be performed at the first consultation, including assessment of blood pressure and routine urine analysis. Careful note should be taken of any signs of anaemia. The distribution of facial and body hair is often important, as hirsutism may be a presenting symptom of various endocrine disorders. Body weight and height should also be recorded.

Breast examination

The opportunity should always be taken to examine the breasts, both in relation to endocrine changes and for the presence of any tumours (Fig. 2.2). The breast reflects the endocrine status of the woman and the signs of pregnancy as have previously been described in Chapter 1. The presence of the secretion of milk at times not associated with pregnancy, known as **galactorrhoea**, may indicate abnormal endocrine status. Systematic palpation with the flat of the hand should be undertaken to exclude the presence of any nodules in the breast or axillae.

Examination of the abdomen

Inspection of the abdomen may reveal the presence of a mass. The distribution of body hair should be noted, and the presence of scars, striae and hernias. Percussion of the abdomen may be used to outline the limits of a tumour, to detect the presence of a full bladder or to recognise the presence of tympanitic loops of bowel. Free fluid in the peritoneal cavity will be recognised by the presence of dullness to percussion in the flanks and resonance over the central abdomen (Fig. 2.3).

Palpation of the abdomen should take account of any guarding and rebound tenderness. It is important to ask the patient to outline the site and radiation of any pain in the abdomen, and palpation for enlargement of the liver, spleen and kidneys should be carried out. Auscultation of bowel sounds is important where obstruction or ileus is suspected.

Pelvic examination

The patient should be examined resting supine with the knees drawn up and separated, or in stirrups in the lithotomy position. Systematic inspection of the vulva should take note of the clitoris, urethral meatus, vulval and labial skin, the fourchette and hymen, and evidence of scarring or distortion of the perineum (Fig. 2.4). The patient should be asked to cough or strain to demonstrate stress incontinence and descent of the vaginal walls. The presence of any ulceration or discharge should also be noted.

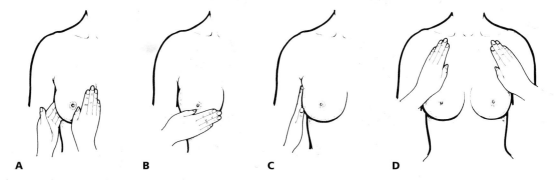

Fig. 2.2 Systematic examination of the four quadrants of the breasts.

A   B   C   D

A

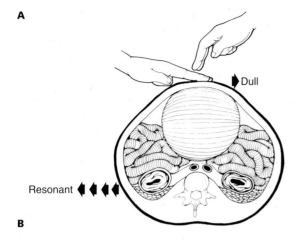

B

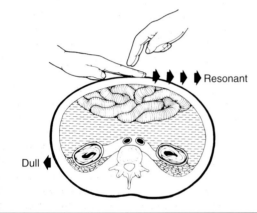

Fig. 2.3 **A** Percussion over a large ovarian cyst – central dullness and resonance in the flanks; **B** percussion in the presence of ascites – dullness in the flanks and central resonance.

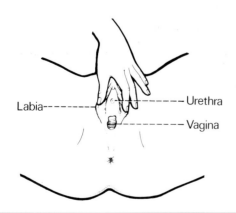

Fig. 2.4 Inspection of the external genitalia.

Speculum examination

Speculum examination should be performed before digital examination to avoid any contamination with lubricant. A bivalve or Cuscoe's speculum is most commonly used, and enables a clear view of the cervix to be obtained (Fig. 2.5). Where vaginal wall prolapse is suspected, a Sims' speculum should be used, as it provides a clearer view of the vaginal walls.

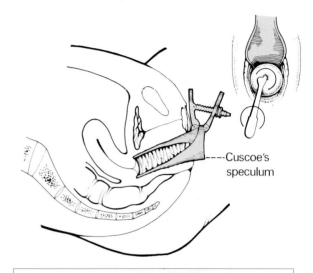

Fig. 2.5 Insertion of a Cuscoe's speculum (left) and collection of a cervical smear (right).

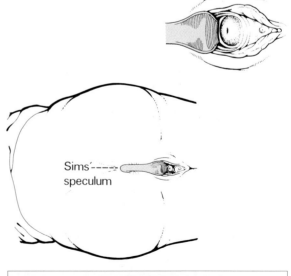

Fig. 2.6 Examination in the lateral semiprone position with a Sims' speculum enables inspection of the vaginal walls.

The instrument is inserted in the direction of the vagina and the blades are opened after full insertion of the instrument. Having noted the appearance of the cervix, a cervical smear is taken with an Ayre's spatula. The spatula is gently scraped across the epithelial surface of the cervix, and the smear is applied to a labelled glass slide, which is immediately placed in preservative fluid. The presence and nature of any vaginal discharge are recorded, and a swab is taken for culture where appropriate.

Where the Sims' speculum is used, it is preferable to examine the patient in the semiprone or Sims' position (Fig. 2.6).

Bimanual examination is performed as previously described in the obstetric section. It must be remembered that the abdominal hand is used to compress the pelvic organs on to the examining vaginal hand.

The size, shape, consistency and position of the uterus must be noted. The uterus is commonly preaxial or anteverted, but will be postaxial or retroverted in some 10% of women. Provided the retroverted uterus is mobile, the position is rarely significant. It is important to feel in the pouch of Douglas for the presence of thickening or nodules, and then to palpate laterally in both fornices for the presence of any ovarian or tubal masses. An attempt should be made to differentiate between adnexal and uterine masses, although this is often not possible. For example, a pedunculated fibroid may mimic an ovarian tumour, whereas a solid ovarian tumour, if adherent to the uterus, may be impossible to distinguish from a uterine fibroid (Fig. 2.7). The ovaries are usually palpable in the normal pelvis, but the Fallopian tubes are only palpable if they are significantly enlarged.

In a child or in a woman with an intact hymen, it may be necessary to perform a single-finger vaginal examination or a rectal examination. It should always be remembered that a rough or painful examination rarely produces any useful information and, in certain situations such as tubal ectopic pregnancy, may be dangerous.

A

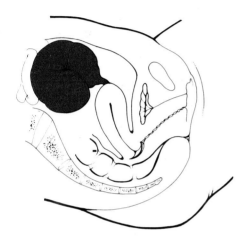

B

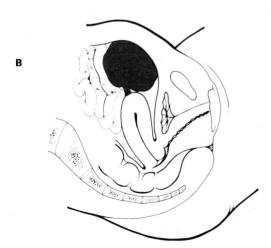

Fig. 2.7   Differentiation between **A** an adnexal mass and **B** a pedunculated fibroid may be difficult.

Gynaecological examination

- Breast examination
- Abdominal palpation
- Inspection of external genitalia
- Speculum examination
- Bimanual examination
- Cervical smear

3 Physiological changes in pregnancy

The recognition of abnormal events in pregnancy demands a clear understanding of the normal processes of maternal adaptation. In all mammalian species, there are extensive biochemical, physiological and structural changes during pregnancy and the puerperium.

From a teleological point of view, there are two main reasons for these changes:

1. To provide a suitable environment for the nutrition, growth and development of the fetus
2. To prepare the mother for the process of parturition and subsequent support of the newborn infant.

The changes that occur in pregnancy in order to achieve these objectives are both visible and subtle.

MATERNAL WEIGHT GAIN

Of the physical changes that occur, the most obvious are the enlargement of the abdomen and the increase in body weight. There are no reliable

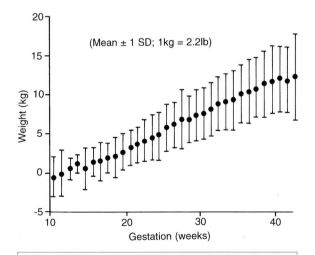

Fig. 3.1 Maternal weight (mean ± 1 SD) in normal pregnancy. (From James et al 1994 High risk pregnancy — management options, Baillière Tindall, with permission.)

data available for weight gain in the first 12 weeks of pregnancy, but in normal pregnancy the average gain is 0.3 kg/week up to 18 weeks, 0.45 kg/week from 18 to 28 weeks and thereafter a slight reduction with a rate of 0.36–0.41 kg/week until term (Fig. 3.1). Failure to gain weight and sometimes slight weight loss may occur in the last 2 weeks. The average weight gain for primigravidae for the whole pregnancy is 12.5 kg, and is probably about 0.9 kg less for multigravidae. Acute excessive weight gain is commonly associated with abnormal fluid retention.

Contributions to weight gain

The individual components affecting weight gain are derived from both maternal and feto-placental factors (Fig. 3.2). Pregnancy is an anabolic state, and thus results in an increase in body fat, the growth of the breasts and the uterus and an expansion of blood volume and extracellular fluid. The contribution to maternal weight gain from the conceptus comes from fetal weight, amniotic fluid and the placenta. Poor weight gain is therefore associated with an increased incidence of low birth weight infants, but the range of weight gain in normal pregnancy may vary from almost zero to twice the mean weight gain.

Although there have been conflicting reports about the status of protein storage in the human, it now seems likely that no more protein is laid down than can be accounted for by fetal and placental growth and by the increase in size in specific target organs such as the uterus and breasts. An increase in fat storage occurs in normal pregnancy, with the deposition of fat occuring principally over the back, upper thighs and abdomen.

Surprisingly, there is a poor correlation between maternal weight gain and energy intake, and it is generally not advisable to inhibit weight gain (or, indeed, to reduce weight) in pregnancy – it often results in simultaneous restriction of essential nutrients, and this may have undesirable effects on fetal growth and development.

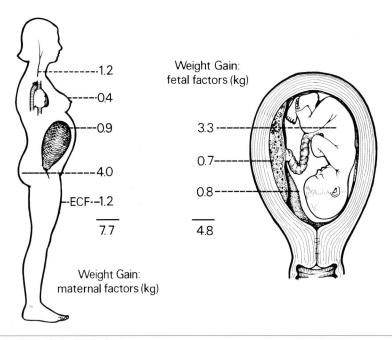

Fig. 3.2 Maternal (left) and fetal (right) contributions to weight gain at term (ECF = extracellular fluid).

Postpartum weight

Following delivery, women tend to retain weight long term, at a level of some 3 kg, compared to their weight before pregnancy. The most rapid weight loss occurs between 4 and 10 days postpartum, and is mainly due to the loss of fluid. After the first 10 days, weight loss is more gradual at about 0.25 kg/week. Eventually the average woman loses most of the weight she gains during pregnancy, taking into account the effects of age and normal weight gain over time.

CHANGES IN BREASTS

As mentioned earlier, some of the first signs of pregnancy are recognized in the breast, with an increase in size, enlargement of the nipples, increased vascularity and pigmentation of the areola.

Breast structure

The breast contains 10–20 lactiferous ducts which branch into a series of ducts and ductules terminating in multiple clusters of milk-secreting alveoli. The alveoli are surrounded by band-like myoepithelial cells which squeeze milk into the duct. The ducts and alveoli are surrounded by fat cells, connective tissue, blood vessels and lymph ducts. The ducts

grow under the stimulus of high oestrogen levels, and the alveoli develop as a result of the action of progesterone and prolactin. From 3–4 months onwards, a thick, glossy protein rich fluid, known as **colostrum**, can be expressed from the breast. Prolactin stimulates the cells of the alveoli to secrete milk by inducing the production of enzymes needed to synthesize milk proteins and lactose (Fig. 3.3).

This effect is blocked during pregnancy by the peripheral action of oestrogen and progesterone, but shortly after delivery the sudden fall in these hormones enables prolactin to act in an uninhibited manner on the breast, and hence lactation begins. Suckling stimulates the release of both prolactin and oxytocin via neurological pathways between the nipple and the hypothalamus, and oxytocin stimulates contraction of the myoepithelial cells and, hence, ejection of milk.

UTERUS

During pregnancy, the uterus undergoes a 20-fold increase in weight from 50 g to 1100 g at term. The uterus consists of bundles of smooth muscle cells separated by thin sheets of connective tissue. The muscle cells are arranged as an innermost longitudinal layer, a middle layer with bundles running in all

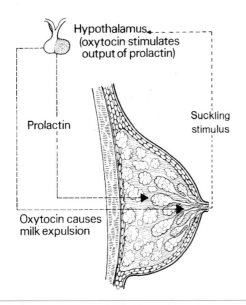

Fig. 3.3 Factors regulating milk production and expulsion.

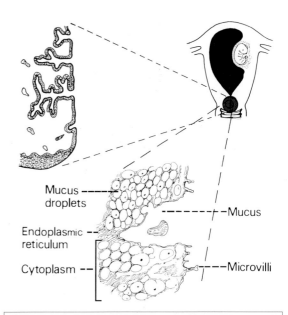

Fig. 3.5 Structure and function of the cervix in pregnancy.

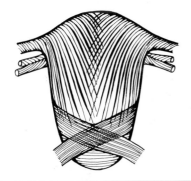

Fig. 3.4 Decussation of muscle fibres in the various layers of the human uterus.

directions and an outer layer of both circular and longitudinal bundles (Fig. 3.4).

The uterus is divided functionally and morphologically into three sections, namely the cervix, the isthmus (later to develop into the lower uterine segment) and the main body of the uterus (corpus uteri).

The cervix

The cervix is predominantly a fibrous organ whose principal function is to retain the conceptus (Fig. 3.5). Eighty per cent of the total protein consists of collagen. In pregnancy it becomes softened, hypertrophied and oedematous, and the changes are characterized by:

1. Changes in stroma
2. Hypertrophy of the cervical glands
3. Changes in cervical secretions.

The connective tissue undergoes hypertrophy and hyperplasia with loosening and dissociation of the fibrils. There is a decrease in the amount of collagen and an alteration in ground structure, which enables the stretching and dilatation of the cervix. Hypertrophy of the cervical glands leads to the production of profuse cervical mucus and to the formation of a thick mucus plug or operculum which acts as a barrier against infection.

The isthmus

The isthmus of the uterus is the junctional area between the cervix and the body of the uterus. It joints the muscle fibres of the corpus to the dense connective tissue of the cervix and constitutes a transitional zone both functionally and structurally. It subsequently develops into the lower uterine segment and becomes more clearly defined from 28 weeks gestation.

Corpus uteri

The body of the uterus has to enlarge to accommodate the growing conceptus and then, at the appropriate time, commence a pattern of rhythmic contractions which will result in expulsion of the fetus. The uterus therefore adapts to these needs by a series of changes:

1. An increase in the size, shape, position and consistency of the uterus. In the latter months of pregnancy, enlargement predominantly occurs in the uterine fundus so that the round ligaments tend to emerge from a relatively caudal point in the uterus. The cavity of the uterus expands from some 4 ml to 4000 ml.

2. Hypertrophy of blood vessels and increased uterine blood flow associated with increased oxygen consumption in both the uterus and the utero-placental bed. Uterine blood flow has been shown to increase from approximately 50 ml/min at 10 weeks gestation to 500–700 ml/min at term (Fig. 3.6).

The blood supply to the uterus is derived from the uterine and ovarian arteries and branches of the superior vesical arteries (Fig. 3.7). All of these vessels undergo massive hypertrophy. Control of blood flow in the arterial tree is dependent on arteriolar vasomotor control, both from the action of the autonomic nervous system and from the direct effect of vasoconstrictor and vasodilator humoral agents. The major control is exerted at an arteriolar level remote from the terminal arterioles, which are invaded by trophoblast and become more passive channels with little regulatory function.

During the first trimester, extravillous cytotrophoblast moves from the tip of anchoring villi to the spiral arteries in the placental bed and migrates down to the intima of the vessels, destroying the normal musculo-elastic tissue and creating flaccid sinusoidal channels. A secondary wave of invasion occurs early in the second trimester which con-

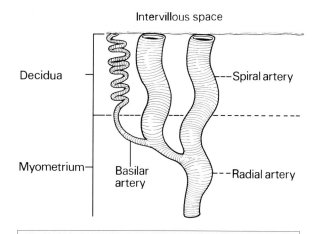

Fig. 3.7 Vascular structure in the utero-placental bed.

solidates these changes and has a long-term effect on the development of uteroplacental perfusion.

Uterine contractility

Myometrial growth is almost entirely due to muscle hypertrophy, although some hyperplasia may occur during early pregnancy. The stimulus for myometrial growth and development is derived from the direct effects of the growing conceptus and from the effect of oestrogens and progesterone produced by the ovary and the placenta.

The pregnant myometrium has a much greater compliance than the non-pregnant myometrium in response to distension. Thus, although the uterus becomes distended by the growing conceptus, intrauterine pressure does not increase although the uterus maintains the capacity to develop maximal active tension.

The continuation of a successful pregnancy depends on the fact that the myometrium remains quiescent until the fetus is mature and capable of sustaining extra-uterine life. Progesterone appears to be the major hormone responsible, and it achieves this effect by increasing the resting membrane potential of myometrial cells whilst at the same time impairing the conduction of electrical activity, and hence limits muscle activity to small clumps of cells.

Development of myometrial activity

Uterine activity occurs throughout pregnancy, and is measurable as early as 7 weeks gestation, when contractions may occur every 20–30 minutes, but reaching a pressure of less than 10 mmHg (Fig. 3.8).

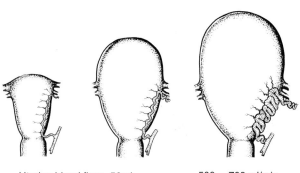

Uterine blood flow: 50 ml ————— 500 – 700 ml/min at term

Fig. 3.6 Changes in uterine blood flow in pregnancy.

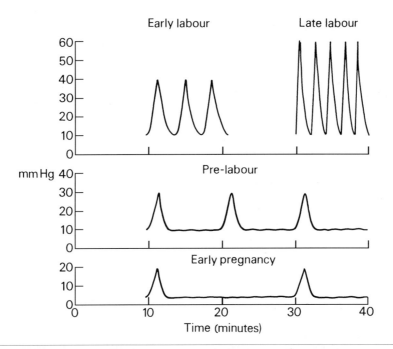

Fig. 3.8   Intra-amniotic pressure reflecting uterine contractions at different stages of gestation.

This pattern gradually changes to one of low frequency and higher amplitude, so that by the third trimester contractions may occur every 10–15 minutes with an amplitude of 20–40 mmHg. These contractions often become noticeable as painless 'tightenings' known as **Braxton–Hicks contractions**. With the onset of labour, the contractions become increasingly more frequent and more painful, eventually reaching amplitudes of up to 100 mmHg in the last phase of the first stage of labour and occurring every 2–3 minutes.

THE VAGINA

The vagina is lined by stratified squamous epithelium which becomes markedly hypertrophic during pregnancy (Fig. 3.9). At the same time, the musculature in the vaginal walls becomes hypertrophied, and the vagina increases in capacity and length. The rich venous vascular network in the connective tissue surrounding the vaginal walls becomes engorged with blood and gives rise to the slightly bluish appearance of the vagina.

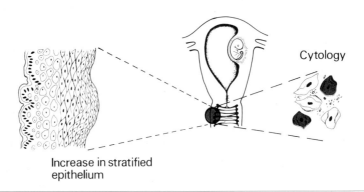

Fig. 3.9   Changes in the vaginal epithelium during pregnancy.

The three layers of superficial, intermediate and basal epithelial cells change their relative proportions, so that the intermediate cells predominate and can be seen in the cell population of normal vaginal secretions. The intermediate cells have a tendency to clump together and curl at the edges, and the epithelial cells generally multiply and enlarge and become filled with vacuoles rich in glycogen. High oestrogen levels stimulate glycogen synthesis and deposition, and the action of lactobacilli on the glycogen in these vaginal cells results in the production of lactic acid. The high acidity of the vagina, with a pH of 3.5–4, provides an acid environment which serves to keep the vagina relatively free of any bacterial pathogens.

CHANGES IN SKIN

Reference has already been made to the development of pigmentation on the face, nipples and abdominal wall in pregnancy. The development of stretch marks or striae gravidarum varies markedly in different populations and in different women. These marks, which often have a distinctly purplish colour in the first pregnancy and later adopt a silvery, thin appearance, represent the effects of disruption of collagen fibres in the subcuticular zone. Although they predominantly occur in the lines of stress of the abdominal wall, they also occur on the lateral aspect of the thighs and breasts, and are as much related to the effect of increased production of adrenocortical hormones in pregnancy as they are to actual stress in the skin folds associated with expansion of the abdomen.

THE CARDIOVASCULAR SYSTEM

Major changes occur in the cardiovascular system in pregnancy, the most significant changes taking place within the first 12 weeks. Although the longer term needs of maternal adaptation are met by alterations in the activity of the cardiovascular system, these changes tend to occur well before the physiological needs of the system arise.

Cardiac output

Cardiac output increases by 40% over the first 14 weeks of gestation and thereafter remains constant (Fig. 3.10). Thus an absolute increase of 1.5 l/min occurs at rest – from 4.5 to 6.0 l/min – under stan-

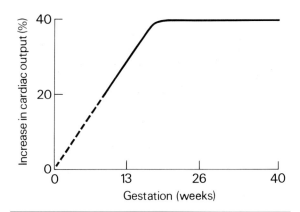

Fig. 3.10 Cardiac output undergoes a massive increase in the first trimester of pregnancy.

dardized conditions of posture and time. During labour, contractions may increase cardiac output by 2 l/min. It has been suggested that this change results from injection of blood from the distended intervillous space. Normally, cardiac output increases because of an increase in both heart rate and stroke volume. As the heart rate increases by 10–15%, the remainder is the result of an increase in stroke volume. Pregnancy is known to proceed normally even when the mother has an artificial cardiac pacemaker, where compensation must occur entirely from increased stroke volume.

Cardiac position and size

With increasing enlargement of the uterus, the diaphragm is pushed upwards and the heart is correspondingly displaced so that the apex beat moves upwards and laterally (Fig. 3.11). The heart enlarges during pregnancy by an increase in volume of 70–80 ml, and this enlargement results both from increased diastolic filling and muscle hypertrophy.

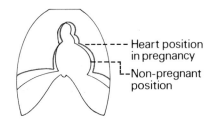

Fig. 3.11 Progressive enlargement of the uterus results in upward displacement of the heart and diaphragm.

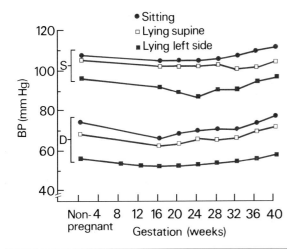

Fig. 3.12 A longitudinal study of the effect of posture on blood pressure in pregnancy.

Myocardial contractility is increased in association with lengthening of myocardial muscle fibres.

Arterial blood pressure

Posture has a profound effect on blood pressure in pregnancy, so that blood pressure is higher when taken with the mother sitting up, lower when she is lying down, and lowest when lying on her side. Longitudinal studies in pregnancy have shown that blood pressure falls during mid pregnancy, but the fall is most noticeable in diastolic pressure (Fig. 3.12) Profound falls in blood pressure may occur in late pregnancy when the mother lies supine on her back, and this phenomenon has previously been described as the **supine hypotensive syndrome**. This results from compression of the inferior vena cava. It must be remembered that aortic compression may also occur, and this will result in a conspicuous difference between brachial and femoral blood pressures in

pregnancy. Thus, when the woman turns from a supine to a lateral supine position, the blood pressure may fall by some 10–15% (Fig. 3.12). Changes in venous pressure are dramatic in some areas. Although central venous pressure remains constant in pregnancy, venous pressure in the arms also remains constant but pressure from the uterus and fetal presenting part results in a marked increase in femoral venous pressure.

Peripheral resistance

In parallel with the increase in cardiac output, peripheral resistance falls to nearly 50% of the non-pregnant values. The factors controlling peripheral resistance are not clearly understood, although there is evidence to suggest that increased production of vasodilator prostaglandins may provide the principal mechanism. The regulation of blood pressure in pregnancy and the development of pregnancy-induced hypertension are determined by the balance of vasoconstrictor and vasodilator factors regulating peripheral resistance.

RESPIRATORY FUNCTION

Alterations to the configuration of the thorax occur in pregnancy. The level of the diaphragm rises, and the intercostal angle increases from 68° in early pregnancy to 103° in late pregnancy, and, because of these changes, breathing tends to be diaphragmatic rather than costal (Fig. 3.13).

Vital capacity is a measure of the maximum amount of gas that can be expired after maximum inspiration. Some pregnant women increase their vital capacity, but this does not always occur. It appears to be related to body build, and the increase is not apparent in obese women.

Inspiratory capacity is a measure of tidal volume plus inspiratory reserve volume, and is increased in

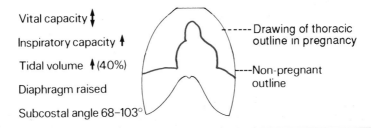

Fig. 3.13 Change in respiratory function in pregnancy.

late pregnancy. This change appears to occur progressively throughout pregnancy.

Respiratory rate does not change during pregnancy, whereas tidal volume, a measurement of the volume of gas inspired and expired in each respiration, does rise by approximately 40%. Minute ventilation therefore also increases. Thus, the resting pregnant woman increases her ventilation by breathing more deeply and not more frequently.

Forced expiratory volume in one second (FEV_1) and peak expiratory flow rate (PFR) are unaffected by normal pregnancy. There is a fall in pCO_2 with a mild respiratory alkalaemia.

CHANGES IN BLOOD

Plasma volume

Sequential studies on plasma volume in pregnancy show a progressive rise until it reaches a plateau at about 32 weeks gestation. Where measurements have been made in the supine position, there is an apparent fall in plasma volume in late pregnancy, which is probably due to poor mixing of dye because of obstructed venous return from the legs. In general terms, multiple pregnancy is associated with a significantly higher increase in plasma volume (Fig. 3.14). Pregnancies exhibiting intrauterine fetal growth retardation are also associated with a poor increase in plasma volume. The actual increase in a singleton

pregnancy is approximately 1250 ml from a non-pregnant mean of 2600 ml.

Red cell mass is a measurement of the total volume of red cells in the circulation, and a steady increase occurs throughout pregnancy. The increase appears to be linear, and the discrepancy between the rate of increase of plasma volume and that of red cell mass results in a decline in the haemoglobin concentration, haematocrit and red cell count during pregnancy and, in particular, in the second trimester. At the same time, the mean corpuscular haemoglobin concentration remains constant.

The white cells

The total **white cell count** rises during pregnancy, and this increase is mainly due to an increase in neutrophil polymorphonuclear leucocytes, which reaches its peak at 30 weeks (Fig. 3.15).

A further massive neutrophilia occurs during labour, with a fourfold increase in the number of polymorphs. Furthermore, there is an increase in the metabolic activity of granulocytes during pregnancy, which may be an effect of oestrogen stimulation.

Eosinophils, basophils and **monocytes** appear to remain relatively constant during pregnancy, but there is a profound fall in eosinophils during labour, and they are virtually absent at delivery. The lymphocyte count remains constant, and the numbers of T and B cells do not alter. However, lymphocyte function and cell-mediated immunity are profoundly

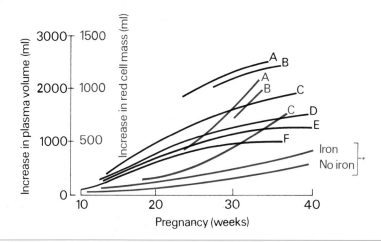

Fig. 3.14 Changes in plasma volume and red cell mass in quadruplets (A), triplets (B), twins (C), healthy multigravidae (D), healthy primigravidae (E) and intra-uterine growth retardation (F); the effect of iron supplement in singleton pregnancy is also shown.

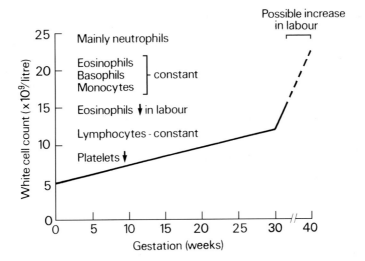

Fig. 3.15 Pregnancy is associated with an increased white cell count; the increase occurs predominantly in polymorphonuclear leucocytes.

depressed by a factor in maternal serum, and this suppression is associated with a lowered resistance to viral infection.

Platelets

Longitudinal studies on platelet counts during pregnancy show a significant fall (Fig. 3.16), and at the same time, after 28 weeks gestation, there is a substantial increase in mean platelet volume. The increase in platelet volume may be associated with the hyperdestruction of platelets in pregnancy, and as young platelets are larger than old platelets, the balance is pushed towards an overall increase in size.

Changes in plasma and serum

Plasma osmolality falls abruptly during the first 8 weeks of pregnancy, and this change is associated with a resetting of the osmoreceptor system to preserve the new low level of osmolality. The ability to excrete a water load is significantly affected by posture, with the upright posture being more antidiuretic than in non-pregnant subjects.

Changes in plasma proteins

The total protein concentration falls from about 7 to 6 g/100 ml during the first trimester and remains reduced throughout pregnancy. This fall is

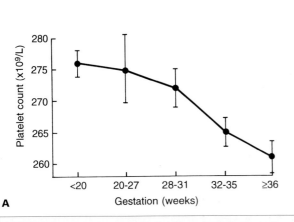

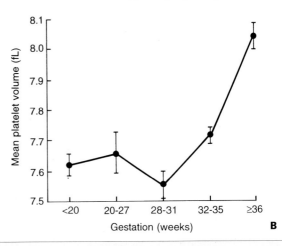

Fig. 3.16 Platelet count and platelet volume in normal pregnancy. (From James et al 1994 High risk pregnancy — management options, Baillière Tindall with permission.)

largely due to the fall in albumin concentration. On the other hand, globulins show a small rise in concentration, but there are marked differences in various globulin fractions. Lipoproteins are classified according to their density into four groups, namely very low-density lipoprotein, intermediate-density lipoprotein, low-density lipoprotein and high-density lipoprotein. α-Lipoproteins generally lie in the high-density fraction, and β-lipoproteins in the low-density fraction. Within the very low-density and intermediate-density lipoprotein fractions, three- to fourfold increases occur in triglyceride, cholesterol and phospholipid concentrations.

Amino acids

With the exception of alanine and glutamic acid, amino acid levels in plasma decrease below the levels found in the non-pregnant state.

Free fatty acids

Levels of free fatty acids (non-esterified fatty acids) are extremely labile in pregnancy and are highly sensitive to fasting, exertion, emotional stress and smoking. Levels of free fatty acids in late pregnancy, however, are consistently elevated above non-pregnant and early pregnancy levels.

Clotting factors in pregnancy

Pregnancy is associated with an increased tendency towards blood clotting, and, in a situation where haemorrhage from the uterine vascular bed may be sudden and life threatening, this increased coagulability has an essential protective and life-saving function. Most clotting factors either remain constant or increase during pregnancy, and this particularly applies to fibrinogen, which exhibits a substantial increase in concentration. Although factor VII and factor VIII:C show a significant increase during pregnancy, factors X, V and II all remain constant or show a small fall (Fig. 3.17). The increased tendency to clot in pregnancy is potentiated to some degree by a decrease in plasma fibrinolytic activity. This decrease disappears within 1 hour of delivery, and it seems likely that it is mediated from the placenta. There is also an increase in circulating fibrin degradation products in the plasma in normal pregnancy.

IMMUNOLOGY OF PREGNANCY

Maternal tolerance

The fetus constitutes an allograft, and if it is not to be rejected it requires the presence of maternal

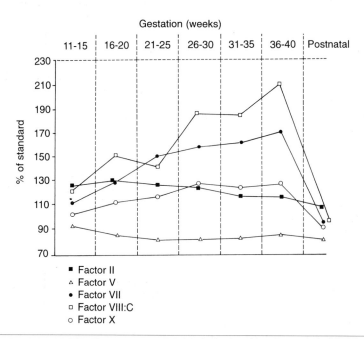

Fig. 3.17 Changes in mean values of factors II, V, VII, VIII and X. (Data from Stirling Y, Woolf L, North W R S, Seghatchian M J, Meade T W 1984 Haemostasis in normal pregnancy. Thrombosis and Haemostasis 52: 176–182.)

tolerance. The mother continues to respond to and destroy other foreign antigens, and confers passive immunity in the newborn, but does not normally reject the fetus. The mechanism by which this apparent anomaly occurs is not completely understood.

The fetus expresses paternal antigens, and these are capable of stimulating the production of maternal antibodies. Although pregnancy may induce blocking antibodies, these do not appear to be vital to the continuation of pregnancy. The placenta is not an impermeable immunological barrier, as shown by the presence of maternal antibodies in the fetus. The uterus is not an immunologically privileged site, as shown by the fact that other tissues implanted there are rejected.

Cell surface antigens

The major histocompatibility complex for cell surface antigens is encoded on chromosome 6. These antigens are central to transplant and cytotoxic responses. They are absent on trophoblast which is central to the feto-maternal interface. Fetal stem vessels and Hofbauer cells are able to bind maternal immunoglobulin, and may therefore act as a filter.

In addition, the fetus has a less well-defined local immunoregulatory capacity, signalling the maternal immune system not to attack via special HLA-like surface antigens expressed by elements of the cytotrophoblast.

Decidual response

The leucocyte response of the decidua is unusual in that lymphoid cells do not appear to be activated and may act as suppressor cells by inhibiting the action of lymphokines essential for cytotoxic and natural killer cell action.

In summary, the fetus appears to avoid attack by the maternal immune system by a combination of having a relatively non-immunogenic interface with the maternal circulation, filtering out harmful antibodies in the placenta, and by a locally mediated manipulation of the maternal immune response.

CHANGES IN THE LYMPHATIC SYSTEM AND THE THYMUS GLAND

Although it is difficult to measure changes in the thymus gland in human pregnancy, there is evidence from animal data that the thymus involutes markedly in pregnancy, probably as a result of the direct action of progesterone on the thymus. At the same time, the lymph nodes draining the uterus increase in size. The number of circulating T-cells probably remains constant, but the number of B-lymphocytes appears to increase. Maternal humoral responses are generally enhanced in pregnancy, with increased antibody synthesis in the IgG fraction. Antibodies to fetal components are frequently found in maternal plasma, but marked variations occur within and between pregnancies. As far as cellular immunity is concerned, the situation is confused, but current evidence suggests that a specific cellular blockade occurs, which is due to immunological enhancement of suppressor cell activity.

RENAL FUNCTION IN PREGNANCY

In line with the increase that occurs in cardiac output, renal blood flow increases by 30–50% in the first trimester and remains elevated throughout pregnancy. The change in renal blood flow is associated with an increase in both the glomerular filtration rate and effective renal plasma flow (Fig. 3.18). These changes are in fact apparent soon after conception and are fully developed by the end of the first trimester. There is evidence that a slight decline in the glomerular filtration rate may occur between 26 and 36 weeks gestation. The increase in the glomerular filtration rate is not associated with any substantial increase in production of creatinine and urea, and therefore plasma levels fall during pregnancy.

Associated with the increase in the glomerular filtration rate, the filtered load of sodium increases by 5000–10 000 mmol/day. Tubular reabsorption increases in parallel with the glomerular filtration rate, with the retention of 3–5 mmol of sodium per

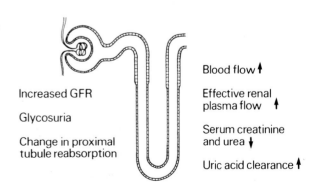

Fig. 3.18 Changes in renal function in pregnancy (GFR, glomerular filtration rate).

day into the fetal and maternal stores. The total net sodium gain amounts to 950 meq*, and this increased sodium load is mainly stored in the maternal compartment.

A similar change occurs with potassium ions, with a net gain of approximately 350 meq*.

Renal tubular function

Renal tubular function also undergoes significant change. Uric acid clearance increases from 6–12 to 12–20 ml/min, with a consequent reduction in plasma uric acid levels. Net tubular reabsorption of uric acid is reduced. With progression of the pregnancy, the filtered load of uric acid increases whilst excretion remains constant, and plasma levels therefore return to non-pregnant values. Glycosuria is a common feature of normal pregnancy, and it exhibits considerable variability from day to day. Glucose reabsorption is not solely dependent on tubular function, although it is linked with proximal tubular reabsorption of sodium and bicarbonate ions. The glomerular filtration rate also plays a significant role in glucose loss through the glomerulus.

The renin–angiotensin system

The renin–angiotensin system shows an early and persistent increase in activity. Renin is a proteolytic enzyme which acts on a substrate of α-2-globulin to produce angiotensin I. Under the action of converting enzyme produced predominantly in the lungs, but also in the placenta, angiotensin I is converted to angiotensin II, which is a potent vasoconstrictor, and also stimulates the release of aldosterone. Renin is produced in the kidney, and also in the uterus and chorion (Fig. 3.19). Approximately 70% of renin in the circulation in pregnancy is biologically inactive. A 2.5-fold increase occurs in plasma renin concentration in the first 12 weeks and then tends to fall slightly as pregnancy progresses. Renin substrate increases gradually throughout pregnancy, and appears to be under the control of oestrogen stimulation. The changes are of particular interest in pregnancy because there is a selective loss of vascular sensitivity to angiotensin II, which does not appear to be the case with adrenaline and noradrenaline.

Aldosterone levels rise gradually throughout pregnancy, but correlate poorly with plasma concentrations of both renin and angiotensin II.

*According to the *1996 Guidance to Authors for Clinical Science*, millimoles should be used in preference to milliequivalents.

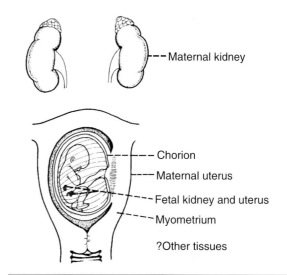

Fig. 3.19 Sources of renin in the mother (above) and fetus (below).

- Maternal kidney
- Chorion
- Maternal uterus
- Fetal kidney and uterus
- Myometrium
- ?Other tissues

Although initial work suggested some blocking agent such as prostacyclin or prostaglandin E$_2$ explained the impaired sensitivity to infused angiotensin II, it now seems that this phenomenon is associated with down-regulation of platelet angiotensin II receptors. These changes reflect the general status of vascular angiotensin AII receptors.

Other changes in the urinary system

Apart from the functional changes in the kidney, various anatomical changes occur in the urinary tract (Fig. 3.20). There is marked dilatation of the calyces and renal pelvis and of the ureters. The changes appear in the first trimester of pregnancy, and it is unlikely that they are due to back-pressure. However, the ureters do not exhibit actual hypotonicity and hypomotility, and there is hypertrophy of the ureteral smooth muscle and hyperplasia of the connective tissue. Vesico-ureteric reflux occurs sporadically, and the combination of reflux and ureteric dilatation is associated with a high incidence of urinary stasis and an increased tendency to urinary tract infection.

THE ALIMENTARY SYSTEM

Heartburn is a common disorder of pregnancy, and this has generally been ascribed to reflux oesophagitis. However, it is known that reflux also occurs in

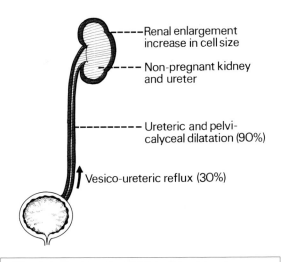

----Renal enlargement increase in cell size

---- Non-pregnant kidney and ureter

-------- Ureteric and pelvi-calyceal dilatation (90%)

↑ Vesico-ureteric reflux (30%)

Fig. 3.20 Changes in the urinary tract include renal enlargement and ureteric dilatation.

women without any symptoms of heartburn. With increased intra-abdominal pressure, there is commonly displacement of the lower oesphageal sphincter through the diaphragm, but this is not necessarily the cause of heartburn. The predominant factors appear to be decreased sphincter tonus and a decreased sphincter response to raised intra-abdominal pressure.

Gastric secretion is reduced in pregnancy, and gastric motility is low. As a consequence, gastric emptying tends to be delayed. Reduced motility also occurs in both the small bowel and the large bowel, and there is also evidence that absorption of sodium and water is increased in the large bowel. This may account for the increased tendency to constipation that characterizes pregnancy.

ENDOCRINE CHANGES

Massive production of sex steroids by the placenta tends to dominate the endocrine picture; these changes will be described in a subsequent chapter on placental function. Significant alterations occur in all maternal endocrine organs.

The pituitary gland

The pituitary gland enlarges in normal pregnancy, and the increase is largely due to changes in the anterior lobe. Prolactin-secreting cells increase in number whilst the number of gonadotrophin cells decreases. Prolactin levels increase substantially, probably as a result of oestrogen stimulation of the lactotrophe. Gonadotrophin secretion is inhibited. The secretion of growth hormone is inhibited whilst

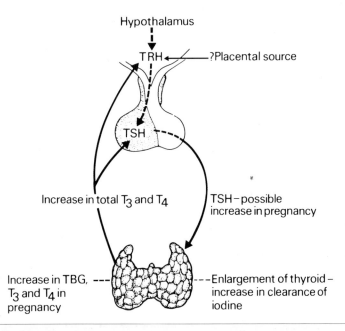

Hypothalamus

TRH ← ?Placental source

TSH

Increase in total T_3 and T_4

TSH – possible increase in pregnancy

Increase in TBG, T_3 and T_4 in pregnancy

Enlargement of thyroid – increase in clearance of iodine

Fig. 3.21 Thyroid function in pregnancy.

plasma adrenocorticotrophic hormone (ACTH) levels increase. Thyrotrophin levels remain constant. The major role of the posterior pituitary lies in the release of oxytocin, and this principally occurs during the first stage of labour and during suckling. Very little is known of vasopressin release.

Thyroid function

The thyroid gland enlarges in up to 70% of all pregnant women, and was relied on by the ancient Egyptians as a sign of pregnancy. There is increased urinary excretion of iodine, and this leads to a relative deficiency in plasma iodide. The thyroid gland triples its uptake of iodide from the blood. Thus, the relative iodine deficiency is probably responsible for the compensating follicular enlargement of the gland.

Thyroxine-binding globulin (TBG) is doubled by the end of the first trimester and remains elevated throughout pregnancy (Fig. 3.21). As a result, total T_3 and T_4 increase in pregnancy, although free T_3 and T_4 rise early in pregnancy and then fall, to remain within the normal non-pregnant range. Thyroid-stimulating hormone (TSH) may increase slightly but tends to remain within the normal range. T_3 and T_4 and TSH do not cross the placental barrier, and there is therefore no direct relationship between maternal and fetal thyroid function. However, iodine and antithyroid drugs cross the placenta, as does long-acting thyroid stimulator (LATS). Hence, the fetus may be affected by the level of iodine intake and by the presence of auto-immune disease in the mother.

The adrenal gland

Plasma cortisol increases throughout pregnancy, and much of this rise is due to binding to corticosteroid-binding globulin. However, the mean unbound cortisol is also elevated in normal preg-nancy. Sex hormone-binding globulin also rises, so that plasma testosterone and androsterone levels rise. 11-Deoxycorticosterone (DOC) shows the greatest percentage increase of all adrenal steroids, and aldosterone, which is predominantly bound to albumin, also increases substantially in normal pregnancy.

Medullary function remains surprisingly constant with little change in plasma levels of adrenaline and noradrenaline.

Changes in maternal physiology in pregnancy

- Weight gain (12.5 kg at 0.4 kg/week; one-third fetal)
- Breast; ducts stimulated by oestrogen, alveoli by progesterone and prolactin
- Uterus increases ×20 in weight, ×10 blood flow
- Hypertrophy of lower genital tract
- Plasma volume increases by 50%
- Cardiac output up 40%
- Increase in tidal volume
- Plasma osmolality falls
- Renal blood flow and glomerular filtration rate increase; creatinine and urea fall
- Ureteric and pelvicalyceal dilatation and reflux
- Reduced bowel motility and sphincter tone
- Endocrine changes in pituitary, thyroid and adrenal glands

BIBLIOGRAPHY

Dawes M G, Grudzinskas J G 1991 Patterns of maternal weight gain in pregnancy. British Journal of Obstetrics and Gynaecology 98: 195–201

Fay R A, Hughes A O, Farron N T 1983 Platelets in pregnancy: hyperdestruction in pregnancy. Obstetrics and Gynecology 61: 238–240

James D K, Steer P J, Weiner C P, Gonik B 1994 High risk pregnancy. W B Saunders, London

Hytten F, Chamberlain G 1991 Clinical physiology in obstetrics. Blackwell, Oxford

Philipp E E, Setchell M 1991 Scientific foundations – obstetrics and gynaecology. Heinemann, London

4 Antenatal care

The concept that the general well-being and reproductive performance of a woman might be improved by antenatal supervision is surprisingly recent and was first introduced in Edinburgh in 1911. In many societies, antenatal care is not available, and for social or religious reasons is not used when it is available.

The basic aims of antenatal care are:

1. To ensure optimal health of the mother throughout her pregnancy
2. To detect and treat disorders arising during pregnancy which relate to the welfare of both mother and fetus and to ensure that the pregnancy results in a healthy mother and healthy infant.

The ways by which these objectives are achieved vary in relation to the efficiency of clinical observation at any given time and to the value of current screening tests, which are designed to detect maternal or fetal problems.

Antenatal examinations are performed at regular intervals, and the recommended timing for visits (Fig. 4.1) is:

1. Monthly visits for the first 28 weeks
2. Bimonthly visits from 28 to 36 weeks
3. Weekly visits for the remaining weeks.

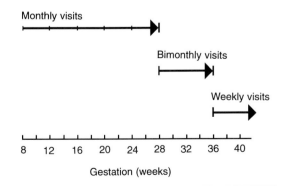

Antenatal Examinations:

Monthly visits

Bimonthly visits

Weekly visits

8 12 16 20 24 28 32 36 40

Gestation (weeks)

Fig. 4.1 Timing of antenatal visits.

These recommendations clearly apply only to apparently normal pregnancies, and need to be modified where circumstances indicate an increased risk to the mother or fetus.

There are differing views about the frequency and pattern of visits during routine antenatal care. Routine observations can be safely managed in local clinics or hospital-based clinics, but observations in high risk pregnancies should be overseen by the specialist obstetric staff.

ROUTINE CLINICAL EXAMINATIONS

The details of antenatal history and routine clinical examinations have been discussed in Chapter 1. The importance of clinical assessment cannot be overemphasized. Routine assessment of blood pressure, urine and body weight and estimates of fetal growth and size form the basis of good antenatal care.

LABORATORY TESTS

At the first visit to clinic, the following routine haematological and urinary investigations are recommended:

1. Haemoglobin concentration and, where indicated, a complete blood picture. This should be repeated on at least two subsequent occasions at 28 weeks and 36 weeks gestation. Estimates of total red cell mass would be more reliable indicators of anaemia, but are generally impracticable in most clinics.
2. Determination of blood groups (ABO and Rh) should be routinely performed and include screening for Rh antibodies in Rh-negative women. If no antibodies are detected, the test should be repeated at 32 weeks gestation. If antibodies are detected, the titre is determined and subsequent samples taken for further titre estimations at appropriate intervals (Fig. 4.2).

Laboratory Tests:

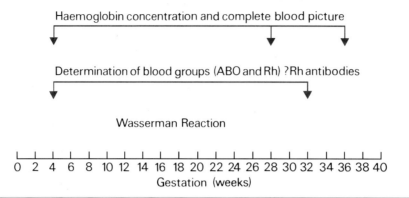

Fig. 4.2 Schedules for routine tests of haemoglobin estimation and detection of Rhesus antibodies.

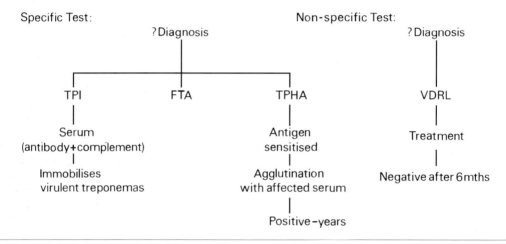

Fig. 4.3 Screening for syphilis.

3. **Screening for syphilis**. Routine screening for syphilis is recommended practice because of the importance of early detection of the disease in pregnancy (Fig. 4.3). The yield is small and the value of the procedure is debatable. There are numerous serological tests available for syphilis, some of which are non-specific, such as the Wasserman reaction, and some of which are specific.

Non-specific tests – The Wasserman reaction, which is a complement fixation test, was the first successful serological test. This test is dependent on the presence of treponemal antibodies in the serum which then unite with a colloidal suspension of lipoids to produce visible flocculation. A similar flocculation test that is widely used is the **veneral disease research laboratory test** (VDRL), which employs a cardiolipin antigen.

The difficulty with these tests is that they may give a false-positive reaction in association with malaria or virus pneumonia, or in auto-immune conditions, such as lupus erythematosus, haemolytic anaemia. Hashimoto's disease or rheumatoid arthritis.

Specific tests – Where there is doubt about the diagnosis, specific tests should be employed. The ***Treponema pallidum* immobilization test** (TPI) is the most specific test available, and is based on the fact that the serum from syphilitic patients contains an antibody which, in the presence of complement, immobilizes virulent treponemas. Positive tests are also found in patients with yaws and other treponemal diseases. Other tests include the **fluorescent treponemal antibody test** (FTA) and the *Treponema pallidum* **haemagglutination test** (TPHA). In the TPHA, the antigen consists of a suspension of turkey red blood cells in formalin and tannin which have been sensitized by contact with virulent treponemas. Positive tests are characterized by agglutination of the sensitized cells on contact with affected serum. The test is easy to perform and is highly specific. The VDRL usually becomes negative within 6 months of treatment, whereas the TPHA remains positive for many years. The VDRL, therefore, assumes the most important role in monitoring treatment.

4. **Screening for HIV infection**. The basis of tests for the detection of HIV infection is the detection of human immunodeficiency virus (HIV) antibodies. The virus can be isolated and grown, but this is difficult. The virus has a predilection for the T-helper subset of lymphocytes. There is an altered T-helper/T-suppressor ratio.

All of these tests can be normal, even with the presence of infection. The most important clinically confounding variable is that HIV antibodies may be absent in the incubation phase. Seropositive mothers always have seropositive babies, but this may not indicate the acquired immune deficiency syndrome (AIDS) in the baby. However, 30–50% of babies have AIDS.

Screening necessitates taking a serum blood sample and repeating after 6 months. Screening is indicated if there are risk factors, i.e. intravenous drugs, a sexual partner who is a drug abuser, or from a high-risk area or who is bisexual, and haemophiliacs. Testing for HIV in an unselected population gives a false positive for every true positive so caution must be exercised. If screening is limited to high-risk groups, selection is much better.

5. **Screening for fetal anomalies**. Structural fetal anomalies account for some 20–25% of all perinatal deaths and for about 15% of all deaths in the first year of life. There is, therefore, a strong case to be made for early detection and termination of the pregnancy where this is appropriate.

The frequency of major structural anomalies is shown in Table 4.1.

Neural tube defects – In 1972, Brock and Sutcliffe described an increase in the concentration of α-fetoprotein in amniotic fluid in the presence of neural tube defects. The likelihood of a major neural tube defect is enhanced where there is a previous history of an affected child. Where there is a history of one affected infant,

Table 4.1 Structural anomalies

Type of anomaly	Frequency
Cardiovascular	8/1000
Craniospinal	2–4/1000
Renal tract	1/1000
Gastrointestinal	1/1000

the risk of a subsequent abnormal child is 1 in 20. This risk is 1 in 10 after two children, and 1 in 5 after three children. There is evidence to show that the maternal ingestion of folic acid supplements will significantly reduce the recurrence rate. Total population screening is now undertaken on serum measurements of α-fetoprotein, but emphasis is now placed on the use of these measurements as a screening measurement for both neural tube defects and Down's syndrome.

Serum α-fetoprotein – Blood samples should be taken between 15 and 19 weeks gestation, and where there is doubt about gestational age, ultrasound assessment should be performed and the serum measurement repeated. If the serum values of α-fetoprotein are abnormally elevated, a detailed ultrasound should be performed. This will identify 95% of neural tube defects. If there is any doubt about the diagnosis, a sample of amniotic fluid can be collected by amniocentesis and tested for levels of α-fetoprotein and acetylcholinesterase (Fig. 4.4). It must be remembered that closed neural tube defects do not give rise to elevated levels of serum α-fetoprotein. They may

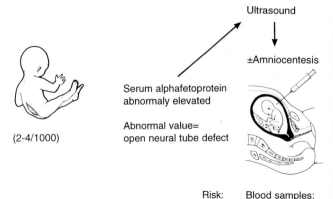

	Risk:	Blood samples:
Previous history of one affected infant	1 in 20	16 and 19 weeks gestation
After 2 children	1 in 10	
After 3 children	1 in 5	

Fig. 4.4 Screening for neural tube defects.

also be difficult to detect on ultrasound scan. However, a 'missed' diagnosis of these lesions is of less significance because these closed lesions are associated with minimal disability.

Several conditions, other than anencephaly or open tube lesions, give rise to raised serum α-fetoprotein levels. These conditions include multiple pregnancy, threatened abortion, intra-uterine death, congenital nephrosis, exomphalos, and duodenal or oesophageal atresia. Where a twin pregnancy is detected, a detailed scan of both fetuses is important. Where one fetus appears to be abnormal, selective termination may be indicated.

Routine ultrasound scan for fetal anomalies – Most hospitals in the UK now offer routine anomaly scans to all mothers between 18 and 20 weeks gestation, although early scans between 10 and 12 weeks may be valuable as 'dating' scans.

Scanning can be provided by trained staff at various levels:

Level 1. A basic, simple scan to establish pregnancy viability, gestational age and the presence of gross anomalies.

Level 2. A detailed scan at 18–20 weeks to establish abnormalities in all systems. This is the standard 18 week scan.

Level 3. If an anomaly is suspected but is of uncertain nature on a level 2 scan, then a level 3 scan will be performed by an obstetrician/radiologist with particular experience in obstetric ultrasound using the highest-quality equipment.

The 18 week scan – Basic measurements to establish gestational age and to exclude abnormality should include:
a. Biparietal diameter
b. Head circumference
c. Anterior and posterior ventricular horns
d. Cerebral hemispheres
e. Femur length
f. Nuchal fold thickness.

For a detailed anomaly scan (Fig. 4.5) the following structures should be identified:
a. The cerebellum
b. Longitudinal and transverse sections of the spine
c. Four chamber view of the heart
d. Chest, diaphragm and stomach to exclude diaphragmatic hernia
e. Abdominal wall and cord insertion
f. Kidneys and bladder
g. Four limbs and the digits.

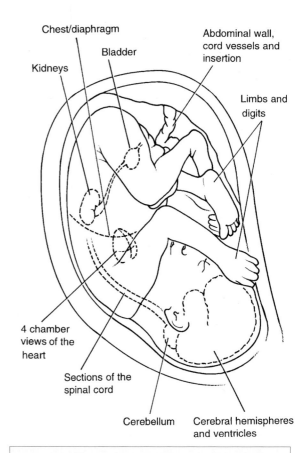

Fig. 4.5 Structures examined by ultrasound imaging in a detailed anomaly scan.

There are also markers that are commonly seen in association with trisomy, 13, 18 and 21, and these include:
a. Choroid plexus cysts
b. Nuchal fat pad in excess of 6 mm
c. Echogenic foci in right and left cardiac ventricles
d. 'Bright' or echo-rich bowel
e. Dilated renal pelvis with width greater than 4 mm.

6. **Screening for chromosomal abnormalities.** Studies in the early 1980s described an association between Down's syndrome and lower levels of maternal serum α-fetoprotein. Whereas screening on the basis of age alone has the virtue of simplicity, it is an ineffective method of screening. Seven per cent of the pregnant population are 35 years or older, and the use of routine amniocentesis in this age group will detect one abnormality for every 125 diagnostic tests. Furthermore, one

chromosomally normal fetus is lost for each chromosomally abnormal fetus detected. In 1984, the first observations were reported that second-trimester maternal serum α-fetoprotein (MSAFP) levels were reduced in chromosomally abnormal pregnancies. Using the combination of age and MSAFP, 40% of all autosomal trisomy pregnancies have been identified with a positive screen group of 7%.

In addition, the measurement of raised levels of human chorionic gonadotrophin (hCG) and low unconjugated oestriol, often known as the triple test, will increase the accuracy of detection to 57%. Such tests can be offered to all pregnant women, and commonly the combination of MSAFP and hCG is used in women over the age of 35 years to provide selection for amniocentesis. In addition to trisomy 21, other trisomies such as 18 and 13 also have lowered MSAFP levels. Other causes for a low MSAFP include fetal death, hydatidiform mole, diabetes, obesity and wrong dates. Further details of screening for chromosomal abnormalities will be presented in a later chapter.

Amniocentesis – This is usually carried out between 15 and 17 weeks. Between 10 and 15 ml of amniotic fluid is aspirated transabdominally using a spinal needle under ultrasound guidance. The procedure carries a 1% risk of causing miscarriage. Fetal cells from the aspirate must be cultured (failure rate 2–5%) before chromosome analysis, and results normally take 3–4 weeks to obtain.

Chorion villous sampling – Fetal cells can also be obtained from chorionic villi by aspirating a small amount of tissue either transabdominally or transcervically. This can be carried out before 12 weeks, and a preliminary karyotype obtained after 48 hours. This allows diagnosis of major chromosome disorders in the first trimester and surgical termination. The procedure is associated with a slightly higher rate of pregnancy loss (1–2%) than amniocentesis.

SCREENING FOR RUBELLA

In 1970, the then Department of Health and Social Security in the UK recommended that rubella vaccination should be offered to all girls between their 11th and 14th birthdays in an attempt to reduce the incidence of congenital rubella defects. However, many women still remain at risk because they have declined, or have not been offered, immunization,

and it has been estimated that approximately 10–15% remain susceptible to the disease at the time of pregnancy. The presence of rubella antibodies in serum is determined by using a technique of radial haemolysis or the haemagglutination inhibition test. The former test is favoured for mass screening programmes.

All women attending antenatal clinics should have serum taken for rubella antibodies unless immunity is already established. Seronegative women should be offered rubella vaccination in the immediate puerperium unless they do not intend to have any further children. Vaccination is performed with a live attenuated rubella virus with vaccines such as Almevax, and involves a single dose of 0.5 ml injected subcutaneously. Although there is little evidence to suggest any significant abnormality rate in women who have conceived immediately before or following rubella vaccination, it is generally recommended that pregnancy should be avoided for 2 months after vaccination.

The diagnosis of rubella during pregnancy can be made on the clinical manifestations of the infection, which include a fine macular rash, lymphadenopathy in the cervical region and a mild pyrexia (Fig. 4.6). The diagnosis can be confirmed in the acute phase by virus isolation from a throat swab or from blood culture, but usually the diagnosis is established by determination of the level of antibodies in the mother. A fourfold rise in antibody titre in consecutive blood samples taken 2 weeks

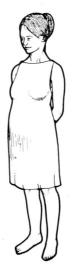

Mild pyrexia

Fine macular rash

Lymphadenopathy

throat swab or blood culture – virus isolation

diagnosis by determination of level of antibodies in mother

Cord blood measurements show similar antibody titres to mother

Fig. 4.6 Clinical manifestations of rubella infection.

apart constitutes evidence of recent rubella infection in the mother. In the infant, cord blood measurements will show similar antibody titres to the mother. However, the presence of raised levels of the immunoglobulin IgM strongly suggests infection acquired in utero.

SCREENING FOR URINARY TRACT INFECTION

Culture of urine is now used as a routine screening procedure. The presence of pathogenic organisms in excess of 10^4 organisms/ml indicates significant bacteriuria, and there is evidence to show that the treatment of asymptomatic bacteriuria of this type will produce a significant reduction in subsequent urinary tract infection.

Clinical examinations and laboratory tests

- Blood pressure, weight, urinalysis
- Abdominal palpation and auscultation
- Hb, Rh antibodies, hepatitis syphilis and rubella
- Detailed scan of fetus
- Serum α-fetoprotein

ANTENATAL EDUCATION

An important part of antenatal care is the preparation for childbirth and the subsequent care of the child. Antenatal education should, ideally, start before pregnancy as part of school education and it should continue throughout pregnancy and the puerperium. Whatever approach is considered preferable, there is a common need to inform the mother of the changes she can expect during pregnancy and of the nature of labour and delivery. The education programme should also include parentcraft and the advice on care of the child should be continued in the puerperium.

DIETARY ADVICE

Diet in pregnancy

There is ample evidence that the outcome of pregnancy can be influenced by dietary intake. Gross malnutrition is known to result in intra-uterine growth retardation, anaemia, prematurity and fetal malformation.

Lesser degrees of malnutrition may also be associated with increased frequency of fetal malformation, and it is therefore important to identify those mothers who have poor dietary intake and provide advice for all mothers during pregnancy. There is also some evidence to suggest that mothers who have experienced complications in a previous pregnancy may benefit from appropriate dietetic advice which may prevent the development of abnormalities. However, this hypothesis remains to be proved.

The incidence of recurrent neural defects appears to be reduced by folic acid supplements given prior to conception and for up to 12 weeks into pregnancy. Women with a previously affected fetus should be advised to take folic acid at a daily dosage of 400 µg whilst trying to conceive and during the first trimester.

Energy intake

A total energy intake of 2000–2500 kcal a day is optimal during the last two trimesters and this requirement may increase to 3000 kcal per day in the puerperium in lactating women.

Protein

First class protein is expensive and therefore is most likely to be deficient in the diet. An average of 60–80 g per day is desirable, and the diet is particularly likely to be deficient in the lower socioeconomic group and in association with vegetarian diets. Animal protein is obtained from meat, poultry, fish, eggs and cheese. Vegetable protein occurs in nuts, lentils, beans and peas (Table 4.2a).

Fats

The importance of fats, particularly essential fatty acids, has been underestimated and, indeed, essential fatty acids may play an important role in preventing the development of hypertension during pregnancy. Fats are an important source of energy, and they provide fat-soluble vitamins, including vitamins A, D and K.

Animal fats are found in meat, eggs and dairy produce, which contain a high percentage of saturated fats. Vegetable fats are also important as they contain unsaturated fats such as linolenic and linoleic acids.

Table 4.2a   Common dietary sources of protein and iron

Sources of protein		Sources of iron	
16 g sources		**5 mg sources**	
Beef, chicken, pork, fish,		Liver, kidney	60 g
Cheddar cheese	60 g	Beef heart	90 g
Cottage cheese	$\frac{1}{2}$ cup	Beans, cooked dry	1 cup
Dried beans (cooked)	1 cup	**3 mg sources**	
Peanuts	$\frac{1}{2}$ cup	Beef, pork	90 g
8 g sources		Spinach, greens	$\frac{1}{2}$ cup
Milk (whole, skim, dried)	1 cup	**2 mg sources**	
Peanut butter	2 table spoons	Peaches or apricots, dried	
Egg	1 large	cooked; raisins, prunes	
Peas (split, dry, cooked)	$\frac{1}{2}$ cup	green peas	$\frac{1}{2}$ cup
4 g sources		Chicken	90 g
Macaroni, rice, oatmeal	$\frac{3}{4}$ cup	**1 mg sources**	
Coconut, shredded (fresh) or		Egg, sweet potato	1 medium
2 cups dried, shredded	$1\frac{1}{2}$ cup	Broccoli, oatmeal, enriched	
Bread	2 slices	macaroni, winter squash	$\frac{1}{2}$ cup
		Orange	1 large
		Bread – enriched	2 slices

Carbohydrates

Carbohydrates are a major source of energy. Our present understanding of fetal biochemistry suggests that there is a close correlation between maternal and fetal blood glucose levels and that glucose is a major source of energy for the fetus.

Minerals and vitamins

The requirements for iron, calcium, iodine and various trace elements such as magnesium and zinc all increase in pregnancy. These elements are found in lean meat, various stone fruits, beans and peas, dairy produce and seafoods (Table 4.2b).

Table 4.2b   Dietary sources of calcium

Sources of calcium	
0.30 g sources	
Milk	1 cup
Cheddar cheese	40 g
0.15 g sources	
Canned salmon (with bones), cottage	
cheese, broccoli	$\frac{1}{2}$ cup
0.05 g sources	
Dried raisins, cooked beans: pinto,	$\frac{1}{2}$ cup
kidney	
Orange	1 medium
Sweet potato	1 medium
Bread – enriched	2 slices

Vitamins A and B are found in kidney, liver and dark green veegetables. Vitamin B_2 is found in whole grain and cereals, and vitamins B_5 in fish, lean meat, poultry and nuts (Table 4.3).

Ascorbic acid is essential for normal fetal growth and maternal health, and is found in citrus fruits,

Table 4.3   General advice on foodstuffs recommended in pregnancy (portions given per day unless otherwise stated)

Foodstuff	Quantity
Dairy	
Milk	600–1000 ml
Butter	150 g
Cheese	1 serving
Meat	
Chicken, pork or beef	2 servings
Liver	Once/week or more
Fish	Once or twice/week
Vegetables	
Potato	1–2 servings
Other	1–2 servings
Salads	Freely
Fruit	
Citrus	1
Other	2–3
Cereals	
Wheat, corn, rice,	
macaroni, spaghetti	4 servings

1 serving = $\frac{1}{2}$ cup.

Brussels sprouts and broccoli. Vitamin D and folic acid are also important, although it is very rare now to see any signs of vitamin D deficiency. Folic acid deficiency is still relatively common, and is associated with the development of megaloblastic anaemia in the mother. Green vegetables, nuts and yeast are all rich sources of folic acid, and it is common practice to give specific supplements during pregnancy.

EXERCISE IN PREGNANCY

Pregnant women should be encouraged to undertake reasonable activity. This will be limited with advancing gestation by the physical restrictions imposed by the pregnancy, but during early pregnancy there is no need to restrict sporting activities beyond the commonsense limits of avoiding excessive exertion and fatigue. Swimming is helpful, particularly in late pregnancy.

COITUS IN PREGNANCY

There is no contraindication to coitus in pregnancy at any stage of gestation, other than the physical difficulties imposed by the changes in abdominal size. It is, however, sensible to advise against coitus where there is evidence of threatened abortion or a history of recurrent abortions. It is also generally contraindicated where there is a history of antepartum haemorrhage or premature rupture of the membranes.

SOCIAL HABITS

Smoking in pregnancy

Smoking has an adverse effect on fetal growth and development (Fig. 4.7):

1. **The effect of carbon monoxide on the fetus.**
   Carbon monoxide has an affinity for haemoglobin 200 times greater than oxygen. Fresh air contains up to 0.5 ppm of carbon monoxide, but in cigarette smoke values as high as 60 000 ppm may be detected. Carbon monoxide shifts the oxygen dissociation curve to the left in both fetal and maternal haemoglobin. Maternal carbon monoxide saturation may rise to 8% in the mother and 7% in the fetus, so that there is specific interference with oxygen transfer.

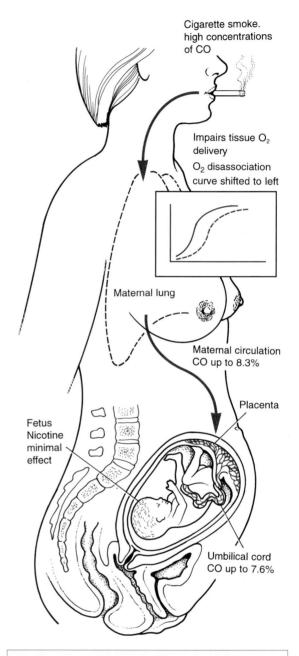

Fig. 4.7 The effects of smoking on the feto-placental unit.

2. **The effect of nicotine on the uteroplacental vasculature as a vasoconstrictor.** Animal studies on the effect of infusions of nicotine on cardiac output and uteroplacental blood flow have shown that high-dose infusions produce a fall in cardiac output and uteroplacental blood flow. However, at

levels up to five times greater than those seen in smokers there are no measurable effects, and it is unlikely that nicotine exerts any adverse effects by reducing uteroplacental blood flow.

3. **The effect of smoking on placental structure**. The placenta largely seems to be spared any significant damage as a result of smoking in pregnancy. Some changes are seen on the placental histology. The trophoblastic basement membrane shows irregular thickening, and some of the fetal capillaries show reduced calibre, but the changes are not consistent or gross and are not associated with any reduction in placental size.

4. **The effect on perinatal mortality**. Smoking during pregnancy reduces the birth weight of the infant, and also reduces the crown–heel length.

It is also now generally agreed that the perinatal death rate is increased as a direct effect of smoking, and this increased risk has been quantified at 20% for those women smoking up to 20 cigarettes per day, and 35% in excess of one packet per day. Mothers should be advised to stop smoking during pregnancy.

Alcohol intake in pregnancy

Excessive alcohol intake is associated with a specific syndrome, the **fetal alcohol syndrome**. The features in the infant include growth retardation, various structural defects, various facial defects, multiple joint anomalies and cardiac defects. However, these problems arise in women who consume 80 g of alcohol per day. This is equivalent to 8 units per day where 1 unit is equivalent to 1 glass of wine or half a pint of beer or lager per day, but fetal growth may be affected on as little as 4 units per day.

There is no evidence to show that such problems arise in association with modest social drinking, so that the occasional glass of wine has not been shown to be associated with risk.

BREAST CARE

Breast feeding should be encouraged in all women unless there is any specific contraindication which would make breast feeding excessively difficult, such as grossly inverted nipples or previous damage to the breasts. It must also be remembered that, although breast feeding is desirable, the reality is that children tend to grow and develop equally satisfactorily on artificial feeding. It is, therefore, wise to do no more than encourage women to

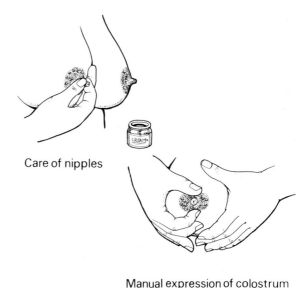

Care of nipples

Manual expression of colostrum

Fig. 4.8 Nipple care and breast preparation.

breast feed, rather than apply any coercion, and the mother's desire must be taken into account.

In the antenatal period, the breasts should be washed daily and carefully dried. The nipples should be massaged with an appropriate cream and the nipple drawn with the fingers if there is any evidence of retraction (Fig. 4.8). The breasts should be supported with an appropriate maternity brassiere. Manual expression of colostrum should be taught and practised from 36 weeks gestation.

COMMON MINOR DISORDERS OF PREGNANCY

Vomiting in pregnancy

Minor degrees of nausea and vomiting are very common in early pregnancy. Nevertheless, this is a symptom complex which appears to have become less significant in recent years. Although it is commonly described as 'morning sickness', it does not always occur in the morning and is often triggered by the smell of food and conditions of stress. The use of anti-emetic drugs has generally fallen into disrepute because of anxiety over taking drugs in early pregnancy. Even a drug such as Debendox, which has been extensively used and investigated in early pregnancy and where there is no evidence of any increase in congenital malformations, has now been withdrawn from the market. There is some evidence to suggest that untreated nausea and vomiting in early pregnancy, with the associated dietary restrictions, may carry risks in their own right.

Most vomiting diminishes or stops by 12–14 weeks gestation and can often be relieved by frequent small meals and the avoidance of highly spiced foods. It also helps to have a sweetened drink before starting activities in the morning. Sometimes the severity of vomiting necessitates hospital admission and intravenous therapy. Reassurance and continued support are essential requirements in management.

In most patients the management of the acute episode of hyperemesis should be treated by intravenous fluid replacement and electrolyte correction, anti-emetic regimes, vitamin supplementation and anti-gastro-oesophageal reflux measures. With this regime, most women will respond, although they may require treatment on more than one occasion. In extreme circumstances, the use of corticosteroids may be effective in controlling the vomiting.

Abdominal pain

Very few women manage to experience an entire pregnancy without an episode of abdominal pain. Most of these episodes are transitory and unaccompanied by any signs of systemic disorder. Nevertheless, it is important to distinguish these from organic disorders such as appendicitis, and yet to avoid unnecessary interference and surgery which may, in themselves, produce disastrous results. The cause for most episodes is never determined.

Heartburn

With the enlargement of the uterus and displacement of the gut, reflux of gastric juices occurs in many women, with resultant heartburn. This is particularly noticeable when the woman is supine and can, to some degree, be avoided by raising the head with pillows when resting and the use of antacids.

Constipation

The increased levels of progesterone in pregnancy appear to reduce bowel motility so that constipation is a common problem. This is sometimes intractable until the pregnancy is completed, but can be helped by increasing dietary fibre intake with bran and green vegetables and by the use of bulk-forming laxatives, or stimulants such as Senokot and milk of magnesia.

Backache

Pregnancy is associated with changes in posture and with increasing lumbar lordosis. The increased laxity of pelvic ligaments induced by high circulating levels of sex steroids also results in some instability of the bony pelvis. Lumbar and sacral backache are therefore very common in pregnancy. Occasionally the pain may be incapacitating and associated with sciatic pain. It may be lumbar or sacro-iliac. In rare cases, it is associated with disc protrusion, and the symptoms may persist after delivery. However, in most women no obvious cause is identified, and the pain disappears after delivery. Pregnant women should be advised to lift objects by flexing their knees and thighs, and not their backs. Sometimes, a supportive corset may be necessary, and rest on a well-supported bed is advisable.

Syncopal episode

'Fainting' in pregnancy is very common, and it is surprising how rarely serious injury ensues. Presumably most pregnant women have sufficient warning signs to avoid dangerous situations. There is little that can be done except to reassure the woman that this is a common problem associated with the general vascular instability of pregnancy and to encourage them to avoid potentially hazardous situations.

Varicosities

Varicose veins and haemorrhoids almost invariably become worse during pregnancy and women should be advised that this is the case. Local support with elastic hosiery can significantly relieve symptoms. In the case of haemorrhoids, constipation should be avoided, and replacement and bed rest recommended where the haemorrhoids have prolapsed. Appropriate vasoconstrictor suppositories should be used.

Common minor disorders of pregnancy

- Vomiting
- Acid reflux
- Constipation
- Backache
- Syncope
- Varicosities
- Carpal tunnel syndrome

Carpal tunnel syndrome

Compression of the median nerve with tingling and paraesthesia in the distribution of the median nerve involving the thumb and the lateral two-and-a-half

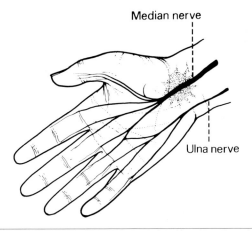

Median nerve

Disturbance of
sensation in skin
Pain on flexion of wrist
Atrophy of thenar muscles
Swelling of fingers

Ulna nerve

Fig. 4.9 Carpal tunnel syndrome is a common complication of pregnancy.

fingers occurs as a complication of pregnancy (Fig. 4.9). It is sometimes relieved by diuretics and occasionally requires splinting of the wrist to produce symptomatic relief. It rarely appears to result in any residual neurological damage and always disappears in the puerperium.

In summary, numerous minor disorders occur in pregnancy. Provided they are recognised as short-term problems, they rarely require more than symptomatic relief and reassurance that the condition will improve with the completion of the pregnancy.

BIBLIOGRAPHY

Brock D J H 1982 Early diagnosis of fetal defects. Churchill Livingstone, Edinburgh

Brock D J H, Sutcliffe R G 1972 Alphafetoprotein in the antenatal diagnosis of anencephaly and spina bifida. Lancet ii: 197–199

Chervenak F A, Isaacson G C, Campbell S 1993 Ultrasound in obstetrics and gynaecology. Little Brown, Boston

Ferguson-Smith M A 1984 Pre-natal diagnosis. Wiley Medical Publications, Chichester

Hall M H 1990 Antenatal care. Clinical obstetrics and gynaecology. Baillière Tindall, London, vol 4(1)

Hobbins J C, Besacerraf B F 1989 Diagnosis and therapy of fetal anomalies. Clinics in diagnostic ultrasound. Churchill Livingstone, Edinburgh

James D K, Steer P J, Weiner C P, Gonik B 1994 High risk pregnancy. W B Saunders, London

Jordan J, Symonds E M 1978 The diagnosis and management of neural tube defects. The Royal College of Obstetricians and Gynaecologists

Poswilla D, Alberman E 1992 Effects of smoking on the fetus, neonate and child. Oxford University Press, Oxford

Rayburn W F, Zuspan F P 1982 Drug therapy in obstetrics and gynaecology. Appleton-Century-Crofts

5 Conception and nidation

OOGENESIS

Primordial germ cells originally appear in the yolk sac and can be identified by the fourth week of fetal development (Fig. 5.1). The cells migrate through the dorsal mesentery of the developing gut and finally reach the genital ridge between 44 and 48 days. Migration occurs into a genital tubercle, consisting of mesenchymal cells, which appears over the ventral part of the mesonephros. The germ cells form sex cords and become the cortex of the gonad. The sex cords break up into separate clumps of cells, and by 16 weeks these clumps of cells become primary follicles which incorporate central germ cells. These cells undergo rapid mitotic activity, and by 20 weeks of intra-uterine life there are about 7 million cells known as oogonia. After this time, no further cell division occurs and no further ova are produced. At birth, the oogonia have begun the first meiotic division and have become primary oocytes. The number of oocytes falls to 1 million by birth and 0.5 million by puberty.

Meiosis

The chromosome number of the gametes is half that of normal cells. With the fusion of the egg and sperm, the chromosome complement is returned to the normal count of 46 chromosomes. In meiosis, two cell divisions occur in succession, each of which consists of a prophase, metaphase, anaphase and telophase (Fig. 5.2). At the end of the first meiotic prophase, the double chromosomes undergo synapsis, producing a group of four homologous chromatids called a tetrad. The two centrioles move to opposite poles, a spindle forms in the middle and the membrane of the nucleus disappears. As the cell enters the metaphase of the first meiotic division, the tetrads line up around the equator of the spindle. Primary oocytes remain in suspended prophase until sexual maturity is reached. Meiotic division resumes as the dominant follicle is triggered by luteinising hormone (LH) to commence ovulation. In anaphase, the daughter chromatids separate and move towards opposite poles. The centrioles divide again, and the haploid number of double chromosomes separate and move to appropriate poles. In the telophase of the second meiotic division, 23 chromosomes arrive at each pole.

Thus, the nuclear events in oogenesis are the same as in spermatogenesis but cytoplasmic division is unequal, resulting in one secondary oocyte. This small cell consists almost entirely of a nucleus, and

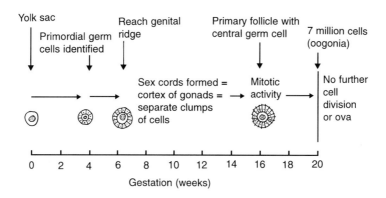

Fig. 5.1 Embryonic and fetal development of oogonia.

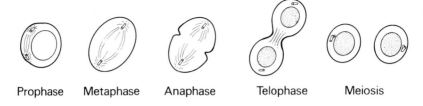

Prophase   Metaphase   Anaphase   Telophase   Meiosis

Fig. 5.2 Nuclear events in oogenesis associated with meiosis.

is known as the first polar body. As the ovum enters the Fallopian tube, the second meiotic division occurs, and a secondary oocyte forms with the development of a small second polar body.

Oogenesis

- Primordial germ cells at 4th week
- Migrate to genital ridge by 48th day
- Primary follicles by 16 weeks
- Oogonia by 20 weeks
- Meiosis starts
- Oocytes by birth
- Follicles mature 11–50 years later
- Meiosis completed by ovulation to give secondary oocytes (haploid)

THE STRUCTURE OF THE MATURE OVARY

The mature ovary in the reproductive era is 3–5 cm in length and weighs 5–8 g. The ovary is suspended from the uterus by the ovarian ligament attached to its medial end. The ovary has a free margin and a hilus through which the blood vessels and lymphatics enter. The ovary is attached to the dorsal aspect of the broad ligament by a fold of peritoneum known as the mesovarium, and to the lateral pelvic wall by the suspensory or infundibulo-pelvic ligament, which contains the ovarian artery and vein. The blood supply to the ovaries comes from the ovarian arteries, which anastomose with the uterine arteries (Fig. 5.3). Both ovarian arteries arise directly from the aorta from a point immediately below the origin of the renal arteries. The right ovarian vein drains into the inferior vena cava, and accompanies the right ovarian artery. The left ovarian vein drains into the left renal vein. The lymphatic capillary plexus accompanies the ovarian vessels, and therefore drains to the middle lumbar lymph nodes and along the uterine vessels to the sacral nodes.

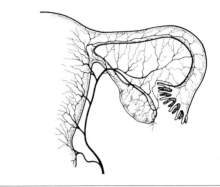

Fig. 5.3 Blood supply to the ovaries formed by anastomosis of uterine and ovarian arteries and veins.

Innervation

The ovary receives innervation from both sympathetic and parasympathetic fibres (Fig. 5.4). The sympathetic fibres arise predominantly from the 10th and 11th thoracic segments and from the lumbo-sacral region. Parasympathetic fibres from the lumbo-sacral region enter the ovary along the vessels of the utero-tubal anastomosis. Sensory fibres to the ovary arise in the lower thoracic area (T_{10}).

The nerves supplying the smooth muscles of intra-ovarian vessels and fibres also terminate in the theca interna and around Graafian follicles, which are surrounded by structures resembling smooth muscle cells. The nerve supply does not penetrate the basement membrane of follicles.

Contractions occur around the follicles and are mediated by adrenergic α-receptors, whereas relaxation is mediated by β-receptors. The function of the nerve supply remains uncertain, but it should be remembered that the suspensory ligaments of the ovary also contain smooth muscle fibres and that contraction of the fibres in the infundibulo-pelvic fold draw the infundibulum of the tube

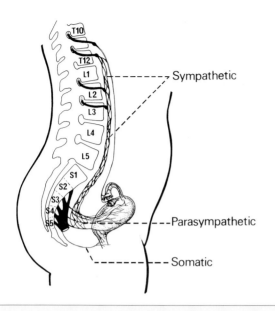

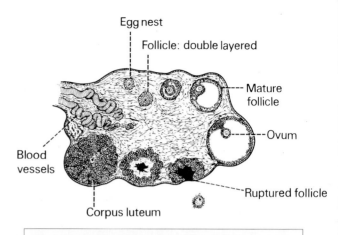

Fig. 5.5 Maturation of the Graafian follicle.

Fig. 5.4 Innervation of the ovaries arises from the lumbar and sacral autonomic outflow.

and the ovary together, thus facilitating oocyte entrapment.

Structure of the ovary

- Length 3–5 cm, weight 5–8 g
- Attached to dorsal aspect of broad ligament
- Blood supply from the ovarian artery
- Left ovarian vein drains into left renal vein
- Middle lumbar lymph nodes
- Sympathetic supply from T_{10} and T_{11}, parasympathetic S_2–S_5, sensory T_{10}

FOLLICULAR DEVELOPMENT IN THE OVARY

The surface of the ovary is covered by a single layer of cuboidal epithelium. The cortex of the ovary contains a large number of oogonia surrounded by follicle cells which become granulosa cells. The remainder of the ovary consist of a mesenchymal core. Most of the ova in the cortex never reach an advanced stage of maturation, and become atretic early in follicular development. At any given time, follicles can be seen in various stages of maturation and degeneration (Fig. 5.5). The first stage of development is characterized by enlargement of the ovum and proliferation of granulosa cells around the ovum with the aggregation of stromal cells to

form the thecal cells. The innermost layers of granulosa cells adhere to the ovum and form the **corona radiata**. A fluid-filled space develops in the granulosa cells, and a clear layer of gelatinous material collects around the ovum, forming the **zona pellucida**. The ovum becomes eccentrically placed, and the Graafian follicle assumes its classical mature form. The mesenchymal cells around the follicle become differentiated into two layers, forming the **theca interna** and **theca externa**.

As the follicle enlarges, it bulges towards the surface of the ovary and the area under the germinal epithelium thins out. The ovum, with its surrounding investment of granulosa cells, escapes through this area at the time of ovulation.

The cavity of the follicle often fills with blood but, at the same time, the granulosa cells and the theca interna cells undergo changes of luteinization to become filled with yellow carotenoid material. The corpus luteum in its mature form shows intense vascularization and pronounced vacuolization of the theca and granulosa cells, with evidence of hormonal activity. This development reaches its peak approximately 7 days after ovulation, and thereafter the corpus luteum regresses unless implantation occurs. This degeneration is characterized by increasing vacuolization of the granulosa cells and increased quantities of fibrous tissue in the centre of the corpus luteum; which finally develops into a white scar known as the **corpus albicans** (Fig. 5.6).

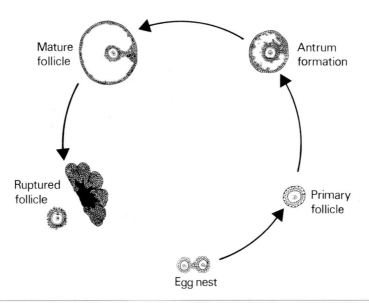

Mature follicle

Antrum formation

Ruptured follicle

Primary follicle

Egg nest

Fig. 5.6 Ovulation and maturation of the corpus luteum.

HORMONAL EVENTS ASSOCIATED WITH OVULATION

The maturation of oocytes, ovulation and the endometrial and tubal changes of the menstrual cycle are all regulated by a series of interactive hormonal changes (Fig. 5.7). The process is in-itiated by the release of LH-releasing hormone, which is a major neurosecretion produced in the median eminence of the hypothalamus. It has been isolated in many sites in the central nervous system, and may act as a neurotransmitter. The hormone is a decapeptide and is released from axon terminals into the pituitary portal capillaries. As the release of both follicle-stimulating hormone (FSH) and luteinizing hormone (LH) are stimulated by this hormone, it is more properly designated as **gonadotrophin-releasing hormone** (GnRH) (Fig. 5.7). The hormone is released in episodic fluctuations but there is no definite association with these surges and LH release. However, there is an increase in the number of surges associated with the higher levels of plasma LH and there is evidence of a decline in the GnRH content of the hypothalamus in mid-cycle in women, but continued ongoing GnRH action is required to initiate the oestrogen-induced LH surge.

The three major hormones involved in repro-duction are produced by the anterior lobe of the pituitary gland or adenohypophysis, and include FSH, LH and prolactin. Blood levels of both FSH and LH appear to remain at a relatively constant level in the first half of the cycle. There is a marked surge of LH 35–42 hours before ovulation and a smaller coincidental FSH peak (Fig. 5.7A). Recent detailed studies suggest that the LH surge is composed of two closely proximate surges. A peak in plasma oestradiol precedes the LH surge and may be the factor that stimulates the hypothalamus to release GnRH (Fig. 5.7B). Plasma LH and FSH levels are slightly lower in the second half of the cycle than in the pre-ovulatory phase. Pituitary gonadotrophins influence the activity of the hypothalamus by a short-loop feedback system.

Prolactin is secreted by lactotrophs in the anterior pituitary gland. Prolactin levels rise at mid-cycle and remain elevated during the luteal phase, and tend to follow the changes in plasma oestradiol-17β. Prolactin tends to control its own secretion through a short-loop feedback on the hypothalamus, which produces the prolactin-inhibiting factor, dopamine, and probably by the production of a hypothalamic-releasing factor (Fig. 5.8). Oestrogen appears to stimulate prolactin release, and various neuro-transmitters such as serotonin, noradrenaline, histamine, morphine and encephalins also stimulate prolactin release by a central action in the brain. Antagonists to dopamine, such as phenothiazine, reserpine and methyl-tyrosine, also stimulate the release of prolactin, whereas dopamine agonists such as bromocriptine have the opposite effect.

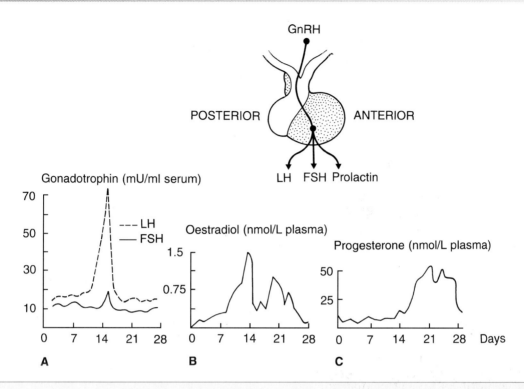

Fig. 5.7 The hormonal regulation of ovulation: GnRH stimulates the release of gonadotrophins from the pituitary; blood levels of **A** gonadotrophins (LH, FSH), **B** oestradiol, and **C** oestradiol and progesterone in the menstrual cycle.

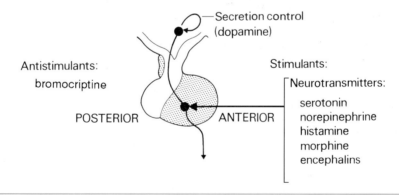

Fig. 5.8 Factors regulating the release of prolactin.

THE ACTION OF GONADOTROPHINS

FSH stimulates follicular growth and development and binds exclusively to granulosa cells in the growing follicle. Of the 30 or so follicles that begin to mature in each menstrual cycle, one becomes pre-eminent. The granulosa cells produce oestrogen, which feeds back on the pituitary to suppress FSH release. At the same time, FSH stimulates receptors for LH.

LH stimulates and sustains development of the corpus luteum, and receptors to LH are found in theca and granulosa cells and in the corpus luteum. There is a close interaction between FSH and LH in follicular growth and maturation. The corpus luteum produces progesterone until the structure begins to deteriorate in the late luteal phase (see Fig. 5.6). Prolactin appears to exert a direct effect on the follicle and to have a role in the initiation and maintenance of luteinization. It stimulates the development of LH receptors and thereby supports the production of high levels of progesterone.

THE ENDOMETRIAL CYCLE

The normal endometrium responds in a cyclical manner to the fluctuations in ovarian steroids. The endometrium consists of three zones and it is the two outer zones that are shed during menstruation (Fig. 5.9).

The basal zone (**zona basalis**) is the thin layer of compact stroma that interdigitates with the myometrium and shows little response to hormonal change. It is not shed at the time of menstruation. The next adjacent zone (**zona spongiosa**) contains the endometrial glands which are lined by columnar epithelial cells surrounded by loose stroma. The surface of the endometrium is covered by a compact layer of epithelial cells (**zona compacta**), which surrounds the ostia of the endometrial glands. The endometrial cycle is divided into four phases:

1. **Menstrual phase**. This occupies the first 4 days of the cycle, and results in shedding of the outer two layers of the endometrium. The onset of menstruation is preceded by segmented vaso-constriction of the spiral arteries. This leads to

necrosis and shedding of the functional layers of the endometrium. The vascular changes are associated with a fall in both oestrogen and progesterone levels, but the mechanism by which these vascular changes are mediated is still not understood.

2. The **phase of repair**. This phase extends from day 4 to day 7, and is associated with the formation of a new capillary bed arising from the arterial coils, and with regeneration of the epithelial surface.

3. The **follicular** or **proliferative phase**. This is the period of maximal growth of the endometrium, and is associated with elongation and expansion of the glands, and with stromal development. This phase proceeds from day 7 until the time of ovulation on day 14.

4. The **luteal** or **secretory phase**. This follows ovulation on day 14 and continues until day 28, when menstruation starts again. During this phase the endometrial glands become convoluted and 'saw-toothed' in appearance. The epithelial cells exhibit basal vacuolation, and by day 20 of the cycle there is visible secretion in the cells. The secretion subsequently becomes inspissated, and as menstruation approaches there is oedema of the stroma and a pseudo-decidual reaction. Within 2 days of menstru-ation, there is infiltration of the stroma by leucocytes.

It is now clear that luteinization of the follicle can occur in the absence of release of the oocyte. This

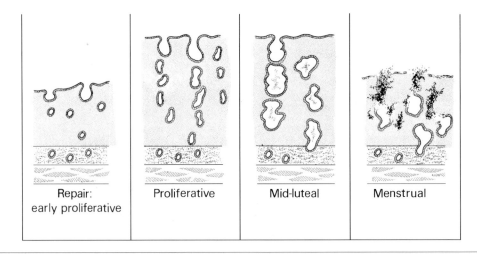

| Repair:
early proliferative | Proliferative | Mid-luteal | Menstrual |

Fig. 5.9 Cyclical endometrial changes in the normal menstrual cycle.

condition is described as **entrapped ovulation** or the LUF (luteinized unruptured follicle) syndrome, and is associated with progesterone production and with a normal ovulatory cycle. Histological examination of the endometrium generally enables precise dating of the menstrual cycle, and is particularly important in providing evidence of ovulation.

Follicular development/ovulation

- 30 follicles begin development under influence of FSH
- Ovum enlarges, granulosa proliferates and thecal cells formed
- Innermost granulosa cells form corona radiata, separated from others by zona pellucida
- Proliferative phase of endometrial cycle
- Plasma oestradiol peaks (stimulating GnRH release)
- LH (FSH) surge 35–42 hours prior to ovulation
- Follicle ruptures, becoming corpus luteum, under influence of LH and prolactin
- Luteal phase of endometrial development

SPERMATOGENESIS

The testis provides a dual function of spermatogenesis and androgen secretion. FSH is predominantly responsible for the stimulation of spermatogenesis and LH for the stimulation of Leydig cells and the production of testosterone (Fig. 5.10). The full maturation of spermatozoa takes 64 days, and all phases of maturation can be seen in the testis. The spermatogonia divide and give rise to primary spermatocytes, which have a diploid number of

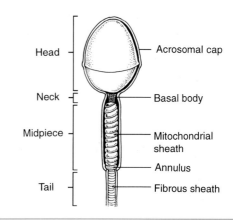

Fig. 5.11 Structure of the mature spermatozoon.

chromosomes. These cells undergo maturation division to secondary spermatocytes (2N haploid), and finally reduction division to form the haploid spermatids, which develop into the mature spermatozoa.

Structure of the spermatozoon

The spermatozoon consists of a head, neck and tail (Fig. 5.11). The entire structure is enveloped in a plasma membrane. The head is flattened and ovoid in shape and is covered by the acrosomal cap, which contains lysins.

The nucleus is densely packed with the genetic material of the sperm. The neck contains two centrioles, proximal and distal, which

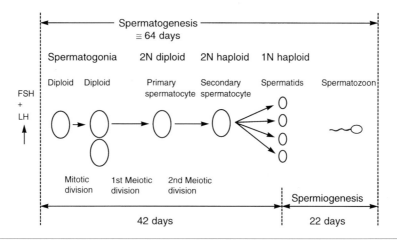

Fig. 5.10 The maturation cycle of spermatozoa.

form the beginning of the tail. The distal centriole is vestigial in mature spermatozoa but is functional in the spermatoid. The body contains a coiled helix of mitochondria, which provides the 'power house'. the tail consists of a central core of two longitudinal fibres. This structure is surrounded by nine pairs of fibres which terminate at various points until a single ovoid filament remains. These contractile fibres propel the spermatozoa.

Seminal plasma

Spermatozoa carry little nutritional reserve and therefore depend on seminal plasma for nutritional support. Seminal plasma originates from the prostate, seminal vesicles, the epididymis, the vas deferens and the bulbo-urethral glands. There is a high concentration of fructose, which is the major source of energy for spermatozoa. The plasma also contains high concentrations of amino acids, particularly glutamic acid, and several unique amines such as spermine and spermidine. The seminal plasma also contains high concentrations of prostaglandins, which have a potent stimulatory effect on the uterine musculature. Normal semen clots shortly after ejaculation but reliquefies within 30 minutes due to fibrinolytic activity during this period.

Spermatogenesis

- Maturation of spermatozoa takes 64 days
- Spermatogonia form primary (diploid) spermatocytes
- Secondary spermatocytes form (haploid) spermatids
- Spermatids form spermatozoa

FERTILIZATION

The process of fertilization involves the fusion of the male and female gametes to produce the diploid genetic complement from the genes of both partners.

Sperm transport

Following the deposition of semen near the cervical os migration of sperm occurs rapidly into the cervical mucus. The speed of this migration depends on the presence of receptive mucus in mid-cycle. During the luteal phase, the mucus is not receptive to sperm invasion and therefore very few spermatozoa reach the uterine cavity. Under favourable circumstances, sperm migrate at a rate of 6 mm/min. This is much

faster than could be explained by the motility of the sperm and must therefore also be dependent on active support within the uterine cavity. Only motile spermatozoa reach the fimbriated end of the tube.

Capacitation

During their passage through the Fallopian tube the sperm undergo the final stage in maturation (capacitation), which enables penetration of the zona pellucida. It seems likely that these changes are enzyme induced, and enzymes such as β-amylase or β-glucuronidase may act on the membranes of the spermatozoa to expose receptor sites involved in sperm penetration. In addition, various other factors that may be important in capacitation have been identified such as the removal of cholesterol from the plasma membrane, and the presence of α- and β-adrenergic receptors on the spermatozoa. Until recently, it was thought that capacitation occurred only in vivo in the Fallopian tube. However, it can also be induced in vitro by apparently non-specific effects of relatively simple culture solutions.

Inhibitory substances in the plasma of the cauda epididymis and in seminal plasma can prevent capacitation, and these substances also occur in the lower reaches of the female genital tract. It seems

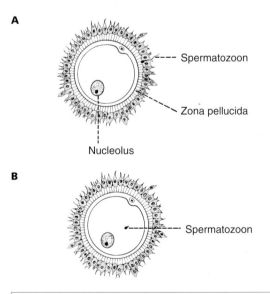

Fig. 5.12 **A** Adherence of the sperm to the oocyte initiates the acrosome reaction; **B** syngamy involves the passage of the nucleus of the sperm head into the cytoplasm of the oocyte, with the formation of the zygote.

likely that these substances protect the sperm until shortly before fusion with the oocyte.

Fertilization

A small number of spermatozoa reach the oocyte in the ampulla of the tube and surround the zona pellucida. The adherence of the sperm to the oocyte initiates the **acrosome reaction**, which involves the loss of plasma membrane over the acrosomal cap (Fig. 5.12A). This process allows the release of lytic enzymes which facilitate penetration of the oocyte membrane. The sperm head fuses with the oocyte plasma membrane and, by phagocytosis, the sperm head and mid-piece are engulfed into the oocyte. The sperm head decondenses to form the male pronucleus, and eventually becomes apposed to the female pronucleus in the fertilized egg – the **zygote**. The pronuclei membranes breakdown to facilitate the fusion of the male and female chromosomes. This process is know as **syngamy**, and is followed almost immediately by the first cleavage division.

During the 36 hours after fertilization, the conceptus is transported through the tube by muscular peristaltic action. The egg undergoes cleavage, and at the 16-cell stage becomes a solid ball of cells known as a **morula**, and then a fluid filled cavity develops to form the **blastocyst** (Fig. 5.13). Six days after ovulation, the embryonic pole of the blastocyst attaches itself to the endometrium,

usually near to the midportion of the uterine fundus. By the seventh day, the blastocyst has penetrated deeply into the endometrium after hatching from the zona.

Endometrial cells are destroyed by the cytotrophoblast, and the cells are incorporated by fusion and phagocytosis into the trophoblast. The endometrial stromal cells become large and pale, and this is known as the **decidual reaction**. Thus, the process of fertilization and implantation is now complete.

Fertilization

- Sperm migration inhibited by luteal phase cervical mucus
- Sperm undergo capacitation in the tube
- Adherence of sperm to oocyte initiates acrosome reaction
- Chromosomes fuse and second polar body expelled
- First cleavage division occurs

THE PHYSIOLOGY OF COITUS

Normal sexual arousal has been described in four levels in both men and women. These levels consist of excitement, plateau, orgasmic and resolution phases. In the male, the excitement phase results in compression of the venous channels of the penis, resulting in erection, which is mediated through the

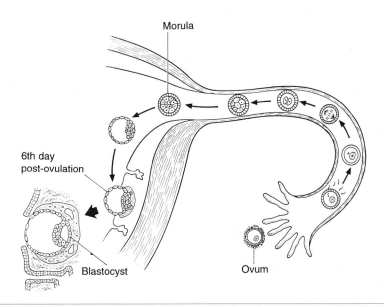

Morula

6th day
post-ovulation

Blastocyst

Ovum

Fig. 5.13 Stages of development from fertilization to implantation.

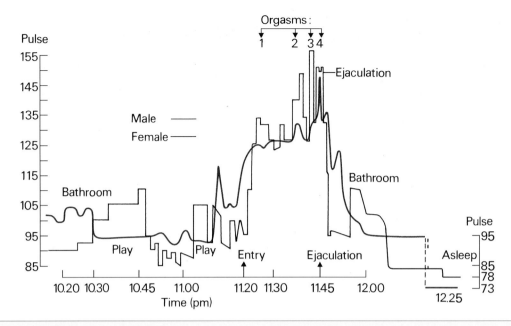

Fig. 5.14 Pulse rate changes during coitus.

parasympathetic plexus through S_2 and S_3. During the plateau phase, the penis remains engorged, and the testes increase in size with elevation of the testes and scrotum. Secretion of the bulbo-urethral glands results in the appearance of a clear fluid at the urethral meatus. These changes are accompanied by general systemic features including carpopedal spasm, increased skeletal muscle tension, hyper-ventilation and tachycardia (Fig. 5.14).

The orgasmic phase is induced by stimulation of the glans penis and by movement of penile skin on the penile shaft. There are reflex contractions of the bulbocavernosus and ischiocavernosus muscles and ejaculation of semen in a series of spurts. Specific musculo-skeletal activity occurs, which is charac-terized by penile thrusting. The systemic changes of tachycardia and rapid respiration persist.

During the resolution phase, penile erection rapidly subsides, as does the hyperventilation and tachycardia. There is a marked sweating reaction in some 30–40% of individuals. During this phase, the male becomes refractory to further stimulation. The plateau phase may be prolonged if ejaculation does not occur.

In the female, the excitement phase involves nipple and clitoral erection, vaginal lubrication, which results partly from transudation through the vaginal walls and partly from secretions from Bartholin's glands, thickening and congestion of the labia majora and the labia minora, and engorgement of the uterus. Stimulation of the clitoris and the labia results in progression to the orgasmic platform with narrowing of the outer third of the vagina and ballooning of the vaginal vault. The vaginal walls become congested and purplish in colour, and there is a marked increase in vaginal blood flow. During orgasm, the clitoris retracts behind the pubic symphysis, and a succession of contractions occur in the vaginal walls and pelvic floor approximately every second for several seconds. At the same time, there is an increase in pulse rate, hyperventilation and specific skeletal muscular contractions. Blood pressure rises, and there is some diminution of consciousness. Both intravaginal and intra-uterine pressure rise during orgasm. The plateau phase may be sustained in the female, and result in multiple orgasm. Following orgasm, resolution of the congestion of the pelvic organs occurs rapidly although the tachycardia and hypertension accompanied by a sweating reaction may persist.

Factors which determine human sexuality are far more complex than the simple process of arousal by clitoral or penile stimulation. Although the frequency of intercourse and orgasm declines with age, this is in part mediated by the loss of interest in the partners. The female remains capable of orgasm until late in life, but this behaviour is substantially determined by the interest of the male partner. Sexual interest and performance also declines with age in the male, and the older male requires more time to achieve excitement and erection. Ejaculation may become less frequent and forceful.

Common sexual problems will be discussed in a separate chapter.

BIBLIOGRAPHY

Moore K 1988 The developing human. Clinically oriented embryology. W B Saunders, London
Philipp E E, Setchell M 1991 (ed) Scientific foundations of obstetrics and gynaecology. Heinemann, London

6 Placental and fetal growth and development

EARLY PLACENTAL DEVELOPMENT

After fertilization and egg cleavage, the morula is transformed into a blastocyst by the formation of a fluid-filled cavity within the ball of cells.

The outer layer of the blastocyst consists of primitive cytotrophoblast, and by day 7 the blastocyst penetrates the endometrium as a result of trophoblastic invasion (Fig. 6.1). The outer layer of trophoblast becomes a syncytium. In response to contact with the syncytiotrophoblast, the endometrial stromal cells become large and pale, a process known as the decidual reaction, and endometrial cells are phagocytosed by the trophoblastic cells.

The nature and function of the decidual reaction remain uncertain, but it seems likely that the decidual cells both limit the invasion of trophoblastic cells and serve an initial nutritional function for the developing placenta.

During development of the placenta, cords of cytotrophoblast or Langhans' cells grow down to the basal layers of decidua and penetrate some of the endometrial venules and capillaries. The formation of lacunae filled with maternal blood presages the development of the intervillous space.

The invading cords of trophoblast form the primary villi, which later branch to form secondary villi and, subsequently, free-floating tertiary villi.

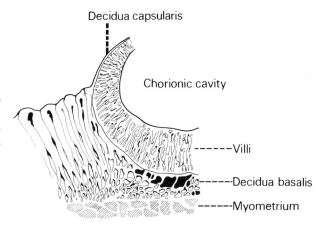

Fig. 6.2 Development of early placentation.

The central core of these villi is penetrated by a column of mesoblastic cells which become the capillary network of the villi. The body stalk, which attaches the developing fetus to the placenta, forms the umbilical vessels, which advance onto the villi to join the villous capillaries and establish the placental circulation.

Although trophoblastic cells surround the original blastocyst, the area which develops into the placenta becomes thickened and extensively branched, and is known as the **chorion frondosum**. However, in the area which subsequently expands to form the outer layer of the fetal membranes, the villi become atrophic and the surface smooth; this structure forms the **chorion laeve** (Fig. 6.2). The decidua underlying the placenta is known as **decidua basalis** and the decidua between the membranes and the myometrium as **decidua capsularis**.

FURTHER PLACENTAL DEVELOPMENT

By 6 weeks after ovulation, the trophoblast has invaded some 40–60 spiral arterioles. Blood from

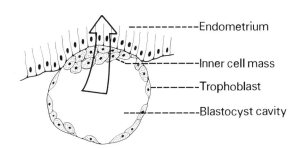

Fig. 6.1 Implantation of the blastocyst.

the maternal vasculature pushes the free-floating secondary and tertiary capillaries into a tent-shaped 'maternal cotyledon'. The tents are held down to the basal plate of the decidua by anchoring villi, and the blood from arterioles spurts towards the chorionic plate and then returns to drain through maternal veins in the basal plate. There are eventually about 12 large maternal cotyledons and 40–50 smaller ones.

Placental development

- Blastocyst penetrates endometrium by day 7
- Primary villi formed by cords of cytotrophoblast invading decidua
- The chorion frondosum and underlying decidua basalis form the placenta
- The chorion laeve forms the membranes

THE VILLUS

Despite the arrangement of villi into maternal cotyledons, the functional unit of the placenta remains the stem villus or fetal cotyledon (Fig. 6.3). There are initially about 200 stem villi arising from the chorion frondosum. About 150 of these structures are compressed at the periphery of the major maternal vascular units and become relatively functionless, leaving a dozen or so large cotyledons, and 40–50 smaller ones as the active units of placental function.

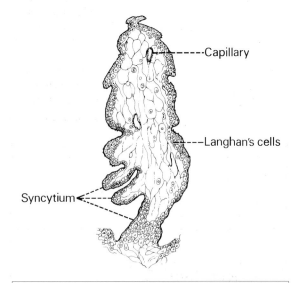

Fig. 6.3 The chorionic villus as the functional unit of the placenta.

The estimated surface area of the chorionic villi in the mature placenta is approximately 11 m^2. The surface area is enlarged by the presence of numerous microvilli. The core of the villus consists of a stroma of closely packed spindle-shaped fibroblasts and branching capillaries (see Fig. 6.5B). The stroma also contains phagocytic cells known as Hofbauer cells. In early pregnancy, the villi are covered by an outer layer of syncytiotrophoblast and an inner layer of cytotrophoblast. As pregnancy advances, the cytotrophoblast disappears until only a thin layer of syncytiotrophoblast remains. The formation of clusters of syncytial cells, known as **syncytial knots**, and the reappearance of cytotrophoblast in late pregnancy, are probably the result of hypoxia.

STRUCTURE OF THE UMBILICAL CORD

The umbilical cord contains two arteries and one vein (Fig. 6.4). The two arteries carry deoxygenated blood from the fetus to the placenta and the oxygenated blood returns to the fetus via the umbilical vein. Absence of one artery occurs in about 1 in 200 deliveries and is associated with a 10–15% incidence of cardiovascular anomalies. The vessels are surrounded by a hydrophilic mucopolysaccharide known as Wharton's jelly, and the outer layer covering the cord consists of amniotic epithelium. The cord length varies between 30 and 90 cm. The vessels grow in a helical shape, which has the functional advantage of protecting the patency of the vessels by absorbing torsion without the risk of kinking or snarling of the vessels. The few measurements that have been made of cord pressures in situ indicate that the arterial pressure is around 70 mmHg systolic and 60 mmHg diastolic, and the venous pressure is exceptionally high at approximately 25 mmHg. This high pressure also tends to preserve the integrity of cord blood flow, and indicates that pressure within the villus capillaries must be in excess of the cord venous pressures. The cord vessels often contain a false knot consisting of a refolding of the arteries; occasionally, blood flow is threatened by a true knot. In a full-term fetus, the blood flow in the cord is approximately 350 ml/min.

PLACENTAL BLOOD FLOW

Trophoblasts invade the maternal arterioles early in pregnancy. Blood enters the intervillous space from

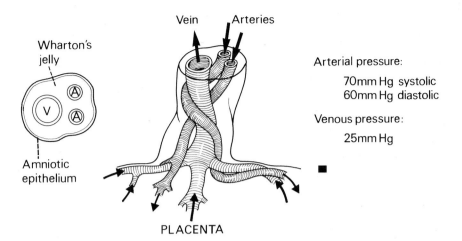

Fig. 6.4 Vascular structure of the umbilical cord: transverse section (left) shows two arteries carrying de-oxygenated blood and one vein carrying oxygenated blood.

the uterine arterioles and spurts towards the chorionic plate and then returns to the uterine venous openings in the placental bed (Fig. 6.5A). The pressure in the intervillous space is estimated at 10 mmHg. Assessments of uterine blood flow indicate values of 500–750 ml/min.

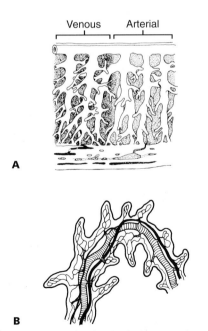

Fig. 6.5 **A** Venous and arterial circulation in the choriodecidual vascular bed; **B** branching of capillary in a terminal villus.

FACTORS WHICH INFLUENCE UTERINE BLOOD FLOW

The regulation of uterine blood flow is of critical importance to the welfare of the fetus, and chronic impairment of flow leads to growth retardation and, in severe circumstances, may result in fetal death. Factors which adversely influence uterine blood flow include haemorrhage, uterine contractions, adrenaline and noradrenaline. Angiotensin II increases uterine blood flow in physiological levels as a result of the direct effect on placental tissue in promoting the local release of vasodilator prostaglandins. In high concentrations it produces vasoconstriction.

Lying in the supine position in late pregnancy may also reduce uterine blood flow by producing compression of the aorta and inferior vena cava.

The placenta

- Stem villi or fetal cotyledons form the functional unit (40–50)
- Surface area 11 m^2
- Blood flow through the cord is 350 ml/min with an arterial pressure of 70/60 mmHg
- Glucose is the main energy source

PLACENTAL TRANSFER

The placenta plays an essential role in growth and

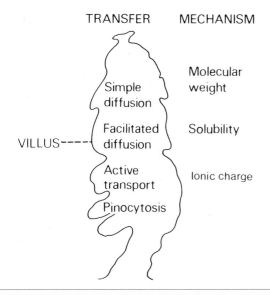

Fig. 6.6 Factors which determine transfer of nutrients and gases across the placenta.

development in the fetus and in regulating maternal adaption to pregnancy.

Transfer of materials across the placental membrane is governed by molecular weight, solubility and the ionic charge of the substance involved. Actual transfer is achieved by simple diffusion, facilitated diffusion, active transport and pinocytosis (Fig. 6.6).

Simple diffusion

Transfer between maternal and fetal blood is regulated by the trophoblast, and it must be remembered that the lining of the chorionic villus is not a simple semipermeable membrane but consists of a metabolically active cellular layer.

Although there are exceptions, small molecules generally cross the placenta by simple diffusion and movement is determined by chemical or electrochemical gradients. The quantity of solute transferred is described by the Fick diffusion equation:

$$\frac{Q}{t} = \frac{KA(C^1 - C^2)}{L}$$

where Q/t is the quantity transferred per unit time, K is a diffusion constant for the particular substance, A is the total surface area available, and C^1 and C^2 indicate the difference in concentrations of solute; L represents the thickness of the membrane. This method is applicable particularly to transfer of gases although the gradient of oxygen, for example, is substantially increased by the fact that oxygen is extracted by the placenta and myometrium.

Facilitated diffusion

Some compounds are transported across the placenta at rates that are considerably enhanced above the rate that would be anticipated by simple diffusion. Transport always occurs in favour of the gradient but at an accelerated rate. This system pertains to glucose transport and can only be explained on the basis of a specific transport system.

Active transport

Transfer against a chemical gradient occurs with some compounds and must involve an active transport system which is energy dependent. This process occurs with essential amino acids and water-soluble vitamins, and can be demonstrated by the presence of higher concentrations of the compound in fetal blood as compared with maternal blood. Such transfer mechanisms can be inhibited by cell poisons and are stereo-specific.

Pinocytosis

Transfer of high molecular weight compounds is known to occur, and involves ingestion or engulfing of microdroplets of material into the cytoplasm of the trophoblast. This process applies to the transfer of globulins, phospholipids and lipoproteins, and is of particular importance in the transfer of immunologically active material. The major source of materials for protein synthesis and for nutrition in the fetus comes from the transfer of amino acids.

Transport of intact cells

Fetal red cells are commonly seen in the maternal circulation, particularly following delivery. Although some maternal red cells may be found in the fetal circulation, this is much less common, as the pressure gradient favours movement from the relatively high pressure of the fetal capillaries to the low-pressure environment of the intervillous space.

Water and electrolyte transfer

Water passes easily across the placenta, and a single pass allows equilibrium. The net water gain to the fetus in late pregnancy is approximately 20–25 ml. The driving force for movement of water across the placenta include hydrostatic pressure, colloid osmotic pressure and solute osmotic pressure.

Sodium

The concentration of sodium is higher in the venous plasma of the fetus than in maternal venous plasma. It therefore seems that the placenta actively regulates sodium transfer, probably through the enzyme Na/K ATPase on the fetal surface of the placenta, and this maintains a negative intracellular potential.

Potassium

The transfer of potassium is controlled, but the mechanism remains obscure. Fetal plasma potassium levels are significantly higher than maternal plasma levels. In particular, fetal plasma potassium levels become significantly raised in the presence of fetal acidosis, whilst remaining normal in the mother. There is evidence for carrier-mediated transfer at the maternal surface of the placenta, and transfer of placental potassium may also be modulated by intracellular Ca^{2+}.

Calcium

Calcium is actively transported across the placenta, and there are higher concentrations in fetal plasma than in maternal plasma.

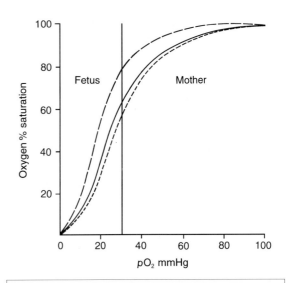

Fig. 6.7   The Bohr effect.

PLACENTAL FUNCTION

The placenta has three major functions:

1. Gaseous exchange
2. Fetal nutrition and removal of waste products
3. Endocrine function.

Gaseous exchange

As the transfer of gases occurs by simple diffusion, the major determinants of gaseous exchange are the efficiency of the fetal and maternal circulations, the surface area of the placenta and the thickness of the placental membrane.

Oxygen transfer

The average difference in oxygen tension across the placenta is about 20 mmHg, and this gradient favours the transfer of oxygen from maternal to fetal circulation. Fetal haemoglobin has a higher affinity for oxygen than does adult haemoglobin, and haemoglobin concentration is higher in the fetus. All these factors favour the rapid uptake of oxygen by the fetus at relatively low oxygen tensions. The extent to which haemoglobin can be saturated by oxygen is affected by hydrogen ion concentration, the increase of which in deoxygenated blood favours the release of maternal oxygen in the feto-placental bed. The oxygen dissociation curve is shifted to the right by increases in H+ ion concentration, pCO_2 and temperature, and this is known as the **Bohr effect** (Fig. 6.7). Oxygen is predominantly transported in the form of oxyhaemoglobin as there is little free oxygen in solution in blood.

Carbon dioxide transfer

Carbon dioxide is readily soluble in blood and transfers rapidly across the placenta. The partial pressure difference is about 5 mmHg. Transport of carbon dioxide may occur in solution as either bicarbonate or carbonic acid. It is also transported as carbaminohaemoglobin. The binding of CO_2 to haemoglobin to form carbaminohaemoglobin is affected by factors which influence oxygen release and, thus, an increase in carbaminohaemoglobin results in the release of oxygen. This is known as the **Haldane effect**.

Fetal nutrition and removal of waste products

Carbohydrate metabolism

Glucose transferred from the maternal circulation provides the major substrate for oxidative metabolism in the placenta. Facilitated diffusion allows for rapid transfer of glucose across the placenta. Animal studies have shown that transfer of sugars is selective; generally, glucose and the monosaccharides cross the placenta readily whereas the placenta is virtually impermeable to disaccharides such as sucrose, maltose and lactose. The placenta is also impermeable to the sugar alcohols such as sorbitol, mannitol, deleitol and meso-inositol.

In the fasting, normal pregnant woman, blood glucose achieves a concentration of approximately 4.0 mmol/l in the maternal venous circulation and 3.3 mmol/l in the fetal cord venous blood. Infusion of glucose into the maternal circulation results in a parallel increase in both maternal and fetal blood glucose levels until the fetal levels reach 10.6 mmol/l, when no further increase occurs regardless of the values in the maternal circulation.

The hormones that are important in glucose homeostasis, namely insulin, glucagon, human placental lactogen and growth hormone, do not cross the placenta, and maternal glucose levels appear to be the major regulatory factor in fetal glucose metabolism. The placenta itself utilizes glucose, and may retain as much as half of the glucose that enters the tissues. In mid-pregnancy, approximately 70% of this glucose is metabolized by glycolysis, 10% via the pentose phosphate pathway, and the remainder is stored by glycogen and lipid synthesis. By full term, the rate of placental glucose utilization has fallen by 30%. Glycogen storage occurs in the placenta and in the fetal liver, muscle and heart. Glycogen levels in the fetal liver increase steadily throughout pregnancy and are twice the adult levels at full term. A rapid fall to adult levels occurs within the first few hours of life.

The reserves are of particular importance in providing an energy source in the asphyxiated fetus when anaerobic glycolysis is activated.

Fat metabolism

Fats are insoluble in water and are therefore transported in blood either as free fatty acids bound to albumin, or as lipoproteins consisting of triglyceride attached to other lipids or proteins, and packaged in chylomicra.

The fetus needs fatty acids for cell membrane construction and for deposition in the adipose tissue. This is particularly important as a source of energy in the immediate neonatal period.

There is evidence that free fatty acids cross the placenta and that this transfer is not selective. Essential fatty acids are also transferred from the maternal circulation and evidence suggests that the placenta has the ability to convert linoleic acid to arachidonic acid. Starvation of the mother increases mobilization of triglycerides in the fetus.

Protein metabolism

Fetal protein is synthesized by the fetus from free amino acids transported across the placenta against a concentration gradient. The concentration of free amino acids in the fetus is higher than in the maternal circulation.

The placenta takes no part in the synthesis of fetal proteins although it does synthesize some protein hormones which are transferred into the maternal circulation, namely, chorionic gonadotrophin and human placental lactogen. By full tern, the human fetus has accumulated some 500 g of protein.

Immunoglobulins are synthesized by fetal lymphoid tissue, and IgM first appears in the fetal circulation by 20 weeks gestation, followed by IgA and finally IgG. IgG is the only γ-globulin to be transferred across the placenta, and this appears to be selective for homologous IgG. There is no evidence of placental transfer of growth-promoting hormones.

Urea and ammonia

Urea concentration is higher in the fetus than in the mother by a margin of about 0.5 mmol/l, and the rate of clearance across the placenta is approximately 0.54 (mg/min)/kg fetal weight at term. It has been suggested that protein provides about 25% of the energy source for the fetus. Ammonia transfers readily across the placenta and it is believed that maternal ammonia may provide a source of some fetal nitrogen.

Placental hormone production

The placenta plays a major role as an endocrine organ and is responsible for the production of both protein and steroid hormones. The fetus is also involved in many of the processes of hormone production and in this capacity the conceptus functions as a feto-placental unit.

Protein hormones

Chorionic gonadotrophin – Human chorionic gonadotrophin (hCG) is produced by trophoblast and has a structure which is chemically very similar to that of luteinizing hormone. It is a glycoprotein with two non-identical α- and β-subunits. hCG reaches a peak in maternal urine and blood between 7 and 8 weeks of pregnancy. A small subpeak occurs between 32 and 36 weeks. The β-subunit of hCG can be detected in plasma within 7 days of conception.

The only known function of the hormone appears to be the maintenance of the corpus luteum of pregnancy. The hormone is measured by agglutination inhibition techniques using coated red cells or latex particles, and forms the basis of the standard pregnancy test. This will be positive in urine by 2 weeks after the period is missed in 97% of pregnant women.

Human placental lactogen – Human placental lactogen (hPL) or chorionic somatomammotrophin is a peptide hormone with a molecular weight of 22 000 which is chemically similar to growth hormone. It is produced by syncytiotrophoblast, and plasma hPL levels rise steadily throughout pregnancy. The function of the hormone remains uncertain although it does appear to reduce blood glucose levels and to increase levels of free fatty acids and insulin.

Plasma hPL levels have been extensively used in the assessment of placental function. In the last 2 weeks of gestation the levels in serum fall. The hormone is measured by radioimmunoassay.

Steroid hormones

Progesterone – The placenta becomes the major source of progesterone production by the 17th week of pregnancy, and the biosynthesis of progesterone is mainly dependent on the supply of maternal cholesterol. In maternal plasma, 90% of progesterone is bound to protein and is metabolized in the liver and kidneys. Some 10–15% of progesterone is excreted in urine as pregnanediol. The placenta produces about 350 mg of progesterone per day by full term, and plasma progesterone levels increase throughout pregnancy to achieve values around 150 mg/ml by full term. The measurement of urinary pregnanediol or plasma progesterone has been used as a method of assessing placental function but has not been proved to be particularly useful as the scatter of hormonal values is so wide that the assessment of abnormality is obscured.

Oestrogens – Over 20 different oestrogens have been identified in the urine of pregnant women but the major oestrogens are oestrone, oestradiol-17β and oestriol. The largest increase in oestrogen excretion occurs in oestriol. Whereas oestrone excretion increases 100-fold, urinary oestriol increases 1000-fold. The ovary makes only a minimal contribution to this increase as the placenta is the major source of oestrogen in pregnancy. The substrate for oestriol production comes from the fetal adrenal gland (Fig.

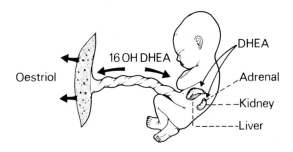

Fig. 6.8 Formation of oestriol by the feto-placental unit.

6.8). Dehydroepiandrosterone (DHEA) synthesized in the fetal adrenal cortex passes to the fetal liver where it is 16-hydroxylated. Conjugation of these precursors with phosphoadenosyl phosphosulphate aids solubility, and active sulphatase activity in the placenta results in the release of free oestriol. Oestradiol and oestrone are directly synthesized by the syncytiotrophoblast. Urinary and plasma oestriol levels increase progressively throughout pregnancy until 38 weeks gestation, when some fall occurs. Oestriol excretion falls as a result of fetal adrenal suppression. This will occur following the administration of corticosteroid to the mother, or in the absence of the fetal adrenal gland as seen in anencephaly. It may also occur in the presence of placental failure, and excretion therefore forms the basis of a placental function test.

Corticosteroids – There is little evidence that the placenta produces corticosteroids. In the presence of Addison's disease or following adrenalectomy, 17-hydroxycorticosteroids and aldosterone disappear from the maternal urine. In normal pregnancy, there is a substantial increase in cortisol production and this is at least partly due to the raised levels of transcortin in the blood, so that the capacity for binding cortisol increases substantially.

Placental function

- Oxygen transfer to fetus occurs by simple diffusion promoted by a 20 mmHg difference in O_2 tension, the higher O_2 affinity of fetal Hb and the Bohr effect
- Carbon dioxide transfer to mother by simple diffusion
- Glucose transport by facilitated diffusion
- Fats transported by pinocytosis of free fatty acids–albumin or as lipoproteins
- Active transport of amino acids
- Synthesis of some fatty acids
- Immunoglobulin transfer (IgG only) by pinocytosis
- Hormone production including hCG, progesterone and various oestrogens (with the fetus)

FETAL DEVELOPMENT

Growth

Up to 10 weeks gestation, a massive increase in cell numbers occurs in the developing embryo but the actual gain in weight is small. Thereafter, a rapid increase occurs until the full-term fetus achieves a weight of about 3.5 kg (Fig. 6.9). Protein accumulation occurs in the fetus throughout pregnancy but fetal adipose tissue does not reach significant levels in the subcutaneous and intra-abdominal stores until after 28 weeks. There is a reduction in the fetal growth rate towards term (Fig. 6.10). Actual growth rate is determined by a variety of factors including the efficiency of the placenta, the adequacy of the utero-placental blood flow and inherent genetic factors in the fetus. Fetal weight is also determined by race, maternal height and weight, and parity.

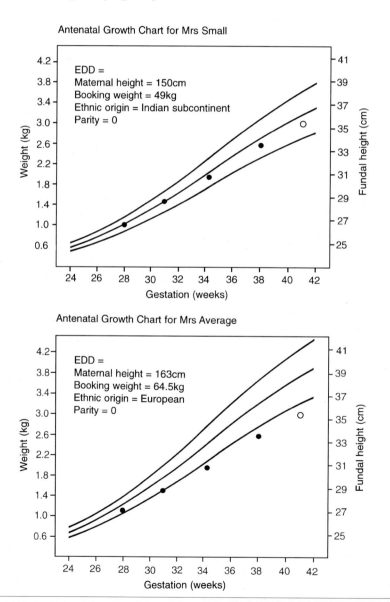

Fig. 6.9 Fetal weight and gestational age plotted on the basis of parity, maternal height and weight, and ethnic group. (By kind permission of J. Gardosi.)

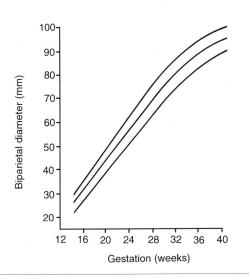

Fig. 6.10 Biparietal diameter (BPD) – mean ± 2 SD and gestational age in normal pregnancy. (From Erikson et al 1985, with permission.)

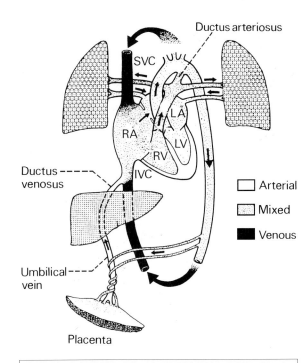

Fig. 6.11 Fetal circulation showing the distribution of arterial, venous and mixed blood.

Cardiovascular system

The heart develops initially as a single tube, and by 4–5 weeks gestation a heartbeat is present at a rate of 65 beats/minute. The definitive circulation has developed by 11 weeks gestation, and the heart rate increases to around 140 beats/minute. In the mature fetal circulation, about 40% of the venous return entering the right atrium flows directly into the left atrium through the foramen ovale (Fig. 6.11). Blood pumped from the right atrium into the right ventricle is expelled into the pulmonary artery, where it passes either into the aorta via the ductus arteriosus or into the pulmonary vessels.

The fetal cardiac output is estimated to be 200 ml/kg body weight per minute. Unlike the adult, fetal cardiac output is entirely dependent on heart rate and not on stroke volume. Autonomic control of the fetal heart matures during the third trimester, and parasympathetic vagal tonus tends to reduce the basal fetal heart rate.

The fetal respiratory system

There is evidence that fetal respiration is present from 12 weeks onwards and that, by 34 weeks gestation, respiration occurs at a rate of 40–60 movements/minute with intervening periods of apnoea. These respiratory movements are shallow, but occasional gasps occur which result in a larger flow of fluid into the bronchial tree. Fetal breathing is stimulated by hypercapnia, but hypoxia tends to reduce breathing movements whilst increasing gasping behaviour. Fetal respiration is inhibited by maternal smoking.

The fetal pulmonary alveoli are lined by two main types of alveolar epithelial cells. Gaseous exchange occurs across the type I cells, and the type II cells secrete phospholipid surfactant, which is necessary to prevent the collapse of the alveoli in neonatal life (Fig. 6.12). The principal surfactants are lecithin and sphingomyelin and production of lecithin begins

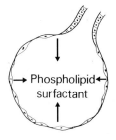

Fig. 6.12 Secretion of phospholipid into the alveoli determines lung expansion at birth.

to increase at about 32 weeks gestation. Measurement of lecithin in amniotic fluid provides a useful method of assessing fetal lung maturity.

Fetal gastrointestinal tract

Mucosal glands appear in the gut by 16–20 weeks gestation, and by 26 weeks most of the digestive enzymes are present. Amylase does not appear until after birth. The fetus swallows amniotic fluid and peristaltic gut movement is established by mid-pregnancy. The digestion of cells and protein in amniotic fluid results in the formation of fetal faeces or meconium. Meconium normally remains in the gut and appears in the amniotic fluid only under conditions of fetal stress and asphyxia.

The fetal kidney

Functional renal corpuscles first appear in the juxta-glomerular zone of the renal cortex at 22 weeks gestation and filtration begins at this time. The formation of the kidney is complete by 36 weeks gestation. Glomerular filtration increases towards term as the number of glomeruli increase and the fetal blood pressure rises.

In the fetus, only 2% of the cardiac output perfuses the kidneys. The fetal renal tubules are capable of active transport before any glomerular filtrate is received and thus some urine may be produced within the tubules before glomerular filtration starts. The efficiency of tubular reabsorption is low, and glucose in the fetal circulation spills into fetal urine at levels as low as 4.2 mmol/l.

Fetal urine makes a significant contribution to the formation of amniotic fluid.

Special senses

The fetus will respond to sound by movement of the limbs and trunk, and by the alteration of the fetal heart rate. Visual perception is more difficult to assess but it seems likely that some perception to light develops in late pregnancy.

Fetal development

- 5 weeks: fetal heartbeat present
- 11 weeks: fetal circulation developed
- 12 weeks: fetal respiratory movements
- 20 weeks: mucosal glands appear in gut, peristalsis established
- 22 weeks: functional renal corpuscles and filtration
- 26 weeks: most digestive enzymes present
- 28 weeks onwards: autonomic control starts to slow basal heart rate
- 32 weeks: lecithin rises

AMNIOTIC FLUID

The formation of amniotic fluid

The amniotic sac develops early in pregnancy, and has been identified in the human embryo as early as 7 days. The first signs of the development of the amniotic cavity can be seen in the inner cell mass of the blastocyst.

Early in pregnancy, amniotic fluid is probably a dialysate of fetal and maternal extracellular compartments. There is some evidence, for example, that up to 24 weeks gestation, when keratinization begins, significant transfer of water may occur across fetal skin. In the last half of pregnancy, fetal urine provides a significant contribution to amniotic fluid volume. Certainly, the absence of kidneys, renal agenesis, in the fetus is invariably associated with minimal amniotic fluid volume – **oligohydramnios**.

The role of the fetus in regulation of amniotic fluid volume is poorly understood, but the fetus swallows amniotic fluid, absorbs it in the gut and later excretes urine into the amniotic sac (Fig. 6.13). Congenital abnormalities which impair the ability to swallow are commonly associated with excessive amniotic fluid volume or **polyhydramnios**.

In summary, amniotic fluid is formed by secretion of fluid from amnion and fetal skin and from the passage of fetal urine into the amniotic sac. Circulation of amniotic fluid occurs by reabsorption of fluid through the fetal gut, skin and amnion.

Amniotic fluid volume

By 8 weeks gestation, 5–10 ml of amniotic fluid has accumulated; thereafter the volume increases

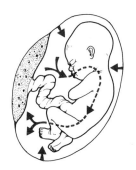

Amniotic fluid volume:

gestation	ml
8 weeks	5–10
38 weeks	1000
>42 weeks	<300

Fig. 6.13 Amniotic fluid secreted in the amnion is swallowed by the fetus, absorbed through the gut and excreted in fetal urine.

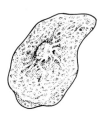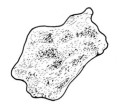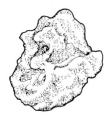

Prominent nucleus   Microtubules on surface   Smooth and microtubular surfaces

Fig. 6.14   Scanning electron microscope image of amniotic fluid cells showing prominent nuclei and surface microtubules.

rapidly in proportion to fetal growth and gestational age to a maximum volume of 1000 ml at 38 weeks gestation. Subsequently, serial diminution in the amount of fluid takes place, so that after 42 weeks the mean volume falls below 300 ml.

Clinical significance of amniotic fluid volume

The fetus exerts a large influence on this fluid space through urine production and swallowing.

Diminution of amniotic fluid volume is associated with reduced placental function, and this is seen particularly in pre-eclampsia and essential hypertension.

Polyhydramnios, or excessive fluid, is commonly associated with oesophageal or duodenal atresia and with central nervous system abnormalities such as anencephaly and hydrocephaly, which interfere with swallowing. In approximately 30% of all cases of polyhydramnios there is a significant congenital anomaly. The distribution of such anomalies is as follows in order of frequency:

- Anencephaly
- Oesophageal atresia
- Duodenal atresia
- Iniencephaly
- Hydrocephaly
- Diaphragmatic hernia.

Cells of the amniotic fluid

Amniotic fluid contains two distinct types of cells. the first group is derived from the fetus, the second from the amnion. Cells of fetal origin are larger and more likely to be anucleate. Those originating from the amnion are smaller, with a prominent nucleolus

contained within the vesicular nucleus, and are found in proportionately greater numbers prior to the 32nd week (Fig. 6.14).

In addition to these groupings by cellular morphological criteria, two other distinct populations of cells in the amniotic fluid are differentiated by haematoxylin and eosin staining. The relative numbers of each cell type vary depending upon the duration of pregnancy. Cells which stain with eosin are most prominent early in gestation, but after the 38th week compose less than 30% of the total cell population. These are probably the cells derived from the amnion.

Basophilic cells increase in number as pregnancy progresses but also tend to decrease after the 38th week. The presence of these cells in large numbers has been correlated with the female fetus, and the fetal vagina is felt to be a possible source.

After 38 weeks gestation, a large number of eosinophilic anucleate polygonal cells appear. These cells stain orange with Nile blue sulphate, and are thought to be derived from maturing fetal sebaceous glands.

Clinical value of tests on amniotic fluid

Both the biochemical and cytological components of amniotic fluid are used for a variety of clinical estimations. Amniotic fluid can be obtained after 16 weeks gestation by **amniocentesis**, which involves the insertion of a fine needle through the anterior abdominal wall into the amniotic sac and the withdrawal of amniotic fluid (Fig. 6.15). This is performed under local anaesthetic, after localization of the placenta by ultrasound in order to avoid any damage from the procedure. The following diagnostic procedures are currently employed in clinical practice.

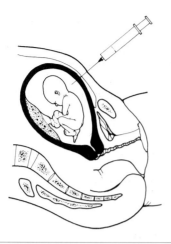

Fig. 6.15 Amniotic fluid is obtained by amniocentesis under ultrasound control.

Prenatal diagnosis

Alphafetoprotein can be measured in amniotic fluid and this is useful in the prenatal diagnosis of neural tube defects – particularly anencephaly and open spina bifida. Elevated levels may also be associated with other abnormalities, such as exomphalos, ectopia vesicae and fetal nephrotic syndrome. The quality of ultrasound imaging is now so clear that most congenital anomalies of the central nervous system can be detected with confidence and accuracy without the need to perform an amniocentesis.

Chromosomal abnormalities and sex-linked diseases

The fetal karyotype can be determined on cells cultured from amniotic fluid. This can reveal chromosome abnormalities such as Down's syndrome, trisomy 21, and will also reveal the sex of the fetus, which may be useful in the management of patients with sex-linked disorders such as haemophilia and muscular dystrophy.

Metabolic disorders

There are a large number of metabolic disorders, all fairly rare, such as Tay–Sach's disease and galactosaemia, which can be diagnosed in utero from tests on amniotic fluid cells.

Rhesus isoimmunization

A spectrophotometric peak at 450 nm representing unconjugated bilirubin is present in amniotic fluid throughout normal pregnancy, the peak becoming smaller and disappearing at about 36 weeks gestation. During pregnancy complicated by rhesus (Rh) incompatibility, the height of the 450 nm peak has been correlated with the severity of the fetal anaemia resulting from intravascular haemolysis.

This discovery has significantly altered the clinical management of Rh disease. When there is evidence of Rh incompatibility, a sample of amniotic fluid is collected at 32 weeks gestation by amniocentesis. The height of the peak at 450 nm gives an indication of the severity of the disease and from this measurement a decision can be made concerning the optimal time for induction of labour, or whether, in very severe disease, intra-uterine transfusion of the fetus is necessary (Fig. 6.16).

Amniotic fluid

- Produced by amnion, fetal skin and fetal urine
- Volume up to 1000 ml at 38 weeks
- Oligohydramnios associated with poor placental function and renal agenesis
- Polyhydramnios associated with significant congenital anomalies in 30% cases
- Contains fetal cells and cells from the amnion
- Clinical estimations of α-fetoprotein, fetal chromosomes, metabolic abnormalities, Rh disease and fetal maturity

---

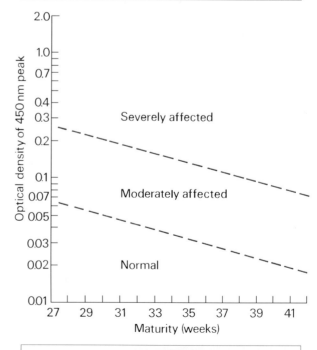

Fig. 6.16 Optical density of amniotic fluid in the prediction of rhesus isoimmunization.

Estimation of fetal maturity

After the 38th week of gestation, large numbers of eosinophilic anucleate polygonal cells appear. These cells stain orange with Nile blue sulphate, and are thought to be derived from maturing fetal sebaceous glands, but may be related to the appearance of increased quantities of phospholipid at this time. After the 40th week of gestation, the orange-stained cells usually constitute more than 50% of the total cellular content of the amniotic fluid. Pior to the 38th week, only 10% or less of the total number of cells are of this type.

The measurement of lecithin or the lecithin/sphingomyelin ratio has been used to measure fetal lung maturity. Lecithin is a major part of the surfactant produced by the fetal alveolar epithelial cells and the presence of concentrations of lecithin in excess of 3 mg/100 ml indicates that the fetal lungs are mature and that there is no risk of the development of respiratory distress syndrome.

The determination of creatinine may also be helpful, since a level greater than 2 mg/100 ml appears to indicate a gestation of longer than 37 weeks. However, the values may also be increased by severe pre-eclampsia, irrespective of length of gestation.

Fetal distress and placental insufficiency

Chronic fetal hypoxia commonly results in the passage of meconium into amniotic fluid. Placental insufficiency is also associated with a reduction in amniotic fluid volume.

Direct examination of the amniotic fluid can be achieved by **amnioscopy**, the passage of an amnioscope through the uterine cervix. This enables inspection of the colour of amniotic fluid, and will also give an impression of amniotic fluid volume. Amnioscopy is a useful adjunct in the management of the 'at risk' pregnancy, but can only be performed where the cervix is sufficiently dilated to allow the passage of the amnioscope. It may sometimes result in the rupture of membranes unless undertaken with care.

BIBLIOGRAPHY

de Swiet M, Chamberlain G V P 1992 Basic science in obstetrics and gynaecology. Churchill Livingstone, Edinburgh

Erikson P S, Secher N J, Weis-Bentson M 1985 Normal growth of the fetal biparietal diameter and the abdominal diameter in a longitudinal study. Acta Obstetrica et Gynecologica Scandinavica 64: 65–70

Gardosi J, Chang A, Kalyan B, Sahota D, Symonds E M 1992 Customised antenatal growth charts. Lancet 339: 283–287

Thorburn G D, Harding R 1994 Textbook of fetal physiology. Oxford University Press, Oxford

7 Infertility

The incidence of infertility varies in different countries and has been recorded to be as high as 50% in some West African communities compared with values of around 12% in Western European societies (Fig. 7.1).

It is important to differentiate between infertility, which is diminished fertility, and sterility, which is absolute infertility. Primary infertility is defined as diminished fertility throughout the reproductive years and secondary infertility infers failure to conceive after one or more successful pregnancies.

If conception does not occur after 12 months of normal sexual activity without contraception, the couple should be considered to be potentially infertile, as 75% of couples normally conceive within 1 year. It is therefore reasonable to proceed with investigations at this time.

Such a definition has to be modified by circumstances. For example, if a woman has had secondary amenorrhoea for 2 years, it would be pointless to wait for 12 months of regular sexual exposure before investigating her subfertility. At the other extreme, if her partner was away for a substantial part of the year, it would be sensible to defer intensive investigations until regular sexual exposure could be established. Both partners must be investigated, as infertility may result from male or female factors and is often associated with a combination of both factors. At the completion of all investigations, about 10% will exhibit no identifiable cause for their infertility, and long-term follow-up studies on these couples have shown that only 30–40% will conceive over a 7 year period after investigation.

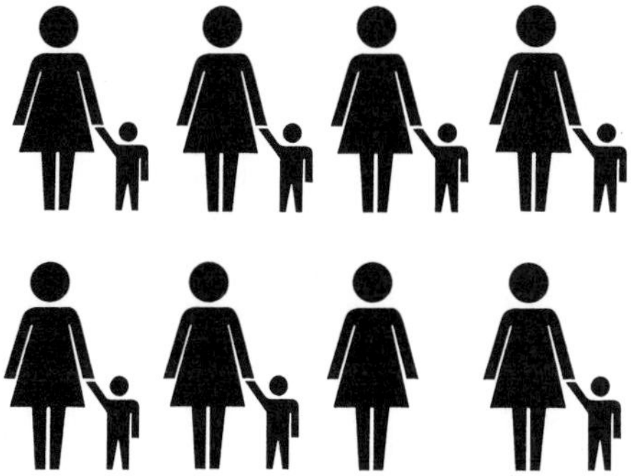

Changes in the socio-economic status of women in Western society has resulted in the deferment of child-bearing. Age undoubtedly affects fertility. Studies on various racial groups show consistently that natural fertility progressively declines from the age of 25 years. Evidence suggests that women who marry at 40 years of age have a 60% chance of not having children, and after the age of 44 years the chances of conception are very poor. The reason for this reduction in fertility may be partly due to a reduction in the frequency of coitus, a reduction in the frequency of ovulation, a reduction in male fertility associated with an increased production of defective sperm and, finally, an increased propensity to miscarry in older women.

The relative incidence of causative factors will vary according to country and whether the problem is primary or secondary. Furthermore, in many couples, there are multiple reasons for the infertility. Figure 7.2 shows the pattern of causative factors of primary infertility in a Western population.

HISTORY AND EXAMINATION

Both partners should be requested to attend at the initial interview. On occasions, the male partner may be reluctant to attend and this should not be considered as a basis for refusing investigation. It should, however, be apparent to the woman that the value of investigation will be seriously limited without the cooperation of the male partner.

The initial interview

The initial interview should take into account the following factors:

Fig. 7.1 The incidence of infertility is estimated at 1 in every 8 couples in Western European societies.

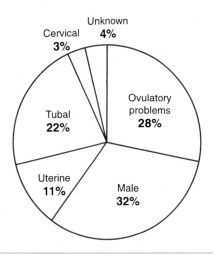

Fig. 7.2 Causes of primary infertility in a Western European population.

1. Age, occupation, religion and educational background
2. Number of years that conception has been attempted and the previous history of contraception.
3. Previous marriages and pregnancies of either partner.
4. Whether the infertility is primary or secondary and, if necessary, the details of any complications associated with previous pregnancies.
5. Coital history including frequency of intercourse. Any history of dyspareunia or of impotence or difficulty in ejaculation may be important.
6. General medical history of any concurrent or previous serious illness and of any surgery, particularly in relation to appendicitis in the female or herniorrhaphy in the male. A history of undescended testes or of orchidopexy may be particularly important.

FEMALE CAUSES OF INFERTILITY

General factors such as the age of both partners, a history of serious systemic illness, inadequate nutrition and emotional stress may all be factors that contribute to infertility but the major defined problems are found in defects of ovulation, tubal disease and cervical hostility.

Disorders of ovulation

Disorders of ovulation are divided into five categories:

1. Primary amenorrhoea – the failure of onset of menstruation by the age of 18 years. This is rarely a presenting symptom in relation to subfertility, and will be considered separately.
2. Secondary amenorrhoea – no menstruation for 6 months or more in a woman with a previous history of menstruation.
3. Oligomenorrhoea (infrequent periods) where the periods occur between 6 weeks and 6 months and may be ovulatory or anovulatory, However, even if the cycles are ovulatory, ovulation is so infrequent that fertility becomes impaired.
4. Anovulatory cycles – cycle length may be within normal limits but ovulation does not occur.
5. Ovulation appears to occur but the ovum is entrapped in the follicle. The corpus luteum may be defective and implantation does not occur.

Endocrine causes of oligomenorrhoea and secondary amenorrhoea

Anovulation is commonly, although not invariably, associated with amenorrhoea or oligomenorrhoea and these conditions may occur as the result of any one of a series of changes in the hypothalamic, pituitary, ovarian axis (Fig. 7.3). Alterations in the menstrual cycle are commonly associated with periods of stress and also with excessive weight gain or obesity and, at the other extreme, with anorexia nervosa or self-inflicted starvation.

Pituitary failure, as in Sheehan's syndrome, is now a rare condition but pituitary tumours in the form of pituitary microadenomas, which are prolactin-secreting, are a relatively common cause of secondary amenorrhoea.

Disorders of adrenal and thyroid function may not be clinically apparent if they are mild and therefore should be excluded by biochemical assessment.

Ovarian failure may occur as a result of premature menopause and the presence of streak ovaries. Polycystic ovaries associated with hirsutism, obesity and oligomenorrhoea commonly result in anovulation. This is due to an enzyme block in the conversion of androstenedione and testosterone to oestrogen and is associated with a high production rate of luteinizing hormone (LH) and follicle-stimulating hormone (FSH).

Anovulatory 'normal cycles'

The presence of a normal menstrual cycle does not necessarily imply that ovulation is occurring and, in recent years, it has been recognized that the oocyte

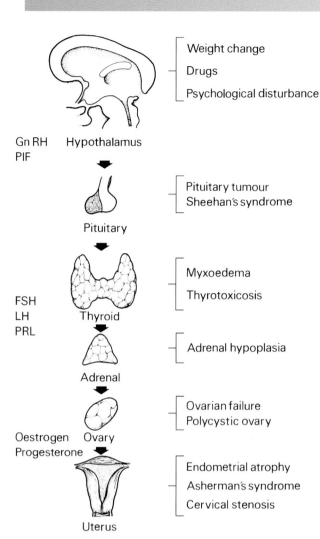

Gn RH Hypothalamus
PIF

— Weight change
— Drugs
— Psychological disturbance

— Pituitary tumour
Sheehan's syndrome

Pituitary

FSH
LH   Thyroid
PRL

— Myxoedema
— Thyrotoxicosis

Adrenal

— Adrenal hypoplasia

Oestrogen Ovary
Progesterone

— Ovarian failure
Polycystic ovary

— Endometrial atrophy
— Asherman's syndrome
— Cervical stenosis

Uterus

Fig. 7.3 Endocrine factors associated with non-ovulation. GnRH, gonadotrophin-releasing hormone; PIF, prolactin-inhibiting factor; FSH, follicle-stimulating hormone; LH, luteinizing hormone; PRL, prolactin.

development of the secretory phase of the endometrium. Luteal phase inadequacy results in either failure of implantation or early abortion. Diagnosis may be difficult and the aetiology is not understood, but there is no doubt that the problem arises in the first half of the cycle with defective follicular development.

Tubal factors

The function of the Fallopian tubes involves both ovum pick-up and transport of the fertilized gamete. Ovum pick-up is dependent on the action of the tubal fimbriae in pulling the tubal ostium over the follicle. The action of the tubal cilia also serves to aspirate the ovum. Subsequent progress and nutrition of the zygote by the tube is determined by the muscular action of the tubal wall, by the ciliated action and secretion of the tubal epithelium.

It is estimated that tubal factors account for about 20% of cases of infertility although this figure will vary considerably according to the population under consideration.

Occasionally congenital anomalies occur but the commonest cause of tubal damage is infection (Fig. 7.4).

Infection may cause occlusion of the fimbrial end of the tube with the collection of fluid, **hydrosalpinx**, or pus, **pyosalpinx**, within the tubal lumen.

Acute salpingitis results from sexually transmitted diseases such as gonorrhoea but may also result from other organisms such as *Escherichia coli*, anaerobic and haemolytic streptococci, staphylococci and *Clostridium welchii*. It may also result

may not be released from the follicle whilst luteinization of the unruptured follicle may still occur. This is known as the **luteinized unruptured follicle (LUF) syndrome**, and is commonly associated with endometriosis. The diagnosis can only really be made by laparoscopic inspection of the ovary to establish whether there is any evidence of an ovulation stigma.

Abnormalities of implantation and the luteal phase

Implantation requires the presence of adequate

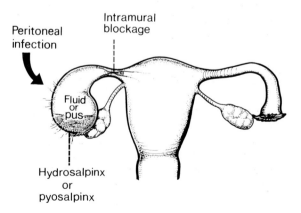

Peritoneal infection

Intramural blockage

Fluid or pus

Hydrosalpinx or pyosalpinx

Fig. 7.4 The pathogenesis of tubal obstruction and subfertility: intramural tubal obstruction results from intra-uterine infections.

from infection with bacteriodes and from myco-plasma and viral infections. Tuberculosis of the tubes may occur in women with pulmonary tuberculosis but has become increasingly rare as a cause of subfertility. Infections arising from intra-uterine contraceptive devices and following abortion or termination of pregnancy and infections in the puerperium commonly result in cornual blockage – often without any other significant change to the remainder of the tube. Pelvic infection from appendicitis associated with peritonitis results in peritubal adhesions and leaves the tubal lining unaffected.

Infections which affect the lumen of the tube result in loss of the ciliated epithelium and damage and fibrosis within the tubal wall, thus impairing the peristaltic function of the tube in promoting movement of the gamete. Therefore, even in the presence of a patent tube, damage to the wall and lumen may result in severe impairment of tubal function.

Lesions of the uterine cavity

Conditions which impinge on the uterine cavity may interfere with implantation and conception. Intramural and submucous fibroids interfere with implantation although pregnancy can occur and continue in the presence of large fibroids (Fig. 7.5).

Severe intra-uterine infections following pregnancy associated with retained products of conception and where uterine curettage is performed may result in complete ablation of the uterine cavity by adhesion of the walls, or partial occlusion of the cavity by the formation of intra-uterine adhesions or synechiae. This condition is known as **Asherman's syndrome**.

Congenital abnormalities of the uterus do not interfere with conception as a rule but may result in recurrent abortions.

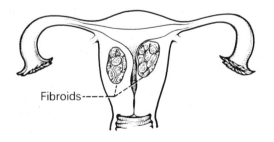

Fig. 7.5 Submucous fibroids cause subfertility by interference with implantations or by causing recurrent abortions.

Cervical factors

Ejaculation occurs into the vagina, and semen is deposited around the cervix. However, the cervix is effectively closed with cervical mucus, and sperm migration occurs by penetration of sperm into the cervical mucus. At the time of ovulation, endocervical cells secrete copious, clear, watery mucus which has a high water content and consists of long chains of polypeptide macromolecules with occasional side chains of carbohydrate. The chains of molecules contain channels which allow a direct passage of the spermatozoa into the uterine cavity. Sperm penetration occurs within 2–3 minutes of deposition. Between 100 000 and 200 000 sperm colonize the cervical mucus and remain at this level for approximately 24 hours after coitus. Approximately 200 sperm eventually reach the Fallopian tube. The vagina is generally hostile to sperm survival, and sperm in the vagina pool soon become immobilized. Mucus produced by the cervix under the influence of progesterone is hostile to sperm penetration.

Thus, poor penetration of sperm may result from cervical infection, from antisperm antibody activity in either cervical mucus or seminal plasma, from production of abnormal mucus by the cervix or from the effect of progestational agents on the mucus.

Female causes of infertility

- Disorders of ovulation
- Luteal phase failure of implantation
- Tubal occlusion or impaired cilia action
- Congenital/acquired lesion of uterine cavity
- Cervical infection, antisperm antibodies

INVESTIGATION OF THE FEMALE

The investigation of the female involves determination of three basic issues:

1. Does ovulation occur on a regular basis?
2. Is there any impairment of tubal function and of implantation?
3. Is there a cervical factor preventing sperm invasion?

Detection of ovulation

Basal temperature

An increase of 0.5°C occurs in basal body temperature in the luteal phase of the menstrual

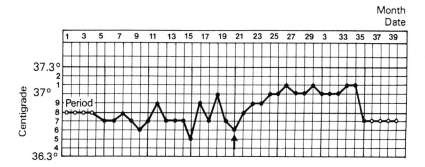

Fig. 7.6 Ovulatory chart in a 35 day cycle. The temperature falls immediately prior to ovulation and rises during the luteal phase of the cycle.

cycle. The temperature should be recorded sublingually before rising each morning, and provides a useful indication of the time of ovulation (Fig. 7.6). However, ovulation may occur in the absence of any temperature shift.

Cervical mucus

The production of mucus increases during the follicular phase to reach a peak at the time of ovulation with profuse production of clear, acellular mucus with low viscosity and high 'stretchability' (Spinnbarkeit) (Fig. 7.7). This mucus can be recognized by the woman herself, and is the best method for self-assessment of the time of ovulation. Some women experience pain in the midcycle (Mittel–Schmertz) associated with ovulation and can therefore estimate the timing of their ovulation. Mid-cycle mucus also dries on a glass slide with a characteristic fern pattern. This pattern presents a granular amorphous appearance which disappears with the influence of progesterone.

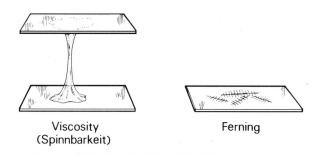

Viscosity
(Spinnbarkeit)

Ferning

Fig. 7.7 Characteristics of cervical mucus: the 'stretchability' can be evaluated between two glass slides (left); mid-cycle mucus shows ferning (right).

Hormonal tests

Serial measurement of FSH and LH in either blood or urine shows a well-defined peak which occurs approximately 20 hours before ovulation and can therefore be used as a technique for timing ovulation. However, the practical difficulties imposed by this approach limit its value.

The measurement of daily oestrogen levels provides a useful technique in assessing follicle maturation but is of limited value in timing ovulation.

The best hormonal evidence that ovulation has occurred is the measurement of serum progesterone in the luteal phase of the cycle. The interpretation of the results depends on the day of the cycle, and values in excess of 32 nmol/l, indicate that ovulation has occurred. However, none of these tests are infallible.

Endometrial biopsy and vaginal cytology

Biopsy of the endometrium can be performed without anaesthesia or formal dilatation and curettage (Fig. 7.8). The presence of secretory phase endometrium is taken as evidence of ovulation.

Examination of vaginal squames using the Papanicolaou stain can also be employed in the assessment of hormonal status (Fig. 7.9). Vaginal cells are shed as three types of cell – parabasal, intermediate and superficial (or cornified) – according to the size and staining characteristics of the cells. Progesterone causes maturation of intermediate cells, which tend to clump together, and the appearance of numerous polymorphonuclear leucocytes.

Ultrasonography

Ultrasound examination of the ovaries can be used to identify follicular growth. Follicular diameter

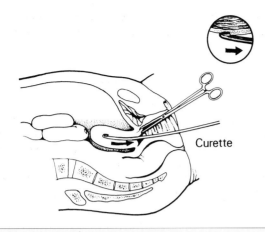

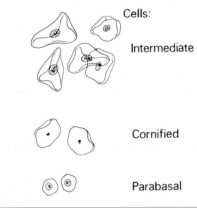

Fig. 7.8 Endometrial biopsy can be achieved without anaesthesia using 'vabra' aspiration or simple endometrial curettage; magnified view (inset).

Cells:

Intermediate

Cornified

Parabasal

Fig. 7.9 Vaginal cytology can be useful in assessing hormone status. Cells from the vaginal epithelium include parabasal, intermediate and superficial squames. The nature and staining features change with the hormonal status.

increases from 11.5 mm 5 days before ovulation to 20 mm on the day before ovulation, and decreases to approximately half this size on the day after ovulation. This is a useful and practical way of monitoring the time of ovulation.

Laparoscopy

Direct visualization of the ovary enables the observer to obtain more definite evidence of ovulation. Even this technique can be fallacious, as it is sometimes difficult to be certain if follicular rupture has occurred.

In summary, there are numerous techniques which provide presumptive evidence of ovulation.

In the initial assessment, basal body temperature charts and serum progesterone measurements are the most widely used techniques. The only definite proof of ovulation is pregnancy.

Investigation of non-ovulation

If there is evidence of non-ovulation, then further investigation should include measurement of:

1. Serum prolactin – to exclude hyperprolactinaemia.
2. FSH and LH levels in secondary ammenorrhoea. High levels of gonadotrophins in the presence of low levels of oestrogen indicate ovarian failure.
3. Assessment of thyroid function and TSH.
4. Radiography of the sella turcica if prolactin levels are raised to search for evidence of a pituitary prolactinoma. Tomography may be necessary if there is any sign of 'double flooring' of the pituitary fossa.

Investigation of tubal function

It is essential to establish tubal patency before embarking on prolonged drug therapy in either partner. Tubal patency is assessed by the following.

Hysterosalpingography

A radio-opaque dye, such as Diodrast or Urografin, is injected into the uterine cavity and Fallopian tubes. This technique can be performed without anaesthesia, provide the approach is gentle and the dye injected slowly. The dye outlines the uterine cavity and will demonstrate any filling defects. It will also show whether there is evidence of tubal obstruction and the site of the obstruction (Fig. 7.10).

Laparoscopy and dye insufflation

Laparoscopy enables direct visualization of the pelvic organs and, in particular, enables the diagnosis of endometriosis (Fig. 7.11). Methylene blue is injected through the uterine cavity to demonstrate tubal patency. It is not always possible to be certain of the site of tubal obstruction.

Gas insufflation

Inflation of the tubes with carbon dioxide has been used to demonstrate tubal patency but involves the risk of gas embolism. It has been replaced by laparoscopy and salpingography.

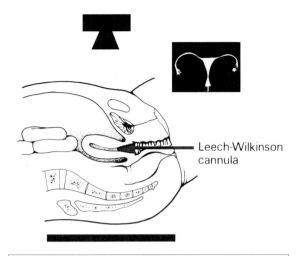

Fig. 7.10 Hysterosalpingography enables assessment of the site of tubal obstruction and the presence of pathology in the uterine cavity. The radio-opaque dye outlines the uterine cavity and Fallopian tubes.

Leech-Wilkinson cannula

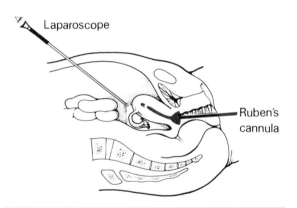

Laparoscope

Ruben's cannula

Fig. 7.11 Dye laparoscopy for evaluation of tubal patency.

Investigation of the cervical factor

It is important to determine that viable sperm penetrate the cervical mucus. A series of tests have been developed to examine this factor.

The postcoital test

This is the most widely used method of assessment and involves asking the couple to have intercourse and to examine the cervical mucus some 2–6 hours after intercourse. The test is best performed at the time of ovulation. The mucus is examined microscopically for the presence of progressive motile sperms. The presence of pus cells in the mucus is also noted as well as evidence of clumped or abnormal sperm.

In vitro sperm penetration tests

A series of in vitro tests have been developed which essentially examine the reaction between cervical mucus and semen from the husband on a slide or in a glass capillary and also the rate of sperm migration and sperm clumping or abnormal motility. Where there is a specific interaction with clumping of sperm, it is useful to test the mucus against donor semen to see if the same effect is obtained.

Investigation of the female

- Temperature chart
- FSH/LH (peaks 20 hours pre-ovulation), day 21 serum progesterone
- Endometrial biopsy
- Ultrasonography to identify follicular development
- Serum prolactin, thyroid function tests, pituitary radiography
- Hysterosalpingography/dye laparoscopy
- Postcoital test, in vitro sperm penetration tests

INVESTIGATION OF THE MALE PARTNER

The simplest and most important investigation of the male partner is the semen analysis. Semen should be collected by masturbation into a sterile container after a period of 2 days abstinence and examined within 2 hours of collection. Special note should be made of:

1. *Volume* – 80% of fertile males ejaculate between 1 and 4 ml of semen. Low volumes may indicate androgen deficiency and high volumes abnormal accessory gland function.
2. *Sperm concentration* – The absence of all sperm (azoospermia) indicates male sterility. However, the lower limit of normality is more difficult to define. It is generally accepted that the lower limit is probably between 15 million and 20 million sperm/ml, but the findings should not be accepted on a single sample. Furthermore, abnormally high values in excess of 200 million sperm/ml may be associated with subfertility.
3. *Total sperm count* – This measurement is sometimes used as an alternative to sperm concentration. The lower limit of normal is accepted as 50 million per ejaculate.

4. *Sperm motility* – Sperm motility is an important measurement of fertility and normal semen should show good motility in 60% of sperm within 1 hour of collection. The characteristic of forward progression is equally important.

The World Health Organization now grades sperm motility according to the following criteria:

Grade 1 – rapid and linear progressive motility
Grade 2 – slow or sluggish linear or non-linear motility
Grade 3 – non-progressive motility
Grade 4 – immotile.

5. *Sperm morphology* – sperm morphology shows great variability even in normal fertile males. It is unusual to see a count with more than 80% normal forms. It is important to look for leucocytes as they may indicate the presence of infection. If pus cells are present, the semen should be cultured for bacteriological growth. In general terms, fertility relates poorly to abnormal sperm morphology. The wide variety of forms that can be demonstrated in the seminal fluid are shown in Figure 7.12.

Spermatogenesis and sperm function may be affected by a wide range of toxins and therapeutic agents. Various toxins and drugs may act on the seminiferous tubules and the epididymis to inhibit spermatogenesis. Chemotherapeutic agents depress sperm function and sulphasalazine reduces sperm motility and density (Fig. 7.13). Otherwise, drugs such as antihypertensive agents cause impotence, and anabolic steroids may produce profound hypospermatogenesis.

In the presence of a normal semen analysis and a normal postcoital test, further tests on the male are unlikely to contribute to subsequent management. In the presence of oligospermia or azoospermia, further studies should include the following investigations:

1. *Hormone measurements* – High levels of FSH indicate severe testicular damage whereas normal levels may indicate obstructive disease. Low or undetectable levels are found in males with hypopituitarism. The presence of high FSH levels and azoospermia obviates the need for further investigation as these findings indicate irreversible failure of spermatogenesis.

LH and testosterone levels are of limited value although low values of both hormones may indicate a pituitary or hypothalamic disorder and high levels of LH with low levels of testosterone are characteristic of Klinefelter's syndrome.

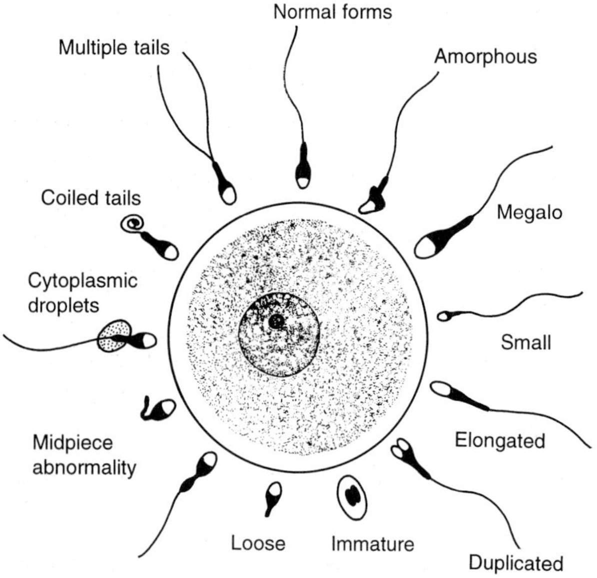

Fig. 7.12 Abnormal forms of spermatozoa commonly seen in seminal fluid.

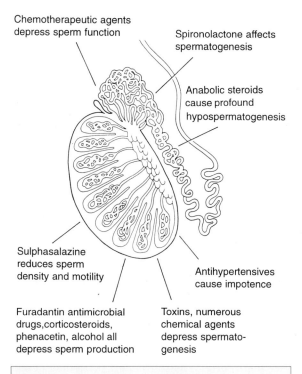

Fig. 7.13 Chemical agents that influence spermatogenesis.

Hyperprolactinaemia may occur in the male in association with a pituitary adenoma and may cause impotence or oligospermia.

2. *Cytogenetic studies* – Chromosome analysis in males with azoospermia may indicate the presence of a karyotype of XXY or XYY and, occasionally, autosomal translocation in the presence of oligospermia. About 2% of infertile males exhibit an abnormal karyotype.

3. *Testicular biopsy* – This should be undertaken only where an obstructive cause of subfertility is suspected. The advent of hormone investigations has greatly reduced the need for this investigation.

Rarely, retrograde ejaculation may cause subfertility and this should be suspected following surgical procedures such as transurethral resection of the prostate. The diagnosis is made by detecting spermatozoa in the urine following orgasm.

Immunological tests for male infertility

Immunity to sperm may occur in the male where autoimmunicity to sperm antigens can be related to infertility. The antigen–antibody reactions may lead to autoimmune infertility by neutralizing sperm decapacitation or by blocking sperm receptors on the egg.

Isoimmune responses to sperm in the female genital tract may be a cause of infertility.

Antibodies may be identified in female serum, or male serum, in cervical mucus and in seminal plasma. Sperm antibodies in seminal plasma appear in the IgG and IgA class, and can be detected using the mixed agglutination reaction (MAR). This test is also used to detect sperm antibodies in serum. This test is based on the formation of mixed agglutinates between polyacrylamide beads sensitized with immunoglobulin and motile test sperm with bound anti-sperm antibodies in the presence of anti-immunoglobulin serum. There are numerous other tests available based on sperm agglutination or sperm immobilization.

Investigation of the male

- Ejaculate volume 1–4 ml
- Sperm concentration 15 million to 200 million/ml
- Total count > 50 million
- Motility at collection 60%
- Morphology
- FSH, serum prolactin, chromosome studies if the above are abnormal

---

TREATMENT OF SUBFERTILITY

The treatment of subfertility is the treatment of the cause.

Anovulation

In the presence of normal gonadotrophin and prolactin levels, the drug of choice is clomiphene or tamoxifen. These compounds are anti-oestrogens and stimulate the release of FSH and LH; they will produce ovulation in 80% of subjects. Clomiphene is administered from the fifth to the ninth day of the cycle with an initial dosage of 50 mg/day increased to 200 mg/day where necessary. It is sometimes necessary to supplement this regimen with a mid-cycle injection of human chorionic gonadotrophin (hCG).

If these compounds are not effective, then it may be necessary to use human menopausal gonadotrophin (hMG) extracted from the urine of menopausal women, as in preparations such as Pergonal, or synthetic hMG. These drugs must be used with great caution as they may result in ovarian hyperstimulation and multiple pregnancy. Daily monitoring of oestrogen levels in blood or urine is advisable, and an injection of hCG is used to trigger ovulation. If anovulation is associated with hyperprolactinaemia, it is essential to exclude a significant pituitary lesion. If there is no major lesion present, treatment is initiated with a dopamine receptor agonist such as bromocriptine. Treatment should be initiated by taking 2.5 mg at night, and can be increased to 5 mg/day, depending on the response as judged by the prolactin levels.

Gonadotrophin-releasing hormone (GnRH) therapy should be administered where there is evidence of hypogonadotrophic hypogonadism. It can be administered by pulsatile subcutaneous injection every 90 minutes. It is important to note that when ovarian stimulation is used in an ovulating woman, follicular development should be monitored and the aim should be to produce one or two follicles in order to minimize the risk of multiple pregnancy.

Tubal pathology

The main method of treatment is by surgical intervention. Success rates are generally poor but have been improved by the use of microsurgery.

Salpingolysis involves the freeing of adhesions around the tubes and generally carries the best prognosis (Fig. 7.14). New techniques involving laser vaporization minimize recurrence of the adhesions.

Salpingostomy in the presence of a hydrosalpinx may re-establish patency but, because of damage to the tubal wall, is successful in only 10–15% of cases (Fig. 7.15). Folllowing all forms of tubal surgery, there is an additional risk of ectopic pregnancy. Tubal obstruction in the intramural portion of the tube is treated by re-implantation of the patent tube into the uterine cavity and localized areas of obstruction, such as pertain following sterilization procedures, can be resected and the tube re-anastomosed.

Indeed, with the possible exception of tubal re-anastomosis after sterilization, in vitro fertilization is the method of choice for the management of tubal obstructive disease.

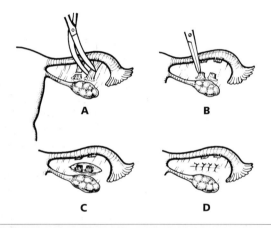

Fig. 7.14 Salpingolysis: **A** division of adhesions; **B** diathermy of adhesions; **C, D,** reconstruction of the peritoneum.

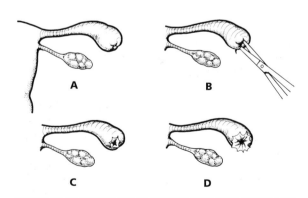

Fig. 7.15 Salpingostomy for fimbrial occlusion and hydrosalpinx: **A** intact hydrosalpinx; **B, C,** opening the fimbriae; **D** position for suturing the opened hydrosalpinx.

IN VITRO FERTILIZATION AND EMBRYO TRANSFER

Extracorporeal fertilization has provided an alternative method of treatment for tubal damage. Oocytes recovered by laparoscopy are fertilized in vitro, and the zygote is transferred back into the uterine cavity. There are a wide range of methods involved in the various techniques of assisted reproduction. Standard in vitro fertilization and embryo transfer involves hyperstimulation of the ovaries followed by the collection of oocytes about 36 hours after adminis-tration of hCG to mimic the LH surge. The eggs are collected from the ovaries by guided aspiration using vaginal ultrasound. Once the oocytes are collected, oocytes and sperm are incubated until fertilization occurs. Embryos at the four to eight cell stage of development are then transferred some 2–3 days after fertilization.

An alternative technique where the tubes are patent is gamete intra-Fallopian transfer (GIFT). This procedure involves immediate transfer of oocytes and sperm into Fallopian tubes using a laparoscopic procedure. There are a variety of alternative techniques which involve procedures such as direct intra-peritoneal insemination (DIPI) or peritoneal oocyte sperm transfer (POST) after oocyte collection. Where the tubes are patent, intra-uterine insemi-nation achieves similar fertilization rates of GIFT.

Fertilization rates with in vitro fertilization vary, but generally approach 80–90%. However, follow-ing transfer of embryos to the uterine cavity, the success rates in achieving delivery of a child fall to approximately 20% in good units.

TREATMENT OF CERVICAL HOSTILITY

This presents a difficult problem, but may be treated by intra-uterine insemination with the husband's semen (AIH). Success rates are low, and the treatment is not without complication as it may result in severe uterine pain. It is contraindicated in the presence of a normal postcoital test. The condition may also be treated by reducing contact with seminal fluid with cervical mucus by using a condom. However, many of these couples will need to be treated with assisted reproduction techniques.

TREATMENT OF THE MALE PARTNER

Specific treatment is possible in only a small proportion of infertile males. Testicular size is important, and in the presence of small testes, azoospermia and high FSH levels it is highly unlikely that any therapy will help.

Where FSH levels are normal and testicular size is normal, ductal obstruction should be suspected and testicular biopsy performed. If normal spermatogenesis is demonstrated, then it is necessary to proceed to vasography and exploration of the scrotum. Surgical anastomosis sometimes allows the re-establishment of fertility.

Ligation of a varicocoele sometime improves semen quality, probably as a result of reducing testicular temperatures. In the presence of idiopathic oligospermia, hCG, clomiphene and bromocriptine are used and sometimes appear to be effective, but the variability in semen analysis makes assessment of efficacy of therapy difficult. Oral androgen therapy has been widely used, but there is little evidence that these compounds are effective.

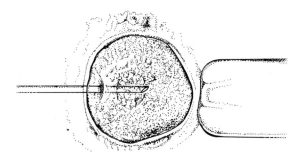

Fig. 7.16 Direct intracytoplasmic injection of spermatozoa or spermatids into the oocyte.

> Case study
> **Sub–fertility**
>
> *Mr and Mrs J. attended their general practitioner complaining of their inability to have a child.*
>
> *Mr J. had been married before, but had no children by his first wife. He was a successful businessman who worked long hours under considerable emotional and physical pressure. His wife worked part-time. She had an irregular menstrual cycle with periods every 3 or 4 months. Coitus occurred infrequently as the husband was occasionally impotent and frequently tired. The semen analysis showed evidence of oligospermia and there was evidence that the wife was anovulatory.*
>
> *There was nothing abnormal to find on physical examination of either partner. The husband was advised to modify his lifestyle, and after appropriate investigation the wife was started on clomiphene. Within 3 cycles, conception was successfully achieved.*
>
> *Subfertility is often multifactorial.*

The most successful treatment for male infertility where there is gross oligospermia now rests with the techniques of micro-assisted fertilization. This includes the techniques of partial zona dissection (PZD), sub-zonal sperm injection (SUZI) and intracytoplasmic sperm injection (ICSI). The last technique involves the direct injection of the immobilized sperm into the cytoplasm of the oocyte (Fig. 7.16). This technique produces pregnancy rates similar to those with standard in vitro fertilization.

DONOR INSEMINATION (AID)

If all evidence suggests that there is no prospect of improving the fertility of the male partner, then the question of donor insemination (AID) should be discussed with the couple.

The implications of the procedure, from both a legal and personal point of view, should be discussed in depth before accepting the woman for donor insemination. The establishment of frozen semen banks has greatly simplified the management and availability of donor insemination and, provided the emotional aspects are thoroughly explored, AID can provide a very satisfactory method of treatment.

All procedures involving manipulation of human gametes are now regulated in the UK by the Human Fertilisation and Embryology Authority. Further reference to their function is made in the final chapter of this book.

OVARIAN HYPERSTIMULATION SYNDROME (OHSS)

This condition is a complication of ovulation induction and is potentially lethal. In its severe form, the condition results in marked ovarian enlargement from the formation of multiple cysts, ascites, pleural effusion, sodium retention and oliguria. Patients may become hypovolaemic and hypotensive and may develop renal failure as well as thromboembolic phenomena and adult respiratory distress syndrome. The pathophysiology of this condition appears to be associated with an increase in vascular permeability, particularly of the ovarian vessels.

Prevention

It is important to monitor follicular development and serum oestradiol levels during treatment with hMG, and it is important to use low doses of hMG when the likely response is uncertain. Even if the ovaries have over-responded and the plasma E_2 level exceeds 1500 pg/ml, OHSS can be avoided if the injection of hCG is withheld. Furthermore, the supplementation of hCG in the second half of the cycle should be withheld.

Treatment

If the haematocrit is below 45% and the signs and symptoms are mild, the patient can be advised to stay at home, but where there is significant ascites as judged by ultrasound examination, she should be hospitalized. Baseline electrolyte values and liver and kidney function should be assessed. Volume expansion can be performed using human albumin, sometimes with crystalloid, and if there is severe ascites or pleural effusion, fluid should be drained to reduce the fluid load. Drugs such as indomethacin and angiotensin-converting enzyme inhibitors may be useful in reducing the severity of the episode. Eventually, the cysts will undergo resorption, and the ovaries will return to their normal size. Further attempts at ovarian stimulation should take into account the dosage regimes used during the episode of OHSS.

Treatment of subfertility

Depends on cause, but options include:
- Stimulation of ovulation with anti-oestrogen $\pm$ hCG
- Treatment of raised prolactin with bromocriptine (having excluded pituitary lesion)
- Tubal surgery
- IVF, GIFT, ICSI, SUZI
- AIH
- AID
- Ligation of varicocoele, surgery to correct obstruction in testis

---

BIBLIOGRAPHY

Brosens J, Gordon A 1990 Tubal infertility. Lippincott, Gover, Philadelphia

Fishel S, Symonds E M (eds) 1986 In-vitro fertilisation: past – present – future. IRL Press, Oxford

Insler V, Lunenfeld B 1986 Infertility, male & female. Churchill Livingstone, Edinburgh

Walters W A W 1991 Clinical obstetrics and gynaecology. Baillière Tindall, London

8 Complications of early pregnancy

Abortion, extra-uterine pregnancy and hydatidiform mole

SPONTANEOUS ABORTION

The definition of spontaneous abortion is the termination of pregnancy before the 24th week of pregnancy. In some countries, such as the USA, this definition is modified to termination of pregnancy before fetal viability or less than 500 g. Most spontaneous abortions occur in the second or third month of pregnancy and account for 10% of all pregnancies. It has been suggested that a much higher proportion of pregnancies abort at an early stage if the diagnosis is based on the presence of a significant plasma level of β-subunit human chorionic gonadotrophin (hCG).

Clinical types of abortion

Threatened abortion

The first sign of an impending abortion is the development of vaginal bleeding in early pregnancy (Fig. 8.1). The uterus is found to be enlarged and the cervical os is closed. Lower abdominal pain is either minimal or absent. About 50% of women presenting with a threatened abortion will continue with the pregnancy irrespective of the method of management.

Incomplete abortion

The threatened abortion may either settle and the

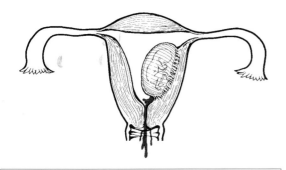

Fig. 8.1 Threatened abortion: blood loss in early pregnancy.

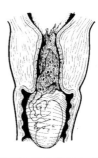

Fig. 8.2 Incomplete abortion: progression to expulsion of part of the conceptus is accompanied by pain and bleeding.

pregnancy continue or proceed to abort. The patient develops abdominal pain, and bleeding becomes worse. The cervix opens, and eventually products of conception are passed into the vagina. However, if some of the products of conception are retained, then the abortion remains incomplete (Fig. 8.2).

Case study
Incomplete abortion

A 32-year-old Asian woman presented with a history of 12 weeks amenorrhoea and vaginal bleeding followed by severe lower abdominal pain. On admission to hospital, she was sweating, pale and hypotensive. Her pulse rate was 68 beats/ minute. She complained of generalized lower abdominal pain. Initially, a ruptured tubal pregnancy was suspected because of the pain and shock, until vaginal examination revealed copious products of conception protruding from an open cervical os. Removal of these products largely relieved the pain and allowed the uterus to contract, thus reducing the blood loss. Subsequent evacuation of retained products of conception was performed after appropriate resuscitation and preparation.

Complete abortion

An incomplete abortion may proceed to completion spontaneously, when the pain will cease and vaginal bleeding will subside with involution of the uterus. Spontaneous completion of an abortion is more likely in abortions over 16 weeks gestation than in those between 8 and 16 weeks gestation, when retention of placental fragments is common.

Septic abortion

During the process of abortion – either spontaneous or induced – infection may be introduced into the uterine cavity. The clinical findings of septic abortion are similar to those of incomplete abortion with the addition of uterine and adnexal tenderness. The vaginal loss may become purulent and the patient pyrexial. In cases of severe overwhelming sepsis, endotoxic shock may develop with profound and sometimes fatal hypotension (Fig. 8.3). Other manifestations include renal failure, disseminated intravascular coagulopathy and multiple petechial haemorrhages. Organisms which commonly invade the uterine cavity are *Escherichia coli*, *Streptococcus faecalis*, *Staphylococcus albus* and *Staph. aureus*, *Klebsiella*, and *Clostridium welchii* and *Clostr. perfringens*.

Early embryonic demise

Sometimes the fetus dies in utero but is not immediately expelled. There is usually some pain and bleeding and the uterus does not increase in size.

There may be bleeding into the choriodecidual space which forms a mass of clot. This becomes organized and laminated and forms what is termed a **carneous mole**.

Recurrent abortions

A patient who has three or more spontaneous abortions is known as a recurrent aborter and should be investigated for the underlying cause.

The aetiology of abortion

In the majority of cases, no definite cause can be found for the abortion.

Feto-placental factors

Genetic abnormalities – Chromosomal abnormalities are a common cause of early abortion and may result in failure of development of the embryo with formation of a blighted ovum or with later expulsion of an abnormal fetus (Fig. 8.4).

Hormone imbalance – Progesterone production is predominately dependent on the corpus luteum for the first 8 weeks of pregnancy, and the function is then assumed by the placenta. Progesterone is essential for the maintenance of a pregnancy, and early failure of the corpus luteum may lead to abortion. However, it is difficult to be certain when falling plasma progesterone levels represent a primary cause of abortion and when they are the index of a dying placenta.

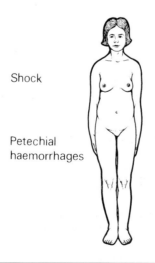

Shock

Petechial haemorrhages

Hypovolaemia

Low output failure

Renal failure
E. coli
Strep. faecalis
Staph. albus and *aureus*
Klebsiella
Clostr. welchii and *perfringens*
Low platelet count

Fig. 8.3 Manifestation of endotoxic shock complicating septic abortion.

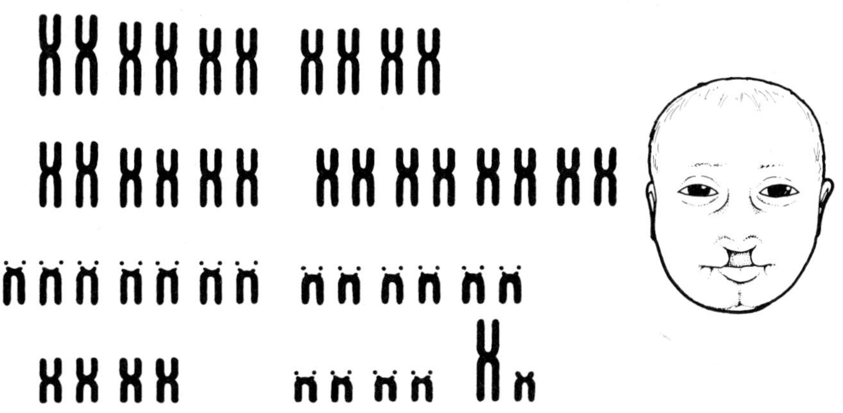

Fig. 8.4 Karyotype of trisomy 13, an example of a chromosomal abnormality. If the fetus survives it has a grossly abnormal face and a poorly developed brain.

Maternal factors

Maternal illness – Severe maternal febrile illnesses associated with infections, such as influenza, pyelitis and malaria, predispose to abortion. Other severe illnesses involving the cardiovascular, hepatic and renal systems may also result in abortion. Specific infections such as syphilis cause abortion, particularly in the second trimester. Pregnancy loss is common in women with systemic lupus erythematosus with a median rate of pregnancy loss of 31%. A disproportionate number of deaths occur in the second and third trimesters compared with other causes of abortion. The role of anti-cardiolipin antibody is discussed under the section 'Recurrent abortion'.

Abnormalities of the uterus – Congenital abnormalities of the uterine cavity, such as a bicornuate uterus or subseptate uterus, may result in abortion and sometimes recurrent abortion (Fig. 8.5). Factors which distort the uterine cavity, such as uterine fibroids and intra-uterine synechiae, interfere with implantation. Cervical incompetence may be congenital but is commonly the result of overvigorous cervical dilatation. There is premature rupture of the membranes and rapid spontaneous abortion in the second trimester of pregnancy.

Criminal abortion

Abortion induced by a variety of techniques makes up a substantial percentage of abortion in some countries. Where the indications for legal abortion are liberal, criminal abortion is infrequent, but in many countries it contributes to a high percentage of apparently spontaneous abortions.

Recurrent abortion

Most women who have had two or more consecutive miscarriages are anxious to be investigated and reassured that there is no underlying cause for the miscarriage. However, it is important to remember that after two consecutive miscarriages the likelihood of a successful third pregnancy is still around 80%. Even after three consecutive miscarriages, there is still a 55–75% chance of success. This implies that recurrent abortion is unlikely to be a random event and that it is necessary to seek a cause.

Genetic factors – In any form of spontaneous abortion, there is a 55% chance of a chromosome imbalance. However, where the chromosome complement of the first aborted conceptus is abnormal, the likelihood of the second conceptus being abnormal is about 80%. If the first conceptus is normal, there is a 70% chance that the second conceptus will be normal. The most common chromosomal defects are autosomal trisomies, which account for half the abnormalities, while polyploidy and monosomy X account for a further 20% each.

Parental chromosomal abnormalities – These are mainly translocations or mosaicisms, and occur in 10% of couples with recurrent abortions. Four or five per cent are translocations and 4–5% are mosaicisms.

There are molecular mutations which may operate in the fetus which has a normal karyotype and these include mutations in genes which code for products critical to development and mutations which lead to fetal metabolic diseases.

Congenital uterine malformations – Uterine anomalies can be demonstrated in 15–30% of women experiencing recurrent abortions. The impact of the abnormality depends on the nature of the anomaly.

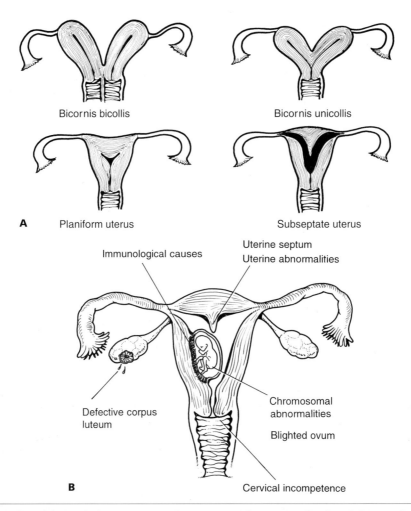

Bicornis bicollis

Bicornis unicollis

A   Planiform uterus

Subseptate uterus

Immunological causes

Uterine septum
Uterine abnormalities

Defective corpus luteum

Chromosomal abnormalities

Blighted ovum

B

Cervical incompetence

Fig. 8.5   **A** Anomalies of the genital tract are sometimes a cause of recurrent abortion; **B** Causes of recurrent abortion.

The fetal survival rate is 86% where the uterus is septate and worst where the uterus is unicornuate. It must also be remembered that over 20% of all women with congenital uterine anomalies also have renal tract anomalies (Fig. 8.5A).

Intra-uterine adhesions – Following damage to the endometrium and inner uterine walls, the surfaces may become adherent, thus partly obliterating the uterine cavity. The presence of these synechiae may lead to recurrent abortion.

Cervical incompetence – Cervical incompetence clinically results in midtrimester spontaneous abortion or early preterm delivery. The abortion tends to be rapid, painless and bloodless. The diagnosis is established by the passage of a Hegar 8 dilator without difficulty in the non-pregnant woman or by ultrasound examination or by a premenstrual hysterogram. Cervical incompetence may be congenital but most commonly results from physical damage caused by mechanical dilatation of the cervix or by damage inflicted during childbirth.

Immunological factors – Research into the possibility of an immunological basis of recurrent abortion has generally explored the possibility of a failure to mount the normal protective immune response or if the expression of relatively non-immunogenic antigens by the cytotrophoblast may result in rejection of the fetal allograft. There is evidence that unexplained spontaneous abortion is associated with couples who share an abnormal number of HLA antigens of the A, B, C and DR loci. Despite attempts to treat women with paternal lymphocytes, which initially appeared to reduce the incidence of recurrent abortion, subsequent studies have failed to confirm the initial findings.

Hormone abnormalities – Recurrent abortion is associated with hypothyroidism and, therefore, hypothyroidism should be treated. However, there is no evidence to suggest that euthyroid women benefit from the administration of thyroxine.

Corpus luteum deficiency may result in spontaneous abortion, and certainly surgical removal of the corpus luteum before 12 weeks gestation commonly results in abortion. However, the frequency of this condition of spontaneous abortion following defective progesterone steroidogenesis remains uncertain.

Infection – Individual pregnancies may be affected by infection, particularly with organisms such as listeria monocytogenes and mycoplasma. *Toxoplasma gondii* also causes abortion, but the evidence that these organisms cause recurrent abortion is limited. The causes of recurrent abortion are summarized in Fig. 8.5B.

Management

Threatened abortion should be treated by rest in bed until the bleeding subsides. Examination of the patient should include gentle vaginal and speculum examination to ascertain cervical dilatation. Some women may prefer not to be examined because of apprehension that the examination may promote abortion, and their wishes should be respected.

In some cases, it may be justifiable to give a progestogen such as 17α-hydroxyprogesterone caproate by intramuscular injection; 19-nor-steroids should not be used as they promote virilization of the female fetus.

An ultrasound scan is valuable in deciding if the fetus is alive and normal, and urinary chorionic gonadotrophin estimation will also provide additional useful information.

If there is pyrexia, a high vaginal swab should be taken for bacteriological culture.

Abortion may be complicated by haemorrhage and severe pain, and may necessitate blood transfusion and relief of pain with opiates.

If there is evidence that products of conception have been passed, the uterus must be evacuated by direct curettage or suction curettage as soon as possible. Products of conception should be submitted for histological examination (Fig. 8.6).

If there is evidence of infection, antibiotic therapy should be started immediately and adjusted subsequently if the organism identified in culture is not sensitive to the prescribed antibiotic.

Septic abortion complicated by endotoxic shock is treated by massive antibiotic therapy, large doses of corticosteroids and adequate, carefully controlled fluid replacement.

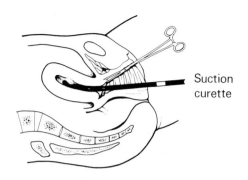

Suction curette

Fig. 8.6   Evacuation of retained products of conception.

Complications of treatment include perforation of the uterus and continuing bleeding associated with incomplete evacuation of the uterus. Intra-uterine infection may result in tubal infection and tubal obstruction with subsequent infertility. If uterine perforation is suspected and there is evidence of intraperitoneal haemorrhage or damage to the bowel, then laparotomy should be performed.

Recurrent abortion should be investigated by examining the karyotype of both parents. Maternal blood should be examined for lupus anti-coagulant, anti-phospholipid antibodies, thyroid function studies and infection screen. The uterine cavity should be examined by hysteroscopy or hysterography. The presence of lupus anticoagulant and anti-cardiolipin antibodies can be treated with low-dose aspirin and corticosteroids.

Spontaneous abortion

- Over 10% pregnancies abort under 24 weeks
- Can be threatened, incomplete, complete, septic, early embryonic demise or recurrent
- Aetiology usually unknown but possible causes include chromosomal abnormalities, hormonal factors, maternal illness, uterine abnormalities and cervical incompetence
- Investigations include hCG, ultrasound and assessment of cervical dilation
- Treatment is expectant for threatened, and curettage for missed or incomplete abortion, with antibiotics, analgesia and transfusion if indicated

---

ECTOPIC PREGNANCY

The term 'ectopic pregnancy' refers to any pregnancy occurring outside the uterine cavity.

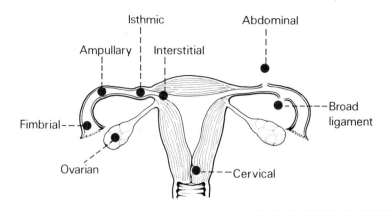

Fig. 8.7   Sites of implantation of ectopic pregnancies.

The most common site of extra-uterine implantation is the Fallopian tube, but it may occur in the ovary as an ovarian pregnancy, in the abdominal cavity as an abdominal pregnancy, or in the cervical canal as a cervical pregnancy (Fig. 8.7).

Tubal pregnancy occurs in 1 in 100 pregnancies in the UK, although this incidence varies substantially in different populations. Tubal pregnancy may occur in the ampulla, the isthmus and the interstitial portion of the tube and the outcome will depend on the site of implantation.

Predisposing factors

The majority of cases of ectopic pregnancy have no identifiable predisposing factor, but a previous history of pelvic inflammatory disease, subfertility and the presence of an intra-uterine device (IUCD) all increase the likelihood of an ectopic pregnancy.

Clinical presentation

Acute presentation

The classical pattern of symptoms includes amenorrhoea, lower abdominal pain and uterine bleeding. The abdominal pain usually precedes the onset of vaginal bleeding, and may start on one side of the lower abdomen, but rapidly becomes generalized as blood loss extends into the peritoneal cavity. Subdiaphragmatic irritation by blood produces referred shoulder tip pain and syncopal episodes may occur.

The period of amenorrhoea is usually 6–8 weeks, but may be longer if implantation occurs in the interstitial portion of the tube or in abdominal pregnancy. Clinical examination reveals a shocked woman with hypotension, tachycardia and signs of peritonism including abdominal distension, guarding and rebound tenderness. Pelvic examination is usually unimportant because of the acute pain and discomfort, and should be undertaken with caution. This type of acute presentation occurs in no more than 25% of cases.

> Case study
> **Acute presentation**
>
> *An 18-year-old woman, para 0, was brought into casualty collapsed with lower abdominal pain. On admission she was shocked with a blood pressure of 80/40, a pulse of 120 beats/minute and a tender, rigid abdomen. Vaginal examination revealed a slight red loss, bulky uterus and marked cervical excitation with a tender mass in the right fornix. At laparotomy, 800 ml of fresh blood was removed from the peritoneal cavity, and a ruptured right tubal ectopic pregnancy was found. Subsequently, a history of recurrent pelvic infections and irregular periods was elicited.*

Subacute presentation

After a short period of amenorrhoea, the patient experiences recurrent attacks of vaginal bleeding and abdominal pain. Any woman who develops lower abdominal pain following an interval of amenorrhoea should be considered as a possible ectopic pregnancy. In its subacute phase, it may be possible to feel a mass in one fornix.

Case study
Subacute presentation

A 22-year-old woman, para 0, was admitted with vaginal bleeding after 8 weeks of amenorrhoea. She had had a positive home pregnancy kit test, and described passing some tissue per vaginam. Ultrasound scan showed an empty uterus, although serum β-hCG was still positive. A presumptive diagnosis of incomplete abortion was made, and evacuation of uterus carried out uneventfully. She was discharged the following day, but readmitted that night with lower abdominal pain; a ruptured ampullary ectopic was found at laparotomy. Some days later, histology of the original curettage was reported as 'decidua with Arias–Stella type reaction, no chorionic villi seen'.

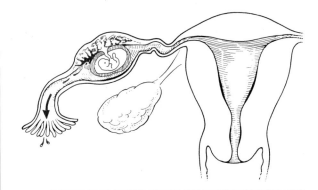

Fig. 8.8 Penetration of the tubal wall by trophoblastic tissue.

Pathology

Implantation may occur in a variety of sites, and the outcome of the pregnancy will depend on the site of implantation.

Abdominal pregnancy may result from direct implantation of the conceptus in the abdominal cavity or on the ovary, in which case it is known as primary abdominal pregnancy, or it may result from extrusion of a tubal pregnancy with secondary implantation in the peritoneal cavity, which is known as secondary abdominal pregnancy. Implantation of the conceptus in the tube results in hormonal changes that mimic normal pregnancy. The uterus enlarges, and the endometrium undergoes decidual change. Implantation within the fimbrial end or ampulla of the tube allows greater expansion before rupture occurs, whereas implantation in the interstitial portion or the isthmic part of the tube presents with early signs of haemorrhage or pain (Fig. 8.8).

Trophoblastic cells invade the wall of the tube and erode into blood vessels. This process will continue until the pregnancy bursts into the abdominal cavity or into the broad ligament, or the embryo dies, thus resulting in a tubal mole. Under these circumstances, absorption or tubal abortion may occur. Expulsion of the embryo into the peritoneal cavity or partial abortion may also occur with continuing episodes of bleeding from the tube.

Differential diagnosis

Ectopic pregnancy should always be suspected where early pregnancy is complicated by pain and bleeding. It is often overlooked if the diagnosis is not con-sidered and may be confused with a threatened or incomplete abortion. It may also be confused with acute salpingitis or appendicitis with pelvic peritonitis. It may sometimes be confused with rupture or haemorrhage of an ovarian cyst.

Management

Diagnosis of the acute ectopic pregnancy rarely presents a problem, and blood should be taken for urgent cross-matching and transfusion. Laparotomy should be performed as soon as possible with removal of the damaged tube.

Diagnosis of tubal pregnancy in the subacute phase may be much more difficult. If sufficient blood loss has occurred into the peritoneal cavity, the haemoglobin level will be low and the white cell count will be usually normal or slightly raised. Serum β-hCG measurement will exclude ectopic pregnancy if negative with a specificity of greater than 99%, and urinary hCG with modern kits that can be used on the ward or in Casualty will detect 97% of pregnancies. In the presence of a viable intrauterine pregnancy, the serum hCG will normally double over a 48 hour period. Thus, serial measurements of serum hCG levels in conjunction with ultrasound diagnosis can be of value in distinguishing early intra-uterine pregnancy from abortion or ectopics. Clinical examination may reveal a mass in one fornix, and needle aspiration of the pouch of Douglas (culdocentesis) will reveal a haemoperitoneum. This technique is now rarely used for diagnostic purposes. Ultrasound scan of the pelvis may demonstrate tubal pregnancy in 2% of cases or suggest it by other features such as free fluid in the peritoneal cavity, but is mainly of help in excluding intra-uterine pregnancy. Intra-uterine pregnancy can usually be identified by transabdominal

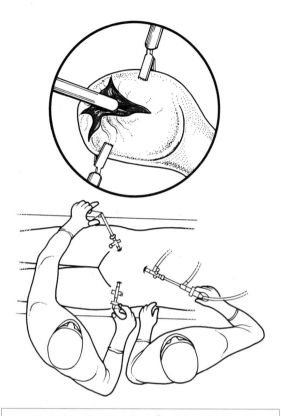

Fig. 8.9 Laparoscopic surgery for tubal disease and tubal pregnancy.

scan at 6 weeks gestation and somewhat sooner by transvaginal scan at 5–6 weeks gestation. Where there is any possibility of an ectopic pregnancy, laparoscopy is essential. Occasionally, there may be no clinical signs of an ectopic pregnancy but if curettings submitted for histopathology show evidence of decidual reaction and the Arias–Stella phenomenon then it is advisable to consider laparoscopy. Once the diagnosis has been established, the ectopic pregnancy must be removed by one of the following techniques:

1. *Salpingectomy* – If the tube is badly damaged the correct treatment is removal of the affected tube. If implantation has occurred in the interstitial portion of the tube, then it may be necessary to resect part of the uterine horn in addition to removing the tube.
2. *Salpingotomy* – Where the ectopic pregnancy is contained within the tube, it may be possible to conserve the tube by removing the pregnancy and reconstituting the tube. This is particularly important where the contralateral tube has been lost. However, there is an increased risk of recurrent ectopic pregnancy in the damaged tube.

3. *Tubal compression* – Occasionally where the tubal pregnancy occurs in the fimbrial end of the tube it may be possible to express the conceptus without opening the tube, but it is essential to be certain that adequate haemostasis is obtained.
4. *Laparoscopic surgery* – Salpingectomy and linear salpingotomy can be performed using minimal access surgery. However, various conditions must be in place. Suitable equipment and a trained operator are essential (see Fig. 8.9) Also, the patient must be haemodynamically stable, the ectopic should be less than 6 cm in diameter and the hCG less than 6000 units. The advantage of this procedure is earlier discharge and return to work. The disadvantage is the persistence of trophoblastic tissue requiring laparotomy in up to 6% of cases, although longer-term fertility and intra-uterine pregnancy rates are comparable to open procedures.
5. *Methotrexate* – Medical treatment of an ectopic pregnancy involves the administration of methotrexate, either systemically or by injection into the ectopic pregnancy by laparoscopic visualization or by ultrasound guidance.

Management of other forms of extra-uterine pregnancy

Abdominal pregnancy

Abdominal pregnancy presents a life-threatening hazard to the mother. The placenta implants outside the uterus and across the bowel and pelvic peritoneum. Any attempt to remove it will result in massive haemorrhage which is extremely difficult to control. The fetus should be removed by laparotomy and the placenta left in situ to reabsorb or extrude spontaneously.

Cervical pregnancy

Cervical pregnancy often presents as the cervical stage of a spontaneous abortion. Occasionally, it is possible to remove the conceptus by curettage but haemorrhage can be severe, and in 50% of cases it is necessary to proceed to hysterectomy to obtain adequate haemostasis.

Ectopic pregnancy

- 1 in 100 pregnancies
- Predisposing factors are previous ectopic pregnancy, or pelvic inflammatory disease, IUCD in situ
- Acute presentation in 25% cases

Ectopic pregnancy (*cont'd*)

- Common features are 6–8 weeks amenorrhoea, anaemia, lower abdominal pain localized to one side and vaginal bleeding
- Pitfalls in diagnosis are negative urinary hCG or ultra-sonography and misdiagnosis as abortion
- Laparoscopy essential to confirm the diagnosis

TROPHOBLASTIC DISEASE

Abnormality of early trophoblast may arise as a developmental anomaly of placental tissue, and results in the formation of a mass of oedematous and avascular villi. There is usually no fetus but the condition can be found in the presence of a fetus. The placenta is replaced by a mass of grapelike vesicles known as a **hydatidiform mole** (Fig. 8.10).

Invasion of the myometrium without systemic spread occurs in about 16% of cases of benign mole, and is known as **invasive mole** or **chorioadenoma destruens**. Frankly malignant change occurs in 2.5%, and is known as **choriocarcinoma**.

Incidence

The overall prevalence of this condition is about 1 in 2000 pregnancies in Western European countries but is much higher in Asia and South-East Asia. It is relatively more common at the extremes of reproductive age. Molar pregnancies are nearly all female, with occasional cases of triploidy.

Pathology

Molar pregnancy is thought to arise from fertilization by two sperm, and can be diploid with no female genetic material or it may exhibit triploidy.

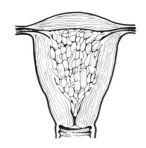

Fig. 8.10   Grape-like vesicles of a hydatidiform mole.

Benign mole remains confined to the uterine cavity and decidua. The histopathology exhibits a villous pattern, which is also found in the invasive mole. However, invasive molar tissue penetrates the myometrium deeply and may result in serious haemorrhage. Choriocarcinoma comprises plexiform columns of trophoblastic cells without villous patterns. Widespread blood-borne metastases are a feature of this disease which, until recent years, carried a very high mortality rate. Metastases my occur locally in the vagina but most commonly appear in the lungs. Theca lutein cysts occur in about one-third of all cases as a result of high circulating levels of hCG. These regress spontaneously with removal of the molar tissue.

About 50% of cases of choriocarcinoma are not associated with molar pregnancy.

Clinical presentation

Molar pregnancy most commonly presents as bleeding in the first half of pregnancy, and spontaneous abortion often occurs at about 20 weeks gestation. Occasionally, the passage of a grape-like villus heralds the presence of a mole. The uterus is larger than dates in about half the cases, but this is not a reliable sign as it may sometimes be small for dates. Severe hyperemesis, pre-eclampsia and unexplained anaemia are all factors suggestive of this disorder. The diagnosis can be confirmed by ultrasound scan and by the presence of very high levels of hCG in the blood or urine.

Management

Once the diagnosis is established, the pregnancy is terminated by suction curettage. Adequate replacement of blood loss is essential, and the procedure is accompanied by the infusion of oxytocin to ensure that the uterus remains well contracted. All cases of molar pregnancy should be followed for 1 year, and further pregnancy during this time is contraindicated. Serial estimations of subunit hCG are followed; where these remain elevated for more than 1 month after uterine evacuation, or where persistent haemorrhage occurs, repeat curettage should be performed.

If the histological evidence shows malignant change, chemotherapy with methotrexate and actinomycin D is employed and produces good results. In the UK, management of these cases is concentrated in specialized centres.

It may occasionally be necessary to remove the uterus where haemorrhage becomes life-threatening. It must be remembered that choriocarcinoma sometimes can occur following an abortion or a normal-term intra-uterine pregnancy.

Pregnancy is contraindicated until 6 months after the serum hCG levels fall to below 2 units, as is the use of the combined oral contraceptive pill. The risk recurrence in subsequent pregnancies is 2–3%.

Case study
Trophoblastic disease

A 27-year-old primigravid woman attended the clinic with a history of 12 weeks of amenorrhoea, complaining of bright vaginal blood loss and lower abdominal discomfort. Abdominal examination revealed that the uterine fundus was 16 weeks in size. There was fresh blood in the vagina, and the cervical os was closed. There was a high titre of hCG in the urine, and an ultrasound scan showed a ground glass appearance in the uterine cavity with no evidence of fetal parts. Suction evacuation of molar tissue was performed the following day, and recovery was uneventful.

Trophoblastic disease

- 1 in 2000 pregnancies in UK
- 16% are invasive mole, 2.5% choriocarcinoma
- Features are large-for-dates uterus, per vaginum bleeding and high hCG
- Curettage should be repeated after 1 month if bleeding has not settled or hCG remains elevated
- Follow-up is by hCG, and advise not to get pregnant for 12 months
- Choriocarcinoma blood-borne metastases, treatment with methotrexate

---

BIBLIOGRAPHY

Beard R W, Sharp F 1988 Early pregnancy loss. Mechanism and treatment. RCOG Press, London

9 Congenital abnormalities and infections in pregnancy

There are a very large number of congenital abnormalities and genetic syndromes documented in the literature, but most clinicians encounter very few of them. Genetic counselling has become an important specialty in its own right. Only those conditions which are encountered relatively commonly will be considered in this section.

CONGENITAL ABNORMALITIES

Incidence

The incidence of serious congenital abnormalities has been estimated at 25–30/1000 births, and this figure has remained relatively constant in England and Wales since 1920. Congenital abnormalities account for 25% of all stillbirths and 20% of all deaths in the first week. The commonest five groups of defect include neural tube defects (3–7/1000), congenital heart disease (6/1000), severe mental retardation (4/1000), Down's syndrome (1.5/1000) and hare lip/cleft palate (1.5/1000) (Table 9.1). Whilst the total number of infants born with congenital defects is small, the overall incidence of

chromosomal abnormalities is high, as about 30% of early abortions show significant chromosomal abnormalities.

Neural tube defects

The neural tube defects are the commonest of the major congenital abnormalities and include anencephaly, microcephaly, spina bifida with or without meningo-myelocele and encephalocele (Fig. 9.1). The incidence is approximately 1 in 200, and the chance of having an affected child after one previous abnormal child is 1 in 20. Infants with anencephaly or microcephaly do not usually survive. Many die during labour, and the remainder within the first week of life. Infants with open neural tube defects often survive – particularly where it is possible to cover the lesion surgically with skin. However, the defect may result in paraplegia and bowel and bladder incontinence. The child often has normal intelligence and becomes aware of the problems posed for the parents.

Although there is some evidence that multivitamin supplementation may reduce the incidence of this condition, the major effort at the present time is directed toward screening techniques (see Chapter 4).

Table 9.1 Major congenital abnormalities

	Approximate incidence per 1000 births
Neural tube defects	3–7
Congenital heart disease	6
Severe mental retardation	4
Down's syndrome	1.5
Cleft lip/palate	1.5
Talipes	1–2
Cerebral palsy	3
Blindness	0.2
Deafness	0.8
Abnormalities of limbs	1–2
Others including renal tract anomalies	2
Total	15–30

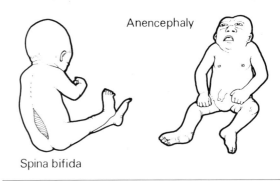

Fig. 9.1 Two common abnormalities of the central nervous system.

Folic acid dietary supplementation is indicated both before and during pregnancy in those women who have experienced a pregnancy complicated by a neural tube defect.

Screening by α-fetoprotein

All women should be offered screening by measurement of serum α-fetoprotein between 16 and 19 weeks gestation. Women who would not accept termination of an abnormal pregnancy should not have the test performed unless it is specifically requested.

An abnormally high value should be investigated by:

1. Repeating the serum measurement on another sample
2. Checking the gestational age by ultrasound scan
3. Checking for multiple pregnancy by scan
4. Screening by scan for neurological abnormality.

Improvements in the precision of ultrasound diagnosis of neural tube defects have meant that scanning procedures have largely replaced the measurement of liquor α-fetoprotein, and hence the need for amniocentesis, although the measurement of amniotic fluid acetylcholinesterase will improve diagnostic precision.

The mother should be advised that there is a risk of abortion which is estimated at about 1%.

Congenital cardiac defects

The next big group is that of congenital cardiac defects. Some of these infants present with intra-uterine growth retardation and oligohydramnios, but in many cases the diagnosis is established after delivery. With improvements in real-time ultrasound imaging, recognition of many cardiac defects has become possible, but early recognition is essential if any action is to be taken.

The most common defects are ventricular and atrial septal defects, pulmonary and aortic stenosis, coarctation and transpositions, including the tetralogy of Fallot. These lesions can generally now be recognized on the four-chamber views recorded during detailed 18 week gestation scans.

Cerebral palsy

This is a disorder of movement and posture caused by a non-progressive insult to the immature brain. There is persistence in infantile behaviour and reflexes, and as the central nervous system matures the manifestations change and the degree of handicap tends to increase. It affects 2/1000 term infants and up to 50/1000 infants with birth weights of below 1500 g. The aetiology is complex but includes disorders of development, intrauterine infection, disturbances of normal fetal nutrition and oxygenation before or during labour as well as postnatal events such as kernicterus, meningitis and trauma. Fewer than 15% of cases are thought to arise from intrapartum asphyxia.

Other conditions amenable to diagnosis by amniocentesis

X-linked diseases

This group includes X-linked diseases such as Duchenne's muscular dystrophy and haemophilia. If the mother is a carrier, and the karyotype demonstrates a male fetus, then the child will have a 50/50 chance of having Duchenne's muscular dystrophy, and therefore abortion should be offered (Fig. 9.2).

However, this diagnostic precision can now be improved by cordocentesis under ultrasound control, and direct blood samples can be obtained from the umbilical and placental blood vessels. Serum creatinine kinase is grossly elevated in the affected infant.

Metabolic disorders

Conditions such as phenylketonuria, which may result in severe mental retardation, are now amenable to prenatal diagnosis by identifying enzyme deficiencies in cultured fetal cells. The conditions which can be reliably diagnosed in this way are listed in Table 9.2.

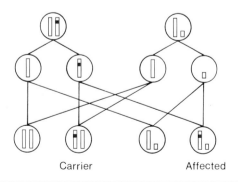

Carrier   Affected

Fig. 9.2 Transmission of a recessively inherited X-linked disorder. The abnormal gene is carried on the female X chromosome.

Table 9.2 Inherited metabolic disorders most commonly diagnosed antenatally

Sphingolipidoses	
Tay–Sachs' disease	Hexoseaminadase A
Gaucher's disease	Glucocerebrosidase
Metachromatic Leucodystrophy	Arylsulphatase
Krabbe's leucodystrophy	Galactocerebroside B Galactosidase
Pompe's disease (glycogen storage)	α-1-4-Glucosidase
Mucopolysaccharidoses	
Hurler disease	α-L-Iduronidase
Hunter disease	Sulpho-iduronide sulphatase
Sanfilippo disease	Heparan sulphate sulphatase
Galactosaemia	Galactose-1-phosphate uridyl transferase
Homocystinuria	Cystathionine synthetase
Maple syrup urine disease	Keto acid decarboxylase
Methylmalonic acidaemia	Methylmalonic CoA mutase

Conditions associated with visible abnormalities such as absent eyes, limb deformities, hare lip and encephalocele may also be diagnosed antenatally by ultrasound scanning.

CHROMOSOMAL ABNORMALITIES

A considerable number of chromosomal abnormalities have been identified from the culture and karyotype of fetal cells in the amniotic fluid, and include structural and numerical abnormalities of the karyotype. The commonest abnormality is that associated with trisomy 21 or Down's syndrome.

Down's syndrome

This syndrome is characterized by the typical abnormal facies, mental retardation of varying degrees of severity and congenital heart disease. The karyotype includes an additional chromosome on group 21, and this presents as a trisomy 21, although it sometimes occurs at number 22. The incidence overall is 1.5/1000 births. However, the risk increases with advancing maternal age, and over the age of 30 years is 1/300, while over the age of 45 years it is about 1/40. The underlying reason may be related to an increased frequency of non-disjunction at meiosis.

About 6–8% of affected infants have the disease as a result of a translocation, and the extra 21 chromosome is carried on to another chromosome, usually in group 13–15. The mother or the father will usually show evidence of being a translocation carrier. If the mother is a carrier the risk of recurrence is 1/10. Thus, all women over the age of 35 years or with a family history of mongolism should be offered amniocentesis with a view to termination of the pregnancy, if the karyotype is abnormal.

Amniocentesis is usually also offered to women who have a previous history of Turner's syndrome (45XO) or Klinefelter's syndrome (47XYY), although the risk of recurrence is low.

Congenital abnormalities

- 25–30/1000 births in England and Wales
- Account for 25% of still-births, 20% of neonatal deaths
- Commonest are neural tube defects (7/1000), followed by cardiac defects (6/1000) and chromosomal defects (1.5/1000)
- Incidence of trisomy 21 increases with age
- Amniocentesis can assist in prenatal diagnosis of neural tube defects, chromosome abnormalities, X-linked disorders and some metabolic defects

---

MATERNAL INFECTIONS WHICH MAY AFFECT FETAL DEVELOPMENT

Rubella

The effect of maternal rubella infection has been discussed in a previous chapter. Congenital malformations include microcephaly, cataracts, deafness, congenital heart disease and osteitis. From 0 to 4 weeks, the risk is 33%, between 5 and 8 weeks 25%, between 9 and 12 weeks 9%, between 13 and 16 weeks 4%, and between 17 and 30 weeks 1% (Fig. 9.3). Injections of γ-globulin where contact with rubella has occurred may help to prevent infections, but the evidence is equivocal. Diagnosis based on the level of rubella antibodies has been previously discussed.

Hepatitis B

There are two types of viral hepatitis – infective hepatitis (virus A) and serum hepatitis (virus B). Virus A is associated with a short incubation period, and virus B with a long incubation time. Hepatitis B surface antigen is known as Australian antigen.

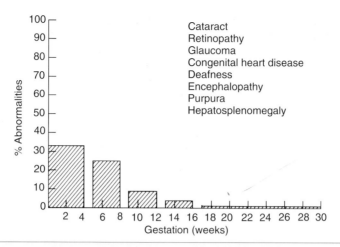

Fig. 9.3 Incidence of congenital defects and rubella in relation to gestational age.

The risk to the fetus of maternal infection appears to be minimal. The infant may become infected by swallowing maternal blood or amniotic fluid during labour and about 25% of these infants subsequently develop hepatitis.

Australia-antigen-positive women are managed with particular precautions as cross-infection may occur from maternal faeces, urine, maternal blood or amniotic fluid. These patients should be managed with barrier nursing, taking especial precautions with the disposal of excreta.

The risk of vertical transmission is substantially reduced by the concurrent administration of immunoglobulin and vaccination after delivery.

Herpes hominis

Herpes infections are due to two antigenic types, 1 and 2. Type 2 is responsible for 95% of genital tract infections, whereas type 1 occurs in non-genital sites such as the mouth, eyes and central nervous system. Type 2 infections are sexually transmitted.

Genital herpes is associated with a fivefold increase in the incidence of abortion during the first 20 weeks. Genital infection at term results in a 40% incidence of infection in the fetus and this may be manifest in skin vesicles, and in infections involving the brain, liver and adrenals.

At the present time, it is generally considered advisable to deliver the infant by Caesarean section to minimize the risk of infection acquired during vaginal delivery if the culture from the vagina remains positive.

Other infections

Cytomegalovirus

It has been estimated that 4% of women acquire this infection during pregnancy. Both the placenta and fetus may be affected by the viraemia which may result in the development of microcephaly and be the cause of mental retardation of infants in the first 6 years of life. The diagnosis can be established by the presence of a rising antibody titre. Newborn screening is based on raised cord blood IgM levels (>20 mg%).

Pregnancy bacteriuria

Bacteriuria in the mother is associated with an increase in low birth weight infants. Urine specimens yielding more than 10^5 colonies/ml are considered bacteriuric and should be treated with appropriate antibiotic therapy.

Toxoplasmosis

Toxoplasma gondii is a protozoal infection which is found throughout the world. The mode of infection involves the domestic cat. Congenital toxoplasmosis may occur if the mother acquires the infection during pregnancy, and its incidence has been estimated in England at 1 in 20 000 births. In France it may be as high as 1 in 2000 births. Maternal infection may be a cause of recurrent abortion.

Chlamydiosis

The intracellular bacterium *Chlamydia trachoma* is a cause of neonatal conjunctivitis and trachoma. The infection can be diagnosed by immunoassay, and treated with 7–14 days of erythromycin.

Herpes zoster

First-trimester infection is associated with an increased risk of abortion and, rarely, embryopathy with intra-uterine growth retardation and limb scarring. The major risk to the fetus comes from neonatal chickenpox, which is most likely to occur when delivery is within 4 days of the onset of symptoms in the mother. This develops 2–3 weeks after delivery and has a 20% mortality. Infants born within this time and mothers who are known not to be immune should be given immunoglobulin.

Listeriosis

Listeria monocytogenes is found in soil, unwashed vegetables, birds, insects and crustaceans. The organism can be transmitted transplacentally or by inhalation of amniotic fluid at delivery. It affects 1/20 000 births. There is an increased risk of intra-uterine death and abortion, and untreated neonatal infection has a 90% mortality rate in the infant. The diagnosis can be established by blood and urine cultures, and should be suspected in any women presenting with a flu-like illness with conjunctivitis, pharyngitis, loin pain and diarrhoea. The organism is sensitive to ampicillin or gentamicin.

HIV infection

Human immunodeficiency virus (HIV) is a retro-virus which affects human lymphocytes and other cells in the central nervous system. There are three levels of manifestation of HIV infection:

1. Asymptomatic – a positive test for HIV but no clinical symptoms
2. Acquired immunodeficiency syndrome (AIDS)-related complex (ARC) – this includes persistent generalized lymphadenopathy, weight loss, lethargy, fever and joint pains
3. AIDS – this includes the clinical symptoms plus opportunistic infections such as *Pneumocystics carinii* and the presence of Kaposi's sarcoma.

Infection is usually asymptomatic, and incubation takes 15–58 months. Transmission is sexual or blood-borne and transplacental. There is no evidence to suggest that airborne infection occurs.

Incidence. In the USA, AIDS is largely confined to homosexual or bisexual individuals (27%). However, 50% of cases occur in intravenous drug abusers and 10% after blood transfusion. Obviously, these clinical incidence figures will continue changing.

In pregnancy, there is no evidence that HIV infection is clinically accelerated. AIDS and ARC depress the T-helper cell population. It does not affect fertility.

There is a higher incidence of pre-term labour and low birth weight infants in affected mothers, but there are complicating social factors. There are three routes of infection of the child:

1. Transplacental
2. At birth
3. Breast milk.

Incidental perinatal transmission occurs in 30–50% of cases.

Fetal AIDS – This syndrome is manifested by intra-uterine growth retardation, microcephaly, prominent forehead and blue sclerae.

Prognosis – The outlook for survival in infected children is very poor, with a high mortality rate. There is some evidence that the extent of maternal illness may determine the risk of infection in the baby.

Care of HIV-seropositive women during pregnancy and in labour – All HIV-positive pregnant women should be managed jointly with a physician who specializes in HIV. It is not considered essential to nurse these mothers in isolation unless there is abnormal haemorrhage or infective complications. Early signs and symptoms include malaise, fevers, night sweats and weight loss. There are numerous gastrointestinal and dermatological symptoms, including Kaposi's sarcoma. There is some evidence to suggest that delivery by elective Caesarean section may reduce the incidence of vertical trans-mission but, as yet, there are insufficient data to justify routine operative delivery.

During the second stage of delivery, staff should wear full protective clothing with face protection and overshoes, with double gloves for suturing.

Fetal blood sampling should be avoided whenever possible.

The placenta should be double-bagged and incinerated. The newborn infant should undergo the following investigations:

1. Full blood count and differential white cell count
2. Urine culture for cytomegalovirus
3. Hepatitis B and C serology
4. HIV serology
5. Virology
6. Immunology including T lymphocyte subsets and immunoglobulin levels.

Breast feeding appears to double the risk of transmission of HIV, and therefore these women should generally be advised against breast feeding.

Maternal infections affecting the fetus

- Incidence of congenital defects in rubella varies in relation to gestational age at time of infection from 33 to 1%
- Hepatitis B transmission is uncommon
- Delivery by Caesarian section is recommended for patients with active herpes (type 2) infection; 40% incidence of neonatal infection
- Cytomegalovirus can cause microcephaly and mental retardation
- Toxoplasmosis affects 1/20 000 births

BIBLIOGRAPHY

Johnstone F D 1992 Clinical Obstetrics and Gynaecology. Baillière Tindall, London
Reed G B, Claireaux A E, Bain A D 1989 Diseases of the fetus and newborn. Chapman & Hall, London

10 Antenatal disorders

HYPERTENSION IN PREGNANCY

Hypertension is the commonest complication of pregnancy in the UK, and occurs in 10–15% of all pregnancies. In its most severe form, the condition is associated with convulsions, proteinuria and oedema and may lead to fetal and maternal death. In its mildest form, hypertension alone in late pregnancy, it appears to be of minimal risk. The association between pregnancy and convulsions has been described in ancient Egyptian and Greek writings, but that between convulsions and hypertension and proteinuria was first described by Vaquez in 1897.

Classification

Numerous attempts have been made to classify hypertension in pregnancy, but the classification should be simple and related to factors which can be clearly defined. Essentially, hypertension may occur as a result of the pregnancy, or it may antedate the pregnancy and be due to underlying renal disease or to essential hypertension. The best classification available at the present time is the one outlined by the American College of Obstetricians and Gynecologists:

Hypertension is defined as a systolic pressure of at least 140 mmHg or a diastolic pressure of at least 90 mmHg on two or more occasions after 20 weeks gestation (Fig. 10.1).

This definition also includes reference to a rise in systolic pressure of at least 30 mmHg or a rise in diastolic pressure of at least 15 mmHg, but it is unlikely that this classification does more than complicate the definition as fetal and maternal risks do not increase if the blood pressure remains less than 140/90 mmHg.

Proteinuria is defined as the presence of urinary protein in concentrations greater than 0.3 g/L in a 24 hour collection or in concentrations greater than 1 g/L on two or more occasions at least 6 hours apart.

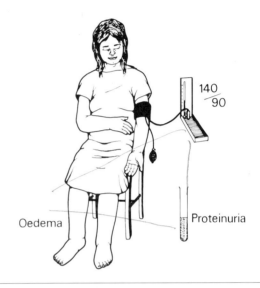

Fig. 10.1 The signs of pre-eclampsia include hypertension, proteinuria and oedema.

Oedema is defined as the development of pitting oedema or a weight gain in excess of 2.3 kg in 1 week. Because oedema of the legs is very common in an otherwise uncomplicated pregnancy, this is the least useful sign and should probably be abandoned in future classifications.

The various types of hypertension are therefore defined as follows:

1. Gestational hypertension
2. Pre-eclampsia
3. Eclampsia
4. Superimposed pre-eclampsia or eclampsia
5. Chronic hypertensive disease
6. Unclassified hypertensive disease.

Gestational hypertension is the development of hypertension alone during pregnancy or within the first 24 hours postpartum in a previously normotensive woman. The blood pressure returns to normal within 10 days after delivery.

Pre-eclampsia is the development of hypertension and proteinuria and oedema after the 20th week of gestation. It is predominantly a disorder of primigravidae.

Eclampsia is the association of convulsions with pre-eclampsia.

Superimposed pre-eclampsia or *eclampsia* is the development of pre-eclampsia in a patient with chronic hypertensive disease or renal disease.

Chronic hypertensive disease is the presence of persistent hypertension before pregnancy or before the 20th week of gestation.

Unclassified hypertensive disease includes those cases of hypertension occurring in pregnancy on a random basis, but where there is insufficient information for classification.

Because of the difficulties in classification, hypertension developing during pregnancy is now often classified simply as pregnancy-induced hypertension with or without proteinuria.

Incidence

Approximately 10–15% of all pregnancies are complicated by hypertension, but in the UK only 1 in 10 of these pregnancies is complicated by proteinuria.

Pathogenesis and pathology of pre-eclampsia and eclampsia

The exact nature of the pathogenesis of pre-eclampsia remains uncertain. However, the pathophysiology (Fig. 10.2) is characterized by:

1. Arteriolar vasoconstriction – particularly in the vascular bed of the uterus and the kidney
2. Disseminated intravascular coagulation.

Blood pressure is determined by cardiac output, blood volume and peripheral vascular resistance. Both cardiac output and blood volume increase substantially in pregnancy, but blood pressure tends to fall in mid-trimester. Thus, the most important regulatory factor is the loss of peripheral vascular resistance that occurs in pregnancy and, as sympathetic tone appears to remain unchanged, the state of peripheral vascular resistance is determined by the balance between humoral vasodilators and vasoconstrictors. There is a specific loss of sensitivity to angiotensin II, which is associated with locally

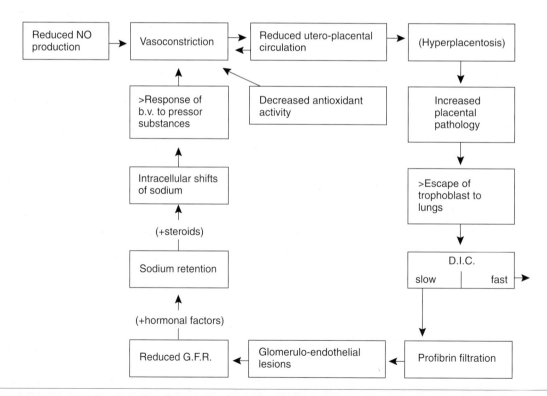

Fig. 10.2 The cycle of pathological changes that occurs in pre-eclampsia.

active vasodilator prostaglandins. Thus, factors which increase the activity of the renin–angiotensin system or reduce the activity of tissue prostaglandins will result in hypertension.

The reduced sensitivity to infused angiotensin II is also associated with down-regulation of vascular and platelet angiotensin AII receptors. There are several alternative mechanisms that may produce vasoconstriction in specific vascular beds. Current hypotheses suggest that pre-eclampsia is a disease of endothelial dysfunction. Nitric oxide (NO) or endothelium-derived relaxing factor (EDRF) is a potent vasodilator. In pre-eclampsia, NO synthesis is reduced, possibly by inhibition of nitric oxide synthetase activity.

The production of anti-oxidants in normal pregnancy limits the damaging effects of lipid peroxides, which are increased in pregnancy. In women who develop pre-eclampsia, anti-oxidant activity is decreased, and this results in endothelial cell damage.

Once vasoconstriction occurs in the utero-placental bed, it results in placental damage and the release of trophoblast into the peripheral circulation. This trophoblast is rich in thromboplastins, which precipitate disseminated intravascular coagulation, giving rise to the pathological lesions in the kidney, liver and placental bed. The renal lesion results in sodium and water retention, with most of this fluid accumulating outside the vascular tree. Plasma volume diminishes as the vascular space is reduced. At the same time, increased sodium retention increases vascular sensitivity to angiotensin II and therefore promotes further vasoconstriction and tissue damage in a vicious circle of events which may ultimately result in cerebral haemorrhage, acute cardiac failure with pulmonary oedema, acute renal failure with tubular or cortical necrosis and hepatic failure with periportal necrosis. The placenta becomes grossly infarcted, and this results in intra-uterine growth retardation and sometimes fetal death. There are many factors which may trigger this sequence of events, including immunological and dietary factors and the pre-existence of underlying chronic renal disease or essential hypertension.

The renal lesion

The renal lesion is the most specific diagnostic feature of pre-eclampsia (Fig 10.3) and features:

1. Swelling and proliferation of endothelial cells to such a point that the capillary vessels are almost obstructed

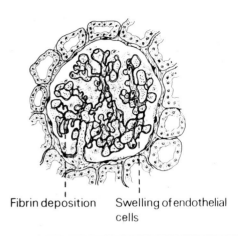

Fibrin deposition   Swelling of endothelial cells

Fig. 10.3 Renal changes in pre-eclampsia include endothelial swelling and fibrin deposition under the basement membrane of the glomerular tuft.

2. Hypertrophy and hyperplasia of the inter-capillary or mesangial cells
3. Fibrillary material (profibrin) deposited on the basement membrane and between and within the endothelial cells.

The characteristic appearance is therefore one of increased capillary cellularity and reduced vascularity. The lesion is present in 71% of primigravidae, whereas it is found in only 29% of multigravidae. There is a much higher incidence of unsuspected chronic renal disease in multigravidae. The glomerular lesion is always associated with proteinuria and with reduced glomerular filtration. Tubular changes result in impaired uric acid secretion leading to hyperuricaemia.

Placental pathology

Placental infarcts occur in normal pregnancy, but are significantly more extensive in pre-eclampsia. The characteristic features in the placenta include:

1. Increased syncytial knots or sprouts
2. Increased loss of syncytium
3. Proliferation of cytotrophoblast
4. Thickening of the trophoblastic basement membrane
5. Villous necrosis.

In the utero-placental bed, the normal invasion of trophoblastic cells along the luminal surface of the spiral arteries does not occur beyond the deciduo-myometrial junction, and there is apparent constriction of the vessels between the radial artery and

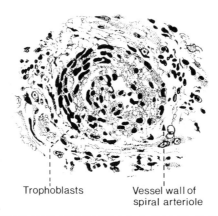

Trophoblasts   Vessel wall of
spraial arteriole

Fig. 10.4 Trophoblast invasion of the spiral arterioles is defective in pre-eclampsia.

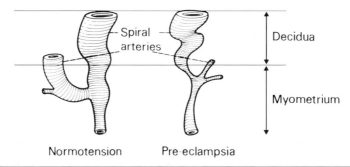

Fig. 10.5 Invasion of the spiral arterioles by trophoblast results in dilatation of the vessels; this process is defective in pre-eclampsia.

the decidual portion (Figs 10.4 and 10.5). These changes may result in reduced uteroplacental blood flow.

Disseminated intravascular coagulation (DIC)

In severe pre-eclampsia and eclampsia, thrombosis occurs in the capillaries. Multiple platelet and fibrin thrombi can be identified in the brain. Similar changes are seen in the periportal areas of the liver and in the adrenal cortex and spleen. In some cases, thrombocytopenia develops, and in 10% of eclamptic women the platelet count falls below 100 000/ml. There is an increase in fibrin deposition resulting both from increased fibrin production and from impaired removal of fibrin. There seems little doubt that coagulation changes play a major role in the pathology of eclampsia.

Immunological aspects of pregnancy hypertension

Pre-eclampsia may be due to an abnormality of the feto-maternal host response. There is a lower incidence of pre-eclampsia in consanguinous marriages and an increased incidence of hypertension in first pregnancies in second marriages.

Indices of cell-mediated immune response have also been shown to be altered in severe pre-eclampsia. However, the incidence of pre-eclampsia differs markedly in different racial groups and climatic conditions, and it also follows a familial pattern.

The HELLP syndrome

A severe manifestation of pre-eclampsia occurs in a variant known as the HELLP syndrome. This syndrome includes the triad of haemolysis (H), raised liver enzymes (EL) and a low platelet count (LP). The thrombocytopenia is often severe, and may result in haemorrhage into the brain and the liver. The syndrome demands intervention and delivery as soon as the acute manifestations are controlled.

Management

Pre-eclampsia and gestational hypertension

The object of management is to prevent the development of eclampsia with its consequent serious sequelae to the mother and to the survival and health of the fetus.

Bed rest – The detection of hypertension is an indication for admission to hospital and bed rest, which results in an improvement in renal and utero-placental blood flow. The improvement in renal blood flow results in a diuresis, loss of weight and a reduction in oedema. In gestational hypertension, there is a case for home management of hypertension with self-assessment of blood pressure and urine testing for proteinuria. The development of proteinuria is an absolute indication for immediate hospital admission. If the blood pressure returns to normal, the patient can be sent home and observations continued on an out-patient basis.

Sedation – Sedation has little part to play in the management of mild hypertension. In the presence of hyperreflexia and cerebral excitability, diazepam 10–20 mg 6-hourly will reduce the risk of convulsions, but has the disadvantage that prolonged treatment will result in placental transfer of diazepam and its metabolite, desmethyl diazepam, and may lead to hypothermia and hypotonia in the fetus – a condition known as the **floppy baby syndrome**.

Whilst diazepam is particularly useful in the management of the pre-convulsive or convulsive state, longer-term prevention of fits may be achieved by the use of sodium phenytoin, intravenously initially and later by the oral route.

Diuretics – Severe pre-eclampsia is associated with hypovolaemia. Further reduction in blood volume with diuretics tends to reduce utero-placental blood flow and renal blood flow. The long-term use of diuretics in pregnancy has been shown to be associated with fetal growth retardation, and has no significant beneficial effect on the development of hypertension or proteinuria. The only positive indications for the use of diuretics are:

1. For the symptomatic relief of oedema
2. In some cases of essential hypertension in pregnancy
3. Use of osmotic diuretics such as mannitol in the immediate postpartum period when oliguria develops.

Monitoring of the feto-placental unit

Pre-eclampsia results in impaired placental function and it is, therefore, important to monitor this function and to assess fetal growth and development. Most commonly used techniques now rely on the assessment of biophysical changes and these measurements include:

1. *Biophysical profile* – The ultrasound assessment of fetal wellbeing has now largely replaced biochemical measurements such as serial oestriol estimations. A biophysical profile involves ultrasound assessment of fetal breathing movements, gross body movements, fetal tone, reactive fetal heart rate and quantitative amniotic fluid volume measurement, and provides an index of fetal health. Further details of this technique are present in the chapter on imaging.
2. *Serial ultrasound measurements* – Assessments of fetal biparietal diameter and abdominal birth are used to examine the role of fetal growth, in association with the assessment of amniotic fluid volume as an index of placental failure.
3. *Doppler flow studies* – The use of pulsed ultrasound enables the measurement of velocity profiles in the fetal and uterine circulation, and from these measurements some estimate can be made of flow rates. A significant reduction in flow in the umbilical arteries or the uteroplacental vessels associated with increased vascular resistance may signify increasing jeopardy to the fetus.
4. *Antenatal cardiotocography* – The antenatal assessment of fetal heart rate and uterine activity provides a useful, but by no means infallible, indication of fetal wellbeing. The presence of episodes of fetal bradycardia, either during the resting phase or during contractions, and the loss of baseline variability of heart rate may indicate fetal hypoxia.

Antihypertensive drug therapy

The role of antihypertensive therapy is currently being explored and re-evaluated. It should be made clear that there is no drug available at the present time that specifically reverses the vascular change of pre-eclampsia. Therefore, the purpose of using antihypertensive therapy is to protect the mother from the effects of the hypertension and to prolong pregnancy to enable greater fetal maturity to be achieved. These objectives can be achieved only if the drug employed has no significant deleterious effects on the mother or infant.

Antihypertensive therapy has its major role in controlling severe hypertension or in treating milder forms of gestational hypertension before 34 weeks gestation.

The drugs most commonly used are:

- Methyl dopa
- Hydralazine
- β-blockers such as oxprenolol, atenolol, metoprolol
- Combined α- and β-blockers such as labetalol
- Calcium channel blockers such as nifedipine.

The most significant sign in late pregnancy is the development of proteinuria, and where this is persistent it is an indication to deliver the patient.

An overall profile of the various management strategies in pregnancy hypertension is shown in Figure 10.6. This flow diagram illustrates the various pathways of progression and their management. Mild gestational hypertension may get better after rest, or may progress to proteinuric hypertension with convulsions in the most extreme cases of eclampsia.

Prevention of pre-eclampsia

Until recently, all practical endeavours have been directed towards preventing eclampsia. However, recently the possibility of preventing pre-eclampsia has been evaluated using low-dose aspirin. Aspirin acts as an inhibitor of cyclo-oxygenase activity and of platelet aggregation. Low-dose aspirin inhibits thromboxane synthesis.

Although there have been conflicting results reported from several large multi-centre studies, it seems reasonable at the present time to recommend that women who have a family history of preeclampsia or eclampsia or who have themselves experienced severe pre-eclampsia should take aspirin using 60 mg daily after 16 weeks gestation until delivery. The Collaborative Low-Dose Aspirin Study in Pregnancy published in 1994 showed that in a large series of women in a randomized controlled trial using low-dose aspirin against a placebo, there was a marginal reduction in the occurrence of pre-eclampsia. There were no significant complications associated with the active treatment.

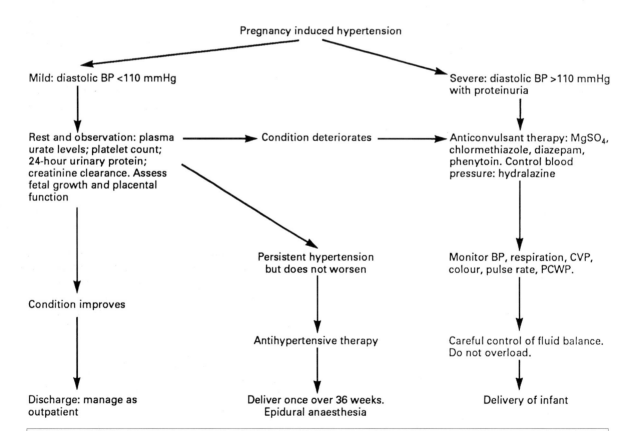

Fig. 10.6   Flow diagram of regression or progression of gestational hypertension and its management (BP, blood pressure; CVP, central venous pressure; PCWP, pulmonary capillary web pressure).

Symptoms of pre-eclampsia and eclampsia

Pre-eclampsia is commonly an asymptomatic condition. However, there are symptoms which must **never** be overlooked as they presage the onset of eclampsia, and these include frontal headache, blurring of vision and epigastric pain (Fig. 10.7). Of these, the most important is the development of epigastric pain – either during the pregnancy or within 24 hours of delivery. It is also extremely important to remember that the most severe forms of pre-eclampsia and eclampsia may occur in the second trimester, despite the fact that the condition most commonly occurs in the third trimester.

Induction of labour

The decision as to when a pregnancy should be terminated is determined by:

1. The maturity of the fetus
2. The severity of the pre-eclampsia and, in particular, the development of persistent proteinuria
3. The presence of additional complications such as placental abruption.

Severe hypertension and proteinuria may sometimes necessitate early induction of labour or Caesarean section to safeguard the health of the mother and because the hazard to the fetus remaining 'in utero' may outweigh the risks of prematurity. No pregnancy should be allowed to proceed past term in the presence of even mild hypertension.

If the cervix is unripe and unsuitable for surgical induction, the cervix can often be ripened by the use of vaginal gel containing prostaglandin E_2. If the cervix is unripe and the condition is severe, it may be necessary to proceed to delivery by Caesarean section, but only after controlling the blood pressure with intravenous hydralazine.

If the cervix is ripe, the labour is induced by:

1. Artificial rupture of the membranes
2. Oxytocin infusion
3. A combination of both procedures.

The fetal heart rate should always be monitored as well as the level of uterine activity.

Complications

1. There is an increased incidence of placental abruption in pregnancies complicated by hypertension.
2. Severe pre-eclampsia is associated with reduced glomerular filtration and this may result in severe oliguria. A diuresis can be induced by the administration of mannitol 500 ml of a 20% solution.
3. Disseminated intravascular coagulation.
4. Maternal complications such as cerebral infarction, heart failure and adult respiratory distress syndrome.

Eclampsia

The onset of convulsions in a pregnancy complicated by pre-eclampsia denotes the onset of eclampsia (Fig. 10.8). Eclampsia most commonly occurs in primigravidae, but may occur in women of high parity who have previously had uncomplicated pregnancies. Eclampsia is a preventable condition and denotes a failure to recognize the early worsening signs of pre-eclampsia. It carries serious risks of intra-uterine death for the fetus and of maternal death from cerebral haemorrhage and

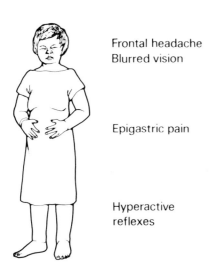

Frontal headache
Blurred vision

Epigastric pain

Hyperactive reflexes

Fig. 10.7 Presenting signs of eclampsia.

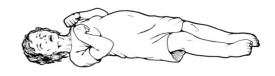

Fig. 10.8 The differentiating feature of eclampsia is the development of convulsions.

renal and hepatic failure. All cases must be managed in hospital. Any woman who is admitted to hospital with convulsions during the course of a pregnancy, or who is admitted in a coma associated with hypertension, should be considered to be suffering from eclampsia until proved otherwise.

Management

The three basic guidelines for management of eclampsia are:

1. Control the fits
2. Control the blood pressure
3. Deliver the infant.

Various drugs are used to control the fits, but the most widely used regimes include:

1. Intravenous injection of diazepam 20–40 mg followed by intramuscular injection of 10 mg according to the state of sedation.
2. Chlormethiazole by continuous intravenous infusion.
3. Magnesium sulphate by intravenous and intramuscular administration. This therapy is widely used in the USA but is not commonly employed in the UK. The drug is effective in suppressing convulsions and inhibiting muscle activity. It also reduces platelet aggregation and hence minimizes the effect of disseminated intravascular coagulation.

It is important to ensure that a clear airway is maintained and that further fits are prevented and, to this end, patients have traditionally been kept under sedation in a darkened room with minimal noise and light. However, there is now evidence to suggest that they may best be managed in an intensive care unit and managed jointly by the obstetric and intensive care unit staffs.

The best method of controlling blood pressure is the intravenous infusion of hydralazine. In a dosage of 25 mg in 500 ml of 5% dextrose or Hartman's solution, the infusion rate can be regulated according to the blood pressure level. Intravenous infusion of labetalol has also been shown to be effective in regulating blood pressure.

Epidural anaesthesia – Epidural anaesthesia relieves the pain of labour and also lowers blood pressure by causing peripheral vasodilatation in the lower extremities. It will also reduce the tendency to fit by relieving the pain and hence reducing the effect of afferent stimuli from that pain.

Clotting studies should be performed before insertion of an epidural catheter because of the risk of spinal cord compression from epidural haematoma formation if there is a clotting defect.

Delivery of the infant – Once convulsions have occurred or, indeed, when severe hypertension and proteinuria are present, then the control of blood pressure can usually be sustained only for a short period unless delivery is effected, as the blood pressure will soon rise again. It is therefore necessary to effect delivery and this can be achieved either by forewater rupture and Syntocinon infusion or by Caesarean section. It is important to remember that delivery should not be attempted until the blood pressure is under control.

Management after delivery

Following delivery, it is important to observe the following points:

1. Maintain the patient in a well-sedated condition in a quiet environment.
2. Special nursing and observation are needed to maintain a clear airway and to avoid further fits.
3. Strict fluid balance charts should be maintained to ensure that fluid overloading does not occur in view of the reduced urinary output.
4. Volume expansion should be achieved using a central venous pressure line or by monitoring pulmonary capillary wedge pressures using a Schwann–Gantz catheter.

Up to 45% of eclamptic fits occur after delivery including 12% after 48 hours. Forty per cent of patients have a fit before the development of both proteinuria and hypertension.

Hypertension in pregnancy

- Occurs in 10–15% pregnancies, of which 1 in 10 have proteinuria
- More common in primigravidae, with a new partner, in certain racial groups and where there is a family history
- Defined by hypertension, oedema and proteinuria of > 0.3 g/l
- May be associated with chronic hypertensive disease
- Characterized by arteriolar vasoconstriction and DIC
- May lead to cerebral oedema or haemorrhage, cardiac or renal failure, placental infarction and DIC
- Management is to prevent eclampsia, monitor feto-placental unit, control hypertension and deliver the infant
- Important signs to watch for are headache, epigastric pain and hyper-reflexia
- During delivery it is important to control blood pressure, monitor fluid balance and urine output; it may be necessary to sedate

---

ANAEMIA IN PREGNANCY

Anaemia is a common complication of pregnancy and in some countries may be a major factor in the cause of maternal death.

Maternal difficulties arise in particular where the anaemia is further complicated by antepartum or postpartum haemorrhage.

The fetus tends to withstand maternal anaemia surprisingly well despite the reduced oxygen-carrying capacity in the mother, but is more likely to be damaged if the anaemia is complicated by other conditions such as pre-eclampsia and placental abruption.

Definition

There is no agreed definition of anaemia, but a haemoglobin level of 10 g/100 ml or less is generally accepted as indicating significant anaemia. Normal haemoglobin levels in pregnancy in UK studies have shown first trimester values of 12.0 g/100 ml, 11.9 g in the second trimester, and 11.4 g in the third trimester. There is a fall in haemoglobin in the second trimester associated with a relatively faster expansion of plasma volume than total red cell mass, but this would not account for a significant degree of anaemia.

Nutritional requirements

Anaemia in pregnancy may arise from any recognized cause, but the most important causes are those related to an imbalance between the demands of maternal adaption and the growing fetus, and the actual supply and absorption of essential nutrients (Fig. 10.9). Essential nutrients for haemoglobin synthesis include protein, iron, vitamin B_6 and B_{12}, folic acid, ascorbic acid and numerous trace elements such as copper. The dietary requirement of iron is estimated at 15 mg per day and, unless the dietary intake is above average, this requirement is unlikely to be met.

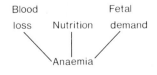

Fig. 10.9 Basic factors in the aetiology of anaemia in pregnancy.

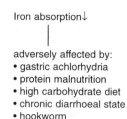

Fig. 10.10 Factors which influence iron absorption.

Iron absorption tends to increase in pregnancy, and iron is absorbed in the ferrous ionized form. Ascorbic acid may assist in absorption because of its reducing action. Iron absorption may be adversely affected by gastric achlorhydria, protein malnutrition and high-carbohydrate diets, chronic diarrhoeal states, and hookworm infestations (Fig. 10.10). Iron loss from the body is generally minimal during pregnancy as menstrual loss ceases, although some loss still occurs from hair, nails and sweat. The major reduction in maternal stores is due to the increased demands of pregnancy.

Investigations

Routine management of pregnancy should include measurement of haemoglobin levels at regular intervals during pregnancy. If the haemoglobin falls to less than 11 g/100 ml, then the following investigations should be performed:

1. Complete blood picture – the important measurements are mean corpuscular volume (MCV) and mean corpuscular haemoglobin concentration (MCHC). MCV gives an index of macrocytosis and megaloblastic anaemia, and MCHC gives the best index for iron deficiency anaemia.
2. Serum iron and iron-binding capacity.
3. Serum folate and serum vitamin B_{12} levels in all cases of persistent anaemia.
4. Other investigations, including culture of the urine to exclude chronic urinary tract infection and examination of the faeces for ova and parasites.
5. Bone marrow analysis where the diagnosis is in doubt.
6. Haemoglobin electrophoresis to exclude haemoglobinopathies.

Treatment

The management of anaemia in pregnancy depends on the identification of the cause. However, the majority of cases are due to nutritional deficiencies associated with an iron intake inadequate to meet the needs of both mother and fetus.

The use of prophylactic oral iron and folic acid is indicated in nutritional anaemia. Iron should be administered in the form of ferrous sulphate, gluconate, succinate or fumarate. Combined preparations commonly contain 150 mg of ferrous sulphate and 0.5 mg of folic acid, and are administered on a once-daily basis.

Where anaemia has become established, oral therapy should always be used first, as the response is as rapid as parenteral therapy, excepting when gut absorption is defective.

Parenteral therapy

Parenteral therapy is indicated where iron deficiency anaemia fails to respond to oral therapy. Iron preparations include saccharated iron oxide and an iron–dextran complex such as Imferon, or an iron–sorbital–citric acid complex such as Jectofer. All of these compounds may cause severe anaphylactic reactions, and a test dose must always be given before a total dose intravenous infusion is given. Intramuscular injections are also sometimes used.

Sickle cell syndrome

These disorders include the heterozygous state for sickle cell haemoglobin (sickle cell trait; HbAS), homozygous sickle cell disease (HbSS), compound heterozygotes for haemoglobin variants such as sickle cell HbC disease and sickle cell thalassaemia.

HbSS – The clinical manifestations of HbSS include chronic anaemia and occasional crises characterised by intravascular sickling leading to vascular occlusion and tissue infarction. Crises are often precipitated by infection and dehydration, and renal complications are common.

Sickle cell HbC disease – This is a milder variant with near-normal haemoglobin levels, but may, on occasions, produce massive sickling crises during pregnancy.

HbAS – This trait rarely causes problems unless there are conditions of extreme anorexia, dehydration and acidosis.

In pregnancy, there are special problems, and therefore screening of all potential high-risk ethnic groups, such as black people of African origin, Indians, Mediterraneans and Saudi Arabians, is important.

Abortion, pre-term labour and fetal loss are high. These risks can be reduced by regular blood transfusions to maintain a high proportion of HbA.

Adequate hydration, prevention of infection and transfusion during pregnancy are all important management factors in reducing the incidence of crises in pregnancy.

The thalassaemias

These conditions are a genetic disorder associated with a reduced rate of production of one or more of the globulin chains of haemoglobin. They fall into two broad disorders of α- and β-thalassaemia.

The **β-thalassaemias** are defined by an inability to synthesize adult β chains; in the heterozygous state they are symptomless. However, in the homozygous state there is severe and persistent anaemia. These conditions are particularly common in the Mediterranean countries and in India and South-East Asia. The major problems in pregnancy are those related to anaemia and the need for repeated transfusions.

The **α-thalassaemias** are characterised by an inability to produce the α-chains common to haemoglobin A. During pregnancy, these women may become very anaemic. Sometimes the fetus may also become anaemic and hydropic and give rise to severe pre-eclampsia.

If routine screening of the parents indicates a risk of carrying a child with α-thalassaemia, the patient should be referred for prenatal diagnosis. Indeed, this is becoming an increasingly important aspect of management of the homozygous forms of either α- or β-thalassaemia.

Anaemia in pregnancy

- Commonly dietary but may be due to sickle cell disease or thalassaemia
- Haemoglobin <10 g/1
- Dietary iron requirement is 15 mg/day
- Assessment should include complete blood picture, serum iron and iron binding capacity, serum folate and B_{12} levels.
- Parenteral therapy is indicated only if oral treatment fails, because of risk of reaction

---

DIABETES IN PREGNANCY

Diabetes affects 0.2–0.3% of pregnancies, and a further 1–2% of pregnant women have evidence of impaired glucose tolerance.

Pregnancy affects maternal diabetes and produces an increase in insulin requirements; at the same time, diabetes has a significant effect on the pregnancy (Fig. 10.11).

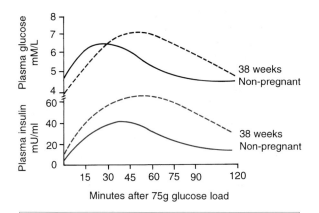

Fig. 10.11 Changes in insulin and glucose levels in normal pregnancy.

With appropriate management and careful regulation of blood glucose levels, perinatal losses can be minimized and will approach levels in the normal population. This management is best undertaken by a combined team of physicians and obstetricians and delivery should always be effected in a major obstetric hospital which has first class neonatal services.

Nomenclature

All forms of diabetes are associated with increased perinatal loss unless properly managed. The degree of risk is related to the severity of the diabetes. The presentation has been defined by the British Diabetic Association as follows:

1. **Potential diabetes** – patients with no evidence of chemical diabetes but who have a family history of diabetes, a previous history of delivering an infant in excess of 4.5 kg, or a history of an unexplained fetal death. Glycosuria is not a reliable sign, but should be investigated if it is persistent.
2. **Latent or gestational diabetes** – Some women who develop overt diabetes in later life develop chemical or clinical diabetes during pregnancy. This condition is known as gestational diabetes.
3. **Chemical diabetes** – these women have an abnormal glucose tolerance test, but no symptoms of diabetes. Perinatal morbidity is significantly increased.
4. **Clinical diabetes** – insulin-dependent diabetes requires careful control throughout pregnancy and should preferably be regulated before pregnancy is commenced.

The American Classification introduced by White in 1965 also linked management and prognosis to further subclassification of the diabetes:

Class A – chemical diabetes only; impaired glucose tolerance.
Class B – diabetes of adult; onset after 20 years of age.
Class C – diabetes of long duration (between 10 and 19 years) with no evidence of vascular disease.
Class D – diabetes present since before the age of 10 years and present for 20 years or more with vascular disease, calcification of leg vessels or benign retinopathy.
Class E – diabetes associated with calcification of limb vessels.
Class F – diabetes-associated nephropathy.
Class G – the presence of proliferating diabetic retinopathy.

In women with suspected abnormalities of glucose tolerance, a glucose tolerance test should be performed. This test involves the oral administration of 75 g of glucose after 3 days of normal food intake and overnight fasting. An abnormal test is defined by the following criteria:

1. A fasting value of blood glucose in excess of 5.5 mmol/l
2. A 1 hour value over 9 mmol/l
3. A 2 hour value over 7 mmol/l

Maternal complications

1. Pregnancy is diabetogenic, and diabetic control therefore becomes difficult. Hyperglycaemia is common, and if uncontrolled leads to the development of ketoacidosis with the risk of both fetal and maternal death.
   Hypoglycaemia may result in fetal death only if it is severe and prolonged, and it is more likely to occur in early pregnancy which is complicated by excessive vomiting.
2. Hydramnios is a common complication of the diabetic pregnancy and may result in an unstable lie and premature rupture of the membranes.
3. Pre-eclampsia is common in diabetics and is made worse by poor control of the diabetes. Both fetal and maternal prognoses are significantly worse where the pregnancy is complicated by diabetic nephropathy.
4. Dystocia and operative delivery – the fetus may be abnormally large and an obstructed and difficult labour (dystocia) is a recognized

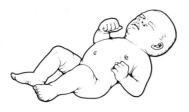

Fig. 10.12 The infant born to the diabetic mother may exhibit macrosomia and abnormal birth weight.

complication. The problem may occur after the head has been delivered because of shoulder obstruction. If there is evidence of potential cephalo-pelvic disproportion, the fetus should be delivered by Caesarean section.

Fetal complication

Babies born to diabetic mothers tend to be larger than normal. There is generalized macrosomia and body fat is commonly increased (Fig. 10.12).

Intra-uterine death tends to occur in the last 3 weeks of pregnancy.

Fetal distress associated with intra-uterine asphyxia and acidosis is a complication of labour.

Neonatal complications

1. *Hypoglycaemia* – there is hyperplasia and hypertrophy of the islets of Langerhans and, as a result, the newborn infant is particularly likely to develop hypoglycaemia. It is therefore important to perform frequent estimations of blood glucose levels in the first 48 hours of life.
2. *Respiratory distress syndrome* – there is higher incidence of respiratory distress syndrome in diabetic infants than in normal infants born at comparable gestational ages.
3. *Congenital abnormalities* – there is a slightly higher incidence of fetal abnormalities in infants born to mothers with diabetes. Congenital abnormalities are found in 7% of all pregnancies.

Management of diabetes

All grades of diabetes carry a significant risk to the fetus. It may be possible to control gestational diabetes with dietary control, but all other forms of diabetes should be controlled with insulin. In general, the aim should be to keep the blood glucose level below 7 mmol/l at all times by appropriate regulation of diet and insulin administration.

Hospital admission is not essential unless there is an additional complication of the pregnancy or it is not possible to control the diabetes at home. It is the policy in Nottingham to train women to measure their own blood glucose levels and to perform profiles every 2 weeks in the first two trimesters, and weekly in the last 12 weeks. Joint management is undertaken by the physicians and obstetricians and by a diabetic clinic sister who visits patients at home and keeps a close check on the glucose profiles.

The measurement of glycosylated haemoglobin levels (HbA) is a useful method of assessing the longer-term stability of the diabetic state; it should normally constitute less than 7% of the total haemoglobin concentration.

Women with insulin-dependent diabetes should have their control optimized prior to conception and be counselled about the maternal and fetal complications of diabetes in pregnancy. Pregnancy should be deferred if the haemoglobin AI is greater than 12% or there is evidence of ischaemic heart disease, untreated proliferative retinopathy, hypertension or proteinuria.

Antenatal assessment

Antenatal progress should be carefully monitored throughout pregnancy. The patient should be seen regularly at fortnightly or weekly intervals, and those women who develop gestational diabetes should receive the same pattern of care as those women with established insulin-dependent diabetes. Regular ultrasound scans identify fetal anomalies, but these scans are of most value in assessing fetal growth and the extent of any hydramnios. The regular monitoring of the fetus should also be pursued by the regular use of biophysical profiles. Placental function tests are no longer used as they are particularly misleading in diabetic pregnancies.

Method of delivery

If good diabetic control is achieved and there are no other complications, it should be possible to allow the pregnancy to proceed to full term, although delivery is usually effected between 38 weeks and term. Induction of labour and vaginal delivery can be achieved with careful regulation of blood glucose levels during labour and continuous intrapartum fetal monitoring. If there is any evidence of fetal distress or delay in labour, Caesarean section should be performed.

Amniocentesis performed before induction or elective Caesarean section to measure the lecithin/sphingomyelin ratio or lecithin concentration will enable the prediction of fetal lung maturity.

Neonatal management

The two major hazards that affect the neonate born to a diabetic mother are:

1. Respiratory distress syndrome
2. Neonatal hypoglycaemia.

These infants should therefore be admitted to the special care neonatal unit to monitor blood glucose levels and to administer oral glucose until feeding is satisfactorily established.

Perinatal mortality

It should be possible to achieve perinatal loss rates that are comparable to the overall perinatal mortality figures. Fetal anomalies occur in 5–6% of cases, and are frequently associated with polyhydramnios.

THYROID DISEASE IN PREGNANCY

Thyroid disorders of various types complicate 0.5% of pregnancies.

Hypothyroidism is more common than hyperthyroidism. The most common causes of hypothyroidism, which complicates 9 in every 1000 pregnancies, are Hashimoto's disease and post-ablative treatment.

Iodine deficiency is commonest in developing countries, and is associated with 30% fetal wastage. The development of cretinism is associated with deafness, mental retardation and spasticity. The diagnosis of hypothyroidism in the mother is made by the presence of low free T_4 and a raised thyroid-stimulating hormone (TSH) level. Treatment is by thyroid replacement therapy.

Hyperthyroidism occurs in 2 in 1000 pregnancies. Graves' disease or toxic goitre is associated with an increased risk of malformation, low birth weight and premature labour. The condition is diagnosed by the presence of high free T_3 and low TSH, or a flat response to thyrotropin-releasing hormone. The condition is treated with carbimazole. or propylthiouracial which inhibits iodination of tyrosine. Propylthiouracil does not cross the placenta and does not cause teratogenesis.

Thyroid-stimulating or -blocking immunoglobulins may cross the placenta and cause fetal thyroid disease.

Diabetes in pregnancy

- Pregnancy may be associated with changes in pre-existing diabetes, the de novo onset of clinical diabetes or an asymptomatic abnormal glucose tolerance
- A glucose tolerance test should be offered if there is a family history of diabetes, previous baby >4 kg, previous unexplained intra-uterine fetal death or glycosuria
- Maternal complications include poor control, hydramnios, pre-eclampsia and obstructed labour
- Fetal complications include macrosomia, increased risks of intra-uterine fetal distress after 37 weeks, intra-partum fetal distress and malformation
- Neonatal complications include hypoglycaemia and respiratory distress syndrome
- Management should be to keep blood sugar <7 mmol/l, monitor fetal growth and placental function
- Delivery should be by Caesarian section if there is evidence of fetal distress or delay

---

CARDIAC DISEASE IN PREGNANCY

Pregnancy is associated with a 30–50% increase in cardiac output and therefore creates considerable hazards for the mother if there is underlying cardiac disease. The maternal risk varies according to the nature of the cardiac lesion.

Low-risk conditions – These include septal defects, patent ductus arteriosus, pulmonary and tricuspid lesions.

Moderate risk – Mitral stenosis, aortic stenosis, Marfan's syndrome, previous myocardial infarction and coarctation are associated with significantly greater risk.

High risk – The conditions with maximum risk include Eisenmenger's syndrome, pulmonary hypertension, Marfan's syndrome involving the aorta and cardiomyopathy.

The risks generally are those of cardiac failure and acute pulmonary oedema. Adequate rest and the avoidance of infection are important. The use of antibiotic cover should be routine during labour. Anticoagulant therapy may also be necessary where there has been a valve replacement. It must be remembered that the risk of cardiac decompensation is maximal during labour and in the first 4 days after delivery.

ASTHMA IN PREGNANCY

Asthma complicates 1% of pregnancies. It does not

have a consistent relationship with pregnancy, as 25% of mothers get better, 25% get worse and the remainder are unaffected by the pregnancy. Severe asthmatic attacks are rare in the last 4 weeks of pregnancy. Sinister signs in the mother include a maternal tachycardia in excess of 120 beats/minute, a respiratory rate in excess of 30/min and a peak flow of less than 120 L/min. Management should be maintained with β-agonists, theophylline, steroids and antibiotics.

EPILEPSY IN PREGNANCY

Pregnancy has no consistent effect on maternal epilepsy, with 50% remaining unchanged, 25% becoming worse and 25% improving. Because of a reduction in absorption of anti-epileptic drugs, a reduction in protein-binding, increased liver metabolism and increased plasma volume, serum levels of drugs tends to fall and dosage needs to be increased.

Status epilepticus is uncommon in pregnancy.

The effect of epilepsy and its treatment on the fetus

There is an increase in perinatal mortality among epileptic mothers. Ten per cent of infants from mothers taking phenytoin and phenobarbitone have vitamin K-dependent clotting problems. Also, the incidence of congenital abnormalities in epileptics both on and off therapy is increased, the commonest abnormalities being orofacial, cardiac and limbal.

Management

The first priority is the control of fits using one drug if possible.

Drug levels should be measured every 2–4 weeks. If possible, a pre-conceptual trial of drug withdrawal should be attempted if the woman has been fit-free for a number of years. If possible, treatment changes should be avoided in pregnancy, apart from the regulation of dosage.

AUTO-IMMUNE DISEASE

Antiphospholipid antibodies are expressed by 15–20% of patients with systemic lupus, and myeloproliferative disorders and are associated with

an increased risk of intra-uterine growth retardation, stillbirth, abortion and thrombosis. Lupus anticoagulant prolongs phospholipid-dependent coagulation, and is associated with an increased risk of fetal loss in all trimesters. Treatment is with prednisolone and low-dose aspirin. Conditions such as rheumatoid arthritis tend to improve during pregnancy, but there is an increased risk of relapse during the puerperium.

LIVER DISEASE IN PREGNANCY

Intrahepatic cholestasis of pregnancy

This condition has a prevalence of 1–2 cases/1000 pregnancies, and is associated with the development of unexplained pruritis and late-onset jaundice in pregnancy. Initially, the patient notices darkening of the urine and pale stools. There is bilirubinuria and high blood levels of bile salts. The condition is not life-threatening, but carries some risk of obstetric haemorrhage, largely due to hypoprothrombinaemia. The pruritis may be relieved by oral dexamethasone. Postnatally, the condition usually resolves within 4–7 days, although the biochemical abnormalities are slow to reverse.

Acute fatty liver of pregnancy

This is a rare disorder involving 1 case in 10 000 pregnancies. It is characterized by microvascular steatosis in pregnancy, and is associated with death from hepatic encephalopathy, genital tract haemorrhage and disseminated intravascular coagulation.

Hepatitis B

Serum hepatitis is a viral liver disease. It may be asymptomatic, but where symptoms occur they may include nausea, anorexia, vomiting and fever. Mothers should be advised about the risk of vertical transmission, and the infant should be protected with Hepatitis B immunoglobulin plus vaccination within 7 days of delivery.

RENAL DISEASE IN PREGNANCY

Chronic renal disease

With the exception of specific disease entities such as systemic lupus, renal polyarteritis nodosa and scleroderma, obstetric outcome is usually successful in the presence of acute or chronic glomerulo-nephritis provided renal function is moderately compromised and hypertension is minimal.

Lupus nephritis

The majority of pregnancies in women with systemic lupus erythematosus (SLE) succeed, particularly where renal function is normal, and two-thirds of women with SLE have no change in their clinical status during pregnancy. Where necessary, therapy with steroids or cytotoxic drugs should not be withheld when there is active disease.

Polycystic kidney disease

These women usually have uneventful pregnancies, but they have a higher incidence of pre-eclampsia and severe pyelonephritis. Genetic counselling is obviously important because the disease is an autosomal dominant syndrome.

During pregnancy, renal deterioration may occur from urinary tract infection. Control of hypertension is important. This condition is not an indication for termination of pregnancy, unless there is severe compromise of renal function.

INFECTIONS IN PREGNANCY

The effects of rubella in pregnancy are well known and are discussed in Chapter 9, but there are many other infections where the effects are not so well known or are often overlooked. Some of these infections are discussed below.

Listeriosis

Listeria monocytogenes is a Gram-positive cocco-bacillus which is widely distributed in the environment. Some exposure is unavoidable, and 1 in 20 people carry the organism in their gut without ill effects. The organism exists in a large number of samples of pre-cooked, ready-to-eat poultry and chilled meats. It is also found in soft, ripened cheeses such as brie, camembert and cheeses of the blue vein type. These cheeses should be avoided by pregnant women, and cook–chilled meals and ready-to-eat poultry should be reheated until they are piping hot.

Clinical manifestations

The mother usually has a short history of a 'flu-like illness' with backache, urinary frequency and fever.

The condition may cause mid-trimester abortion or premature labour, and the infant develops respiratory distress, sepsis, petechial rash and hepatosplenomegaly. There is a high mortality rate. Late onset of the condition may occur 2–5 weeks after delivery, with lethargy, irritability, feeding difficulties and meningitis. Diagnosis is made by culture of the organism from blood or cerebrospinal fluid. The antibiotic treatment of choice consists of ampicillin or amoxycillin in combination with gentamicin.

Mumps

Mumps appears to have no significant adverse effect on the outcome of pregnancy. There is a slight increase in the rate of spontaneous abortions but no increase in the incidence of premature labour. There is an association with the condition of endomyocardial fibro-elastosis, but basically the condition is benign.

Measles

This infection is a paramyxovirus with droplet transmission. Placental transmission does occur and may result in neonatal death and an increased abortion rate, but the organism is not teratogenic.

Varicella

This is caused by a herpes virus. It may occur in pregnancy, and there is evidence of placental transmission. If the infection occurs between 8 and 20 weeks, there is a 5% risk of congenital malformations, including muscular atrophy, microcephaly, cerebellar or cortical atrophy, cataracts and chorioretinitis.

BIBLIOGRAPHY

Brudenell M, Doddridge M C 1989 Current reviews in obstetrics and gynaecology. Churchill Livingstone, Edinburgh
de Swiet M 1995 Medical disorders in obstetric practice. Blackwell, Oxford
Rubin P 1988 Handbook of hypertension. Elsevier, Amsterdam, vol 10

11 Antepartum haemorrhage

Haemorrhage from the vagina after the 24th week of gestation is classified as antepartum haemorrhage. The factors which cause antepartum haemorrhage may be present before 24 weeks, but the original distinction between a threatened abortion and an antepartum haemorrhage was based on the potential viability of the fetus.

Vaginal bleeding may be due to:

1. Haemorrhage from the placental site and uterine cavity
2. Lesions of the vagina or cervix.

UTEROPLACENTAL HAEMORRHAGE

The major causes of uterine bleeding are:

1. Placenta praevia
2. Abruptio placentae or accidental haemorrhage
3. Uterine rupture
4. Unknown aetiology.

Placenta praevia

The placenta is said to be praevia when all or part of the placenta implants in the lower uterine segment and therefore lies in front of the presenting part (Fig. 11.1).

Incidence

Approximately 1% of all pregnancies are complicated by clinical evidence of a placenta praevia. Unlike the incidence of placental abruption, which varies according to social and nutritional factors, the incidence of placenta praevia is remarkably constant.

Aetiology

Placenta praevia is due to delay in implantation of the blastocyst so that this occurs in the lower part of the uterus. It is commoner in high parity, and in conditions where the placental area is large, such as multiple pregnancy or placenta membranacea.

Classification

From the point of view of management, there are three degrees of severity of placenta praevia (Fig. 11.1):

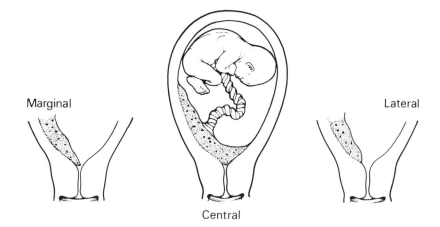

Fig. 11.1 Classification of placenta praevia.

1. Lateral – the placenta encroaches on the lower uterine segment, but does not reach the internal cervical os. This is sometimes known as first-degree placenta praevia.
2. Marginal – the placenta encroaches on or covers the internal cervical os before cervical dilatation occurs. This includes both second- and third-degree placenta praevia.
3. Central – the placenta completely covers the os even with cervical dilatation. This was previously described as fourth degree placenta praevia.

The classification is important in relation to management because spontaneous delivery is extremely rare where there is central placenta praevia, but normal labour and delivery may occur with lateral or marginal implantation.

Bleeding results from separation of the placenta as the formation of the lower segment occurs and the cervix effaces. This blood loss occurs from the venous sinuses in the lower segment. Occasionally, fetal blood loss may occur, particularly where one of the placental vessels lies across the cervical os – a condition known as **vasa praevia**.

Symptoms and signs

The main symptom of placenta praevia is painless vaginal bleeding. There may sometimes be lower abdominal discomfort where there are minor degrees of associated placental abruption.

The signs of placenta praevia are:

1. Vaginal bleeding
2. Malpresentation of the fetus
3. Uterine hypotonus.

Development of the lower uterine segment begins at 28 weeks gestation, and thus bleeding is likely to occur during the second trimester. Bleeding is unpredictable and may vary from minor shows to massive and life-endangering haemorrhage.

The presence of the placenta in the lower segment tends to displace the presenting part and when the placenta is posterior the head is pushed forward over the pelvic brim and is easily palpable. When the placenta is anterior, the presenting part is difficult to feel. Lateral placement of the placenta results in contralateral displacement of the presenting part. Where there is a central placenta praevia, the fetal head is held away from the pelvic brim and the lie may be transverse or oblique. If the head does not approach the pelvic brim when the erect posture is adopted, it is strongly suggestive of a placenta praevia.

> Case study
> **Placenta praevia**
>
> *A 29-year-old woman, para 3, was admitted at 32 weeks gestation in her fourth pregnancy with a history of sudden onset of fresh, red vaginal blood loss not associated with pain. On examination the fetal heart beat was present and a breech presentation was diagnosed. Ultrasound scan showed an anterior placenta extending down to, and covering, the internal os. The bleeding settled and the mother was delivered by elective Caesarean section at 37 weeks.*

Diagnosis of placenta praevia

1. Clinical findings – painless bleeding occurs suddenly and tends to be recurrent. When labour starts, and the cervix dilates, profuse haemorrhage may occur, although sometimes in a lateral placenta praevia the presenting part compresses the placental site and bleeding is controlled.
2. Abdominal examination –
   a. Displacement of the presenting part – the lie may be oblique or transverse. If the placenta lies on the posterior uterine wall, the presenting part will be easily palpable. If the placenta is anterior, the presenting part is difficult to palpate.
   b. Flaccidity of the uterus – uterine muscle tone is usually low and the fetal parts are easy to palpate.
3. Diagnostic procedures –
   a. Ultrasonic scanning – this is predominantly used to localize the placenta and has largely replaced other techniques. Errors in diagnosis are most likely to occur in posteriorly situated placentae because of difficulties in identifying the lower segment. Anteriorly, the bladder provides an important landmark for the lower segment and diagnosis is more accurate. Localization of the placental site in early pregnancy may result in inaccurate diagnosis as fundal development may lead to an apparent upward displacement of the placenta.
   b. Magnetic resonance imaging – this is the most accurate method of placental localization because the internal cervical os can be clearly visualized. However, it is not, as yet, widely available or used.

Management

When antepartum haemorrhage of any type occurs, the diagnosis of placenta praevia should be suspected and hospital admission advised. The diagnosis should be established by ultrasound imaging. Vaginal examination should be performed only in an operating theatre prepared for Caesarean section with blood cross-matched. There are only two indications for performing a vaginal examination:

1. Where there is serious doubt about the diagnosis
2. Where bleeding occurs in established labour.

It is, in fact, often difficult to establish a diagnosis of placenta praevia by vaginal examination where the placenta is lateral, and there is a serious risk of precipitating massive haemorrhage if the placenta is central. If the placenta is lateral, then it may be possible to rupture the membranes and allow spontaneous vaginal delivery.

Conservative management of placenta praevia involves keeping the mother in hospital with blood cross-matched until fetal maturity is adequate, and then delivering the child by Caesarean section. Providing no active bleeding is occurring, there is no need to keep the mother in bed and she should remain ambulant, as she is as likely to bleed lying supine. Blood loss should be treated by transfusion where necessary, so that an adequate haemoglobin concentration is maintained.

Postpartum haemorrhage is also a hazard of the low-lying placenta.

There is an increased risk of placenta accreta where placental implantation occurs over the site of a previous uterine scar.

Placenta praevia

- Complicates 1% of pregnancies
- Commoner in multigravidae and multiple pregnancies
- Painless vaginal bleeding with soft uterus
- Malpresentation
- Lateral, marginal or central grades

Abruptio placentae

Abruptio placentae or accidental haemorrhage is defined as haemorrhage resulting from premature separation of the placenta. The term 'accidental' implies separation as the result of trauma, but most cases do not involve trauma and occur spontaneously.

Aetiology

Placental abruption tends to occur more frequently under conditions of social deprivation, in association with dietary deficiencies. Folic acid deficiency, in particular, has been implicated.

The incidence of placental abruption is increased in the presence of pre-eclampsia or essential hypertension. It must be remembered that hypertension and proteinuria may develop as a result of abruption.

Whatever factors predispose to placental abruption, they are well-established before the abruption occurs. The fetus is more likely to be male, and the birth weight is often low, indicating pre-existing growth retardation. Trauma is a relatively uncommon cause of abruption and, in the majority of cases, no specific predisposing factor can be identified.

Case study
Abruptio placentae

A 19-year-old primigravida was admitted at 39 weeks with sudden onset of constant abdominal pain. On admission her blood pressure was 160/100 mmHg, pulse 100 beats/minute and uterine tone increased with marked tenderness to palpation. The fetal heart beat was present, but shortly after admission it fell to 60 beats/minute, and the baby was delivered by emergency Caesarean section. At operation, a large retroplacental blood clot was noted.

Clinical types and presentation

Three types of abruption have been described (Fig. 11.2):

1. Revealed
2. Concealed
3. Mixed, or concealed and revealed.

Unlike placenta praevia, placental abruption presents with pain, vaginal bleeding and increased uterine activity.

1. *Revealed haemorrhage* – The major haemorrhage is apparent externally, as haemorrhage occurs from the lower part of the placenta and blood escapes through the cervical os. Under these circumstances, the clinical features are less severe.

   Abruption tends to occur after 36 weeks gestation, with the fetal lie longitudinal and the presenting part sitting well into the pelvic brim. In revealed placental abruption, uterine activity may be increased, but this finding is not consistent.

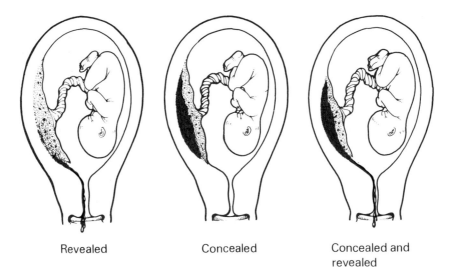

Revealed   Concealed   Concealed and revealed

Fig. 11.2 Types of placental abruption.

2. *Concealed haemorrhage* – In this case, the hae-morrhage occurs between the placenta and the uterine wall. The uterine content increases in volume and the fundal size appears larger than would be consistent with the estimated date of confinement. Uterine tonus is increased and pain and shock are common features. The uterus may become broad, rigid and tender.

It is important to realize that initially the blood pressure may be raised and the pulse rate slowed but, eventually, the patient becomes shocked, with the development of tachycardia, hypotension and oliguria. The peripheral circulation becomes vasoconstricted and there may be physical signs of this condition even before hypotension develops.

It is most important to remember that initially, even in the presence of substantial intra-uterine haemorrhage where the blood loss is concealed, the blood pressure may remain normal or raised and the pulse rate slow, until collapse suddenly occurs. The estimate of blood loss must there-fore be based on uterine size and, in revealed haemorrhage, assessment of external loss. In some severe cases, haemorrhage penetrates through the uterine wall, and the uterus appears bruised. This is described as a **Couvelaire uterus**. On clinical examination, the uterus will be tense and hard and the uterine fundus will be higher than is normal for the gestational age. The patient will often be in labour, and in approximately 30% of cases the fetal heart sounds will be absent and

the fetus will be stillborn. The prognosis for the fetus is dependent on the area of placental separation.

3. *Mixed, or concealed and revealed haemorrhage* – In most cases, the haemorrhage is both concealed and revealed. Haemorrhage occurs close to the placental edge and, after an interval when the haemorrhage is concealed, blood loss soon appears vaginally.

Differential diagnosis

The diagnosis is made on the history of vaginal bleeding, abdominal pain, increased uterine tonus, proteinuria and the presence of a longitudinal lie. This must be distinguished from placenta praevia where the haemorrhage is painless, the lie unstable and the uterus hypotonic.

The diagnosis should also be differentiated from other acute emergencies such as acute hydramnios where the uterus is enlarged and tender and tense, but there is no haemorrhage. Concealed placental abruption may simulate other acute abdominal emergencies such as perforated ulcer, volvulus of the bowel and strangulated inguinal hernia, but these problems are rare during pregnancy.

Management

The patient must be admitted to hospital, and the diagnosis established on the basis of the history and examination findings (Fig. 11.3). Mild cases may be

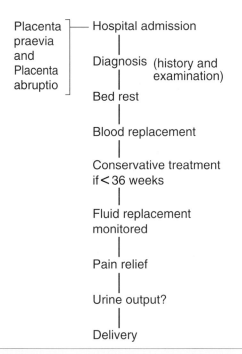

Placenta praevia and Placenta abruptio

— Hospital admission
|
Diagnosis (history and examination)
|
Bed rest
|
Blood replacement
|
Conservative treatment if < 36 weeks
|
Fluid replacement monitored
|
Pain relief
|
Urine output?
|
Delivery

Fig. 11.3 Differential diagnosis and management of antepartum haemorrhage.

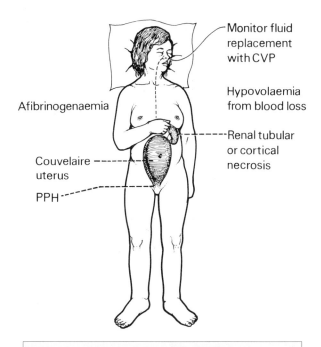

Afibrinogenaemia

Couvelaire uterus

PPH

Monitor fluid replacement with CVP

Hypovolaemia from blood loss

Renal tubular or cortical necrosis

Fig. 11.4 Complications of placental abruption.

treated conservatively and the placental site localized to confirm the diagnosis. If the haemorrhage is severe, resuscitation is the first prerequisite.

It is often difficult to assess the amount of blood loss accurately and intravenous infusion should be started with normal saline, Hartman's solution or blood substitutes until blood is cross-matched and transfusion can be commenced. Fluid replacement should be monitored by the use of a central venous pressure line. Unlike placenta praevia, any significant abruption should be treated by delivering the fetus as soon as possible.

If the fetus is alive and there are no clinical signs of fetal distress, or if the fetus is dead, surgical induction of labour is performed as soon as possible, and where necessary, uterine activity is stimulated with a dilute Syntocinon infusion. If the fetus is alive, it should be monitored, and Caesarean section should be performed if signs of fetal distress develop. If induction is not possible because the cervix is closed, then delivery should be effected by Caesarean section. Pain relief is achieved by the use of opiates.

Complications (Fig. 11.4)

Afibrinogenaemia – Severe placental abruption results in significant placental damage and the release of thromboplastin into the maternal circulation. This is turn may lead to intravascular coagulation and to defibrination with the development of hypo- or afibrinogenaemia. The condition may be treated by the infusion of fresh frozen plasma, platelet transfusion and fibrinogen transfusion, but can only be reversed by deliverying the fetus. It may lead to abnormal bleeding if operative delivery is attempted, or may result in uncontrollable postpartum haemorrhage.

Renal tubular or cortical necrosis

This is a complication that must always be considered as a possibility, and it is essential to keep careful fluid balance charts and to take particular note of urinary output. It may, on occasion, necessitate haemodialysis or peritoneal dialysis, but this complication is one of increasing rarity.

Abruptio placentae

- Associated with social deprivation, pregnancy-induced hypertension, male fetus, intra-uterine growth retardation
- Pain ± bleeding, increased tone
- Revealed, concealed or mixed
- Deranged clotting

Other causes of antepartum haemorrhage (Fig. 11.5)

Unexplained antepartum haemorrhage

In many cases, it is not possible to make a definite diagnosis of abruption or placenta praevia. These cases involve a significant increase in perinatal mortality and it is therefore important to monitor placental function and fetal growth. The pregnancy should not be allowed to proceed beyond term.

Vaginal infections

Vaginal moniliasis or trichomaniasis may cause blood-stained discharge and, once the diagnosis is established, should be treated with the appropriate therapy.

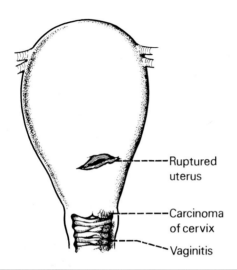

Fig. 11.5 Non-placental causes of antepartum haemorrhage.

CERVICAL LESIONS

Benign lesions of the cervix such as cervical polyps are treated by removal of the polyp. Cervical erosions are best left untreated.

Carcinoma of the cervix is occasionally found in pregnancy. If the pregnancy is early, termination is indicated. If the diagnosis is made late in pregnancy, the diagnosis should be established by biopsy and the lesion treated according to the staging.

12 Multiple pregnancy

Multiple pregnancy presents a series of special problems in obstetric practice. It also has significant implications for the children after birth and during development. The great majority of multiple pregnancies are associated with twins, but the increasing use of in vitro fertilization has now changed the incidence of higher multiple pregnancies as well as affecting the incidence of twinning. Most of the contents of this chapter will specifically relate to twins.

PREVALENCE OF MULTIPLE PREGNANCY

It is difficult to be precise about the natural prevalence of twins, partly because the diagnosis of twins in early pregnancy is often uncertain and partly because the figure varies considerably from one country or race to another. It would be reasonable to assume that the prevalence of twin pregnancies subject to therapeutic abortion would follow the overall incidence, but the prevalence in spontaneous abortion may be higher.

The figures vary from as low as 5.8/1000 pregnancies in Japan to 66.5/1000 in some parts of Nigeria. From 1971 to 1975 the prevalence of twinning in England and Wales was 12.3/1000 pregnancies.

Triplet pregnancy in Japan is 5.6/100 000, in Nigeria up to 177.8/100 000 and in the UK it is 10.2/100 000. Higher multiple births such as quadruplets and quintuplets are commonly associated with the use of fertility drugs, but if one excludes this cause, figures for England and Wales suggest a pregnancy rate of 1.7/million maternities.

The highest naturally occurring multiple pregnancy recorded so far is nontuplets.

TYPES OF TWINNING (Fig. 12.1)

Twins may be monozygotic, derived from one fertilized egg, or dizygotic, derived from two different eggs. With very rare exceptions, all pairs discordant for sex are dizygotic. About one-third of all twin pairs are of unlike sex.

Monochorionic twins are never completely identical but are frequently indistinguishable to the casual observer. Difference in hair and eye colour indicate dizygosity. Thus, it is possible to assign zygosity with reasonable accuracy in most twin pairs by sex, placentation and physical appearance.

The determination of blood group may also help assign zygosity. Discrepant blood groups indicate dizygosity. However, up to 18% of dichorionic twins have similar blood types and therefore concordance of blood group does not determine zygosity.

Monochorionic placentae can be determined by direct examination at the time of delivery or by submitting a sample of the dividing membranes for histological examination. The further approach to confirmation of monochorionicity involves the injection of a contrast liquid into a clamped cord. In monochorionic placentae, positive transfer will occur through the placental circulation, whereas in dichorionic placentae, transfer does not occur. Precise allocation of zygosity can be enhanced by a comparison of blood groups, serum protein and enzyme polymorphism.

THE AETIOLOGY OF TWIN PREGNANCY

Familial factors

Twins tend to occur in families, although there is some debate as to whether this occurs through both female and male partners. The familial tendency is apparent in dizygotic twinning, but this appears to be on the maternal side only. In a study of records at Salt Lake City, the twinning rates of women who were themselves dizygotic twins was 17.1/1000 maternities compared with 11.6/1000 maternities for the general population, but the rate for males who were themselves dizygotic twins was only 7.9/1000 maternities.

A familial tendency to monozygotic twinning is rare but transmission can occur through both maternal and paternal lines.

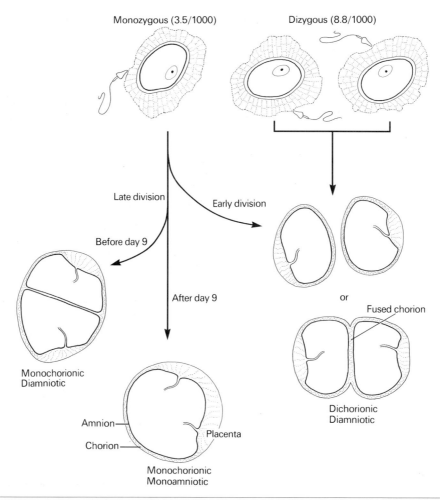

Fig. 12.1 Types of twinning indicating the structure of the membranes and placenta. Note that twins of different sexes are always dizygous and those with a single chorion always monozygous. Dichorionic twins of the same sex can be either monozygous or dizygous.

Parity and maternal age

Twinning rates increase with parity but this increase seems only to apply to dizygotic twinning. Studies in Aberdeen have shown that the rate increases from 10.4/1000 in primigravidae to 15.3/1000 in the para 4+ group.

Dizygotic twinning rates are also age linked, with an increase in twinning in the older mothers.

Ovulation induction

Multiple pregnancy is common following the use of drugs to induce ovulation. It is important to note that the use of gonadotrophin therapy commonly results in twin and triplet pregnancy. To some degree this can be avoided by monitoring ovarian follicular development and withholding the injection of human chorionic gonadotrophin if excessive numbers of follicles develop.

The use of fertility drugs accounts for 10–15% of all multiple pregnancies, and has therefore significantly altered the incidence of multiple pregnancy.

In vitro fertilization and embryo transfer

The above principles also apply to in vitro fertilization where the ovaries are hyperstimulated to enable collection of multiple oocytes. Pregnancy rates are enhanced by replacement of a number of embryos, but the risk of this procedure is that it results in a much higher incidence of twin and triplet pregnancy. In ovulation induction and in vitro fertilization programmes, twin pregnancies are dizygotic but there are also documented cases of monozygotic twins or of quadruplets where only three embryos were replaced.

COMPLICATIONS OF TWIN PREGNANCY

The normal processes of maternal physiological adaptation are exaggerated in multiple pregnancy. Total weight gain is, on average, 3.5 kg greater than in singleton pregnancy. Plasma volume expansion is significantly greater with twin pregnancy. Between 37 and 40 weeks gestation, the expansion is 17% greater in twin pregnancy. Cardiac output does not seem to be different but there is a greater increase in red cell mass; however, a relative anaemia may develop related to haemodilution in twin pregnancy.

It is thus to be expected that the increased strain put on the system by carrying more than one fetus will result in a higher incidence of complications.

Abortion

Resorption of a fetus in twin pregnancy is a common event in early gestation, and on this basis the incidence of 'partial' abortion is high. The incidence of spontaneous abortion is higher in twins, and evidence from Aberdeen has shown that threatened abortion occurs in 26% of twin pregnancies and 20% of singleton pregnancies.

Antepartum haemorrhage

The incidence of antepartum haemorrhage (APH) has been found by some studies to be 'approximately twice as high in twin pregnancies'. However, not all studies have reported this difference. Despite a general belief that bigger placental size should be associated with a higher incidence of placenta praevia, the differences are marginal. The Aberdeen twin study suggested an overall incidence of 0.70% for twins and 0.42% for singleton pregnancies.

Polyhydramnios

Polyhydramnios is a common finding with multiple pregnancy, and complicates 6% of twin pregnancies. Management is difficult and often unsatisfactory. Amniocentesis commonly leads to premature labour and in any case only produces short-term relief of symptoms. Bed rest may help to relieve the physical discomfort, but the condition is often associated with premature rupture of membranes and premature labour.

Pre-eclampsia

There is an increased incidence of both gestational hypertension and pre-eclampsia in twin pregnancies, even allowing for the influence of parity. The incidence of eclampsia is also significantly greater in twin pregnancy. The condition may progress rapidly and is commonly associated with intra-uterine growth retardation.

Preterm labour

The occurrence of premature labour is the most important complication of twin pregnancy. The onset of labour before 37 weeks gestation occurs in 40% of twin pregnancies. The phenomenon appears to be associated with overdistension of the uterus associated with the presence of more than one fetus and the associated increase in amniotic fluid volume. The incidence of preterm labour is also significantly higher in monozygotic twins than dizygotic twins.

Zygosity

Monozygotic twins have a higher perinatal mortality rate than dizygotic twins and a higher incidence of congenital abnormalities, intrauterine growth retardation and preterm delivery. There is also an increased risk of polyhydramnios in monozygotic pregnancies.

Twin pregnancies

- Incidence in England and Wales 12.3/1000 births, increasing because of in vitro fertilization (10–15% of twin pregnancies)
- Familial tendency
- Dizygotic twins increase with age and parity
- Increase weight gain, plasma, volume
- Increase risk of spontaneous abortion, APH, polyhydramnios and pregnancy-induced hypertension
- Intra-uterine growth retardation common

MANAGEMENT OF TWIN PREGNANCY

Multiple pregnancies exhibit every type of pregnancy complication at a greater frequency than occurs in singleton pregnancy. Early diagnosis is therefore essential and provides a convincing argument for routine early pregnancy ultrasound scanning. The commonest clinical sign of twin pregnancy is the greater size of the uterus, which is easier to detect in early, rather than late, pregnancy. There are, of course, other reasons why the uterus may be abnormally enlarged, such as hydramnios and uterine fibroids.

Treatment of any antenatal complication is the same as in singleton pregnancies, but remember that the onset of complications tends to be earlier and of greater severity. Routine hospital admission from 28 weeks gestation for bed rest has been advocated in the past, but clinical trials have failed to demonstrate efficacy. However, careful antenatal supervision and more frequent antenatal visits are indicated. It is important that women with multiple pregnancies are booked for confinement in hospitals where there are suitable special care baby units.

Intra-uterine growth retardation is common, and therefore serial ultrasound measurements to assess fetal growth are important. If there is evidence of growth retardation in one or both fetuses, then early induction of labour should be considered.

MANAGEMENT OF LABOUR AND DELIVERY

Delivery poses many complexities in twin pregnancy because of the variety and complexity of presentations and because the second twin is at significantly greater risk from asphyxia because of placental separation and cord prolapse.

Presentation at delivery

There are a number of permutations for presentation in twin pregnancy at delivery which are partly influenced by the management of the second twin. Rounded-up figures for these presentations are shown in Figure 12.2. By far the commonest presentation is cephalic/cephalic (50%), followed by cephalic/breech (25%), breech/cephalic (10%) and breech/breech (10%). The remaining 5% consist of cephalic/transverse, transverse/cephalic, breech/transverse, transverse/breech and transverse/transverse.

Method of delivery

A decision about the method of delivery should be made as far as possible before the onset of labour.

Caesarean section

Delivery by elective Caesarean section is indicated for the same indications that exist for singleton pregnancies. However, the threshold to intervene is generally lower. Where an additional complication exists, such as a previous Caesarean scar, a long history of subfertility, severe pre-eclampsia or diabetes mellitus, most obstetricians will opt for elective section. Premature labour between 28 and 34 weeks gestation is an indication for Caesarean delivery, as also is malpresentation of the first twin.

Vaginal delivery

When labour is allowed to proceed normally, it is advisable to establish an intravenous line at an early stage. Labour normally lasts the same time as a singleton labour.

The first twin can be monitored with a scalp electrode or by abdominal ultrasound and, if possible, both infants should be monitored. When the first twin is delivered, the lie and presentation of the second twin must be immediately checked and the fetal heart rate recorded.

For delivery of the second twin, the membranes should be ruptured and cord prolapse excluded. If the uterus does not contract within a few minutes, an oxytocin infusion should be started. If fetal distress occurs, then delivery should be expedited by forceps delivery or breech extraction. Under very exceptional circumstances, it may be necessary to deliver the second twin by Caesarean section. It is important to use oxytocic agents with delivery of the second twin as there is an increased risk of post-partum haemorrhage.

Case study
Vaginal delivery

A 22-year-old woman in her first pregnancy with twins presented at 37 weeks gestation in spontaneous labour. The presentation of both babies was cephalic. An epidural catheter was sited for analgesia, and labour progressed uneventfully with the first twin delivering spontaneously. The presentation of the second twin was confirmed as cephalic with a longitudinal lie. As the presenting part was still above the pelvic brim, a Syntocinon infusion was commenced to maintain uterine contractions, and the membranes were left intact awaiting descent of the presenting part. Shortly afterwards, external monitoring of the fetal heart beat showed a bradycardia of 60 beats/minute. Delivery of the second twin was expedited by reaching inside the uterus with the membranes still intact (internal podalic version), locating the feet of the fetus and rotating the fetus to the breech position before rupturing the membranes and delivering the infant by breech extraction.

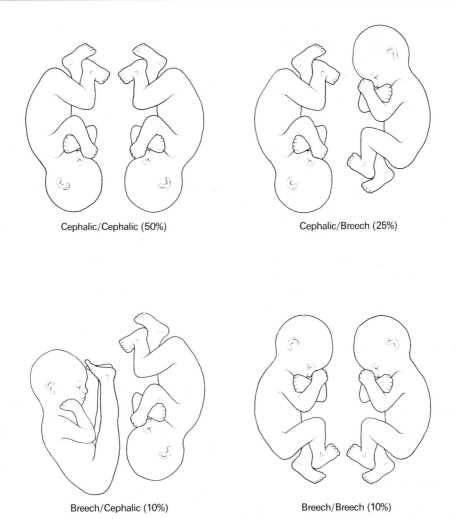

Cephalic/Cephalic (50%)

Cephalic/Breech (25%)

Breech/Cephalic (10%)

Breech/Breech (10%)

Fig. 12.2 The four major presentations of twin pregnancy. The 5% of other variations are not listed in these major groups.

COMPLICATIONS OF LABOUR

There are several complications of labour, some of which are associated with malpresentation. Babies may become obstructed, particularly where there is a transverse lie presenting and that is, in fact, an indication for delivery by Caesarean section. If Caesarean section is performed in the presence of an obstructed transverse lie, it may be preferable to perform a vertical incision in the lower and upper segment rather than a transverse incision because of the possibility of extension of the lower segment scar

into the lower part of the uterus and broad ligaments.

Failed diagnosis

This is now uncommon because of the widespread use of ultrasound imaging in early pregnancy. However, if the diagnosis is made after delivery of the first twin, it is important to withhold syntometrine. If an oxytocin agent is given and the second twin becomes obstructed, delivery must be expedited either by Caesarean section or by reversing the contractions with sympathomimetic agents or deep anaesthesia with delivery of the child by breech extraction or forceps delivery.

Locked twins

This is a very rare complication, where the first twin is a breech presentation and the second is cephalic. Clinically, the twins lock chin to chin. The condition is usually not recognized until delivery of part of the first twin has occurred, and survival of the first twin is unlikely. It may sometimes be possible to disempact the locked twins, but if this fails a destructive operation may be necessary to the first twin to stand any chance of saving the second child.

Conjoined twins

The union of twins results from the incomplete division of the embryo after formation. It is a rare complication, with a calculated frequency of 1 in 546 twin pregnancies. Union may occur at any site, but commonly is head to head or thorax to thorax.

If the union is recognized by ultrasound or radiology before the onset of labour, then the twins should be delivered by Caesarean section, as a significant number of these infants can be surgically separated. If the abnormality is not recognized before the onset of labour, then the labour will usually obstruct.

Perinatal mortality

The perinatal death rate is significantly higher for multiple pregnancies. In general, the mortality rate increases with the number of fetuses. The mortality rate for twins is approximately four times higher than for singleton pregnancies, and the mortality rate for second twins is 50% higher than for the first twin.

The commonest cause of death in both twins is prematurity. Second-born twins are more likely to die from intrapartum asphyxia with separation of the placenta following delivery of the first twin, or where cord prolapse occurs in association with a malpresentation or a high presenting part when the membranes are ruptured.

Twin delivery and labour

- Onset of labour before 37 weeks in 40%
- Second twin at greater risk of asphyxia
- Labour same length as singleton
- Increased risk of post-partum haemorrhage and malpresentation
- Mortality rate four times higher than for singleton, and 50% higher for second twin than for first

---

Twin-to-twin transfusion occurs in 15% of monochorionic twins, and two-thirds of the infants die in utero. There is progressive transfusion from one infant to the other, resulting in one baby with the signs of intra-uterine growth retardation and anaemia whilst the other infant is plethoric and sometime hydropic. Early delivery to save the growth-retarded twin risks death of both infants from complications of prematurity. In utero death of both infants may also occur as a result of acute haemodynamic changes should one fetus die in utero. Death may also occur from lethal congenital malformations, trauma, antepartum haemorrhage and infection.

BIBLIOGRAPHY

MacGillivray I, Campbell D M, Thompson B 1988 Twinning and twins. Wiley, Chichester

13 Normal labour

Labour is the process whereby the products of conception are expelled from the uterus after the 24th week of gestation.

Premature labour is defined as labour occurring before the 37th week of gestation.

Prolonged labour is defined as labour lasting in excess of 24 hours in a primigravida and 16 hours in a multigravida.

THE STAGES OF LABOUR

Labour is divided into three stages, which are defined as follows:

1. The **first stage** commences with the onset of labour and terminates when the cervix has reached full dilatation.
2. The **second stage**, or stage of expulsion, begins at full cervical dilatation and ends with the expulsion of the fetus.
3. The **third stage**, or placental stage, begins with the delivery of the child and ends with expulsion of the placenta.

THE ONSET OF LABOUR

It is often difficult to be certain of the exact time of onset of labour; however, it is defined as the development of regular, painful uterine contractions producing progressive dilatation of the cervix. There are exceptions to this definition, such as cervical stenosis where labour contractions do not produce dilatation of the cervix. This condition is rare and does not interfere with the general definition. The clinical signs of the onset of labour may include:

1. The onset of regular painful contractions which produce progressive cervical dilatation
2. The presence of a 'show' – the passage of blood-stained mucus
3. Rupture of the membranes.

INITIATION OF LABOUR

The cause of the onset of labour remains uncertain despite extensive research. The subject is of considerable importance particularly in relation to premature labour, which remains the major cause of neonatal death.

Many factors play a part in the initiation of parturition and it is unlikely that any one factor is sufficient to explain the phenomenon. It is more likely that there is a cascade of biochemical events regulated and controlled by the fetus. The fetus increases its production of cortisol towards term, and this reduces the production of progesterone by the placenta and increases the production of oestrone and oestradiol. Progesterone inhibits uterine activity and oestradiol increases it. At the same time, these changes lead to an increased production of prostaglandins by the placenta and myometrium, which stimulate increased myometrial activity and also oxytocin release from the posterior lobe of the pituitary gland, which in turn also stimulates myometrial activity. The direct mechanism involved in increasing myometrial contractility is probably related to a release of calcium ions, which increases the activity of the myometrium, and this causes splitting of adenosine triphosphate (ATP) thus stimulating the action of actomyosin.

Uterine activity in labour

The uterus contracts at all times during pregnancy. As full term approaches, the activity increases in frequency and strength. Intra-uterine pressure rises to 20–30 mmHg initially, and contractions occur every 10–15 minutes and last approximately 30–40 seconds. Normal resting tonus in labour starts at 10 mmHg and increases slightly during the course of labour. Contractions increase in intensity to reach pressures of 50 mmHg in labour; in the second stage, with voluntary expulsive efforts, they may reach pressures in excess of 100 mmHg. Contractions produce effacement and dilatation of the cervix and

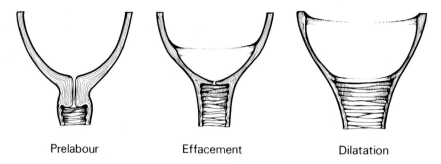

Prelabour | Effacement | Dilatation

Fig. 13.1   Effacement and dilatation of the cervix in labour.

shorten myometrial fibres in the upper uterine segment (Fig. 13.1). This process is known as
retraction. The lower uterine segment becomes
elongated and thinned as labour progresses, and the
conjunction between upper and lower segment rises
in the abdomen. Where labour becomes obstructed,
the junction between upper and lower segments may
become visible near the level of the umbilicus, and is
known as a **retraction ring**. Contractions are
initiated from a pacemaker in the left uterine cornua,
and spread downwards through the myometrium.
The contractions occur first in the fundus of the
uterus, where they are stronger and last longer than
in the lower segment. The phenomenon is known as
fundal dominance, and is essential to progressive
effacement and dilatation of the cervix. As the uterus
contracts, its axis appears to straighten and the fundus
pushes forward against the anterior abdominal wall
(Fig. 13.2). The round ligaments also contract and

pull the uterus forward, and this brings the uterus
into line with the inlet of the pelvis so that the fetus is
pushed straight down into the birth canal.

Pain in labour

Contractions in labour are commonly associated
with pain, particularly as they increase in strength
and frequency (Fig. 13.3). The cause of the pain is
uncertain, but may be due to compression of nerve
fibres in the cervical area, or to anoxia of compressed muscle cells. Pain is felt as lumbar backache and
as pain in the lower abdomen.

The passages

The shape of the bony pelvis has previously been
described. Due to softening of pelvic ligaments, some
expansion of the pelvic cavity can occur. The soft

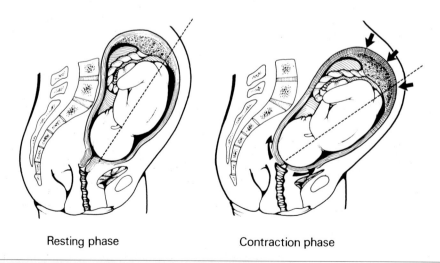

Resting phase | Contraction phase

Fig. 13.2   Change in direction of the fetal and uterine axis during contractions in labour.

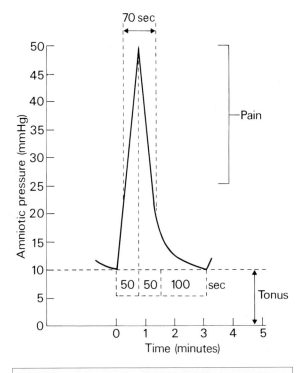

Fig. 13.3 Uterine contractions become painful when the intra-amniotic pressure exceeeds 25 mmHg.

tissues also become more distensible, and substantial distension of the pelvic floor and vaginal orifice occurs during descent and birth of the head. This may result in tearing of the perineum and of the vaginal walls.

The mechanism of labour

The head usually engages in the transverse position, and the passage of the head and trunk through the pelvis follows a well-defined pattern. Not all diameters of the fetal head can pass through a normal pelvis. The process of labour therefore involves the adaption of the fetal head to the various segments of the pelvis, and the following processes occur (Fig. 13.4):

1. *Descent* – descent occurs throughout labour and is a requisite for the birth of the child. Engagement may not occur until labour is well established, but descent of the head is a measure of progress in labour.
2. *Flexion* – flexion of the head occurs as it descends and meets the pelvic floor bringing the chin into contact with the fetal thorax. Flexion produces a smaller diameter of presentation, changing to the sub-occipito-bregmatic diameter from the occipito-frontal diameter.

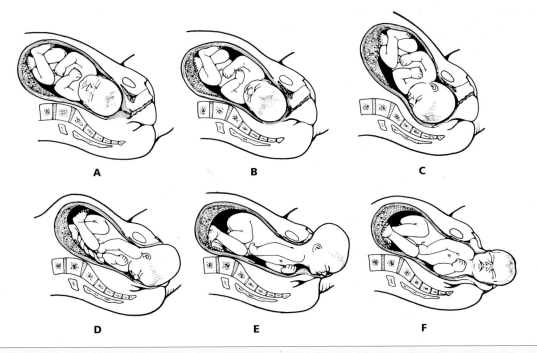

Fig. 13.4 The mechanisms of normal labour involves: **A** descent of the presenting part; **B** flexion of the head; **C** internal rotation; **D** distension of the perineum and extension of the fetal head; **E** delivery of the head; **F** delivery of the shoulders.

3. *Internal rotation* – the head rotates as it strikes the pelvic floor and, normally, the occiput gradually moves from its original lateral position towards the pubic symphysis; occasionally it moves posteriorly towards the hollow of the sacrum.

4. *Extension* – the sharply flexed head descends to the vulva and the base of the occiput comes into contact with the inferior rami of the pubis. The head now extends until it is delivered. The maximal distension of the perineum and introitus is followed rapidly by final expulsion of the head, a process that is known as **crowning**. The head now extends again following delivery.

5. *Restitution* – following delivery of the head, it rotates back to its original position in relation to the shoulders.

6. *External rotation* – when the shoulders reach the pelvic floor, they rotate into the anteroposterior diameter. This is followed by rotation of the fetal head so that the face looks laterally at the thigh.

7. *Delivery of the shoulders* – final expulsion of the trunk occurs following delivery of the shoulders. Lateral flexion of the trunk, first posteriorly to deliver the anterior shoulder under the pubic symphysis, and then anteriorly to disengage the posterior shoulder, is followed by rapid expulsion of the remainder of the trunk.

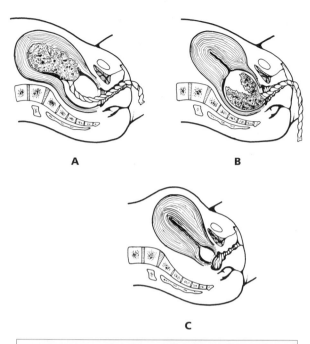

Fig. 13.5 The normal third stage: **A** separation of the placenta from the uterine wall; **B** expulsion into the lower uterine segment and upper vagina; **C** complete expulsion of the placenta from the genital tract.

THE THIRD STAGE OF LABOUR

The third stage of labour starts with the completed expulsion of the infant and ends with the delivery of the placenta and membranes (Fig. 13.5). A fourth stage is sometimes described as the time interval following expulsion of the placenta up to 6 hours after delivery. The only implication of this stage is the possibility of relaxation of the uterus followed by abnormal haemorrhage, which may happen during this time interval.

Once the child is delivered, the uterine muscle contracts, shearing off the placenta and pushing it into the lower uterine segment or upper part of the vagina. The classical signs of placental separation include a show of bright blood, lengthening and descent of the umbilical cord, and raising of the uterine fundus. This becomes tent-shaped instead of globular, and sits on top of the placenta as it descends into the lower segment. The placenta is accompanied by the fetal membranes, although these often become torn and require additional traction for their removal. The whole process lasts between 5 and 10 minutes. If the placenta is not expelled within 30 minutes the third stage should be considered abnormal. The signs of placental separation may be compressed and obscured by oxytocic drugs administered at the crowning of the head.

Mechanism of labour

- Initiated by falling progesterone and rising oestradiol, prostaglandins and oxytocin
- Presenting part undergoes descent, flexion on pelvic floor and rotation
- Head extends on reaching the vulva, then rotates back to original position after delivery
- Shoulders rotate into anterior-posterior diameter and deliver anterior first
- Uterine muscle contracts and shears off placenta

MANAGEMENT OF NORMAL LABOUR

The management of normal labour begins well before the onset of labour, with proper preparation of the mother. This primarily involves education about what actually happens in the various stages of labour. In addition, there are a variety of methods involving controlled respiration, known generally as psychoprophylactic methods, which enable the mother to control pain to some degree and to regulate expulsive efforts during the second stage of labour.

The mother should be advised to come in to hospital when the contractions are at regular 10–15 minute intervals, when there is a show, or if the membranes rupture. If the patient is in early labour, she is given a shower. Shaving of pubic hair is not necessary unless there is likely to be a delivery by Caesarean section. It is also advisable to give a small enema if the bowel is loaded, but this should be left to the discretion of the midwife or doctor attending the patient.

Examination during labour

On admission, the following examinations should be undertaken:

1. *Full general examination* – including temperature, pulse, respiration, blood pressure and state of hydration. The urine should be tested for protein, glucose and ketone bodies.
2. *Obstetrical examination of the abdomen* – inspection, palpation and auscultation to determine fetal lie, and position, station of the presenting part.
3. *Vaginal examination* – in labour, vaginal examination should be performed only after cleansing the vulva and introitus and using aseptic technique with sterile gloves and an antiseptic cream.

Once the examination is started, the fingers of the examining hand should not be withdrawn from the vagina until the examination is completed.

The following factors should be noted:

1. The consistency, effacement and dilatation of the cervix.
2. Whether the membranes are intact or ruptured and, if ruptured, the colour of the amniotic fluid.
3. The nature and presentation of the presenting part and the position of the fetal head. The descent or station of the presenting part is also noted in relation to the level of the ischial spines.
4. Assessment of the bony pelvis, particularly of the pelvic outlet.

GENERAL PRINCIPLES OF MANAGEMENT OF THE FIRST STAGE OF LABOUR

The guiding principles of management are:

1. Observation and intervention if the labour becomes abnormal

2. Pain relief and emotional support for the mother
3. Adequate hydration throughout labour.

Observation – the use of the partogram

The introduction of graphic records has proved to be a major advance in the active management of labour. The partogram is a single sheet of paper which graphically represents progress in labour (Fig. 13.6). The partogram is started as soon as the patient is admitted to the delivery suite, and this is recorded as zero time regardless of the time at which the contractions started. The advantage of this record is that it draws attention visually to aberration from normal progress.

Fetal condition

The fetal heart rate is charted as beats per minute, and deceleration in heart rate which occurs during contractions is shown by an arrow down to the lowest heart rate recorded.

The time of membrane rupture and the nature of the fluid are also noted. Moulding of the fetal head and the presence of caput are also noted.

Progress of labour

Progress in labour is measured by assessing the rate of cervical dilatation and descent of the presenting part. Vaginal examination and assessment of cervical dilatation should be performed on admission to hospital and every 4 hours during the first stage of labour. Cervical dilatation is recorded in centimetres along the 0–10 scale of the cervicograph, and a slope of cervical dilatation is constructed. A normal graph is drawn on to the partogram. Dilatation of the cervix occurs in two well-defined phases. The **latent phase** starts at the onset of labour and ends at about 3 cm dilatation. This takes about two-thirds of the time of labour. This is followed by the **active phase**, which extends from the end of the latent phase until delivery. If the dilatation of the cervix lags more than 2 hours behind the expected rate of dilatation, the labour is considered abnormal. The rate of dilatation increases rapidly during this active phase, although it slows down near full dilatation. The head level is also charted on the cervicograph using the following definition (see Fig. 1.22):

1. If the head is high, the level is five-fifths above the pelvic brim.
2. If the head is just descending into the brim, it is four-fifths above the brim.

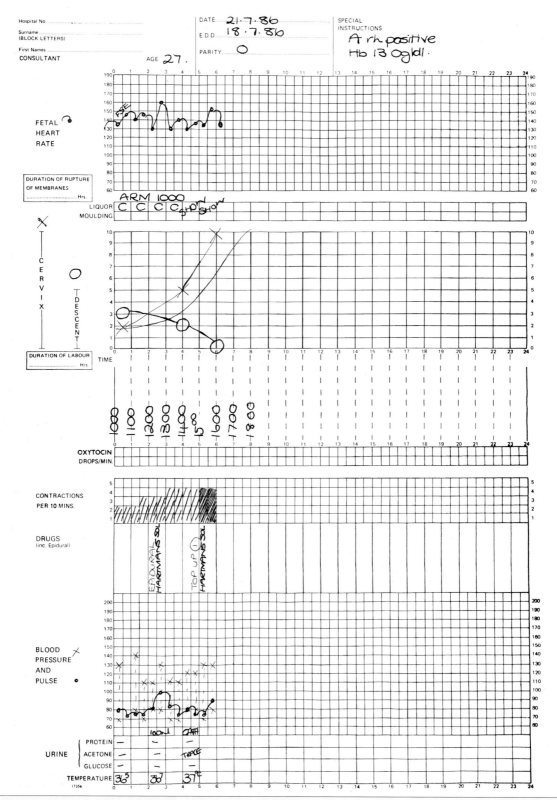

Fig. 13.6 The partogram is a complete visual record of measurements made during delivery.

3. If less than half the head is in the brim, it is three-fifths above the brim.
4. If more than half the head is through the brim, it is two-fifths above the brim.
5. If just the sinciput is palpable, one-fifth is above the brim.

The head level in fifths is plotted on the 0–5 gradations on the cervicograph.

Descent is also assessed in relation to the height of the presenting part above or below the level of the ischial spines. The nature and frequency of the contractions are recorded on the chart by shading in the number of contractions per 10 minutes. Dotted squares indicate contractions of less than 20 seconds duration, cross-hatched squares are contractions between 20 and 40 seconds duration, while contractions lasting longer than 40 seconds are shown by complete shading of the squares.

Management of labour
- Begins with antenatal education
- Normally consists of support, pain relief and observation of fetal condition and cervical dilatation
- Intervention indicated if dilatation lags > 2 hours behind expected rate

---

Pain relief in labour

Narcotic analgesia agents

A variety of narcotic agents have been used for pain relief in labour. The most commonly used agents at present include pethidine 50–150 mg, omnopon 10–20 mg, diamorphine 5–10 mg, pentazocine 30–60 mg, phenazocine 1–2 mg or oxymorphone 1–1.5 mg by intramuscular injection. These drugs are commonly used in conjunction with the phenothiazines or diazepam. The drugs are easy to administer, but have the disadvantage of being relatively ineffective in 30–40% of patients. They also tend to cause nausea and vomiting, and may result in respiratory depression of the neonate – particularly if given when they are most needed, i.e. late in the first stage of labour. Despite the tendency to avoid narcotic analgesics in present-day practice, they are still a valuable part of pain relief and are widely used.

Inhalational agents

These are commonly reserved for use in the later part of the first stage and in the second stage of labour. The three agents in common use are nitrous oxide and oxygen 50:50 (Entonox), trichloroethylene 0.35–0.5% and methoxyflurane 0.35% in air. Nitrous oxide has a low solubility in blood, and only about 10% of women obtain complete pain relief. If optimal effects are to be obtained, patients should be trained to self-inhale Entonox at least 30 seconds before a contraction starts, and that is not always easy to judge.

Trichloroethylene and methoxyflurane

These agents have a high degree of solubility in body fat, and it therefore takes longer to achieve adequate analgesic concentrations. Inhalation should at first be continuous for 10–15 minutes and thereafter only during contractions. After 30 minutes, inhalation should be necessary only every third or fourth contraction. Nausea and vomiting are common side effects.

Regional analgesia

Epidural analgesia – The most widely used form of regional analgesia is epidural analgesia. The procedure may be instituted at any time during labour. A fine cathether is passed into the lumbar epidural space and local anaesthetic such as Marcain or bupivacaine injected (Fig. 13.7). This will reduce and usually eliminate the pain of labour but does not affect uterine activity.

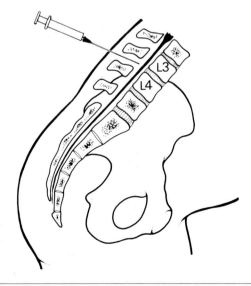

Fig. 13.7 Epidural anaesthesia is induced by injection of local anaesthetic agents into the lumbar epidural space.

The procedure involves the following:

1. Insertion of an intravenous infusion to expand plasma volume, thus reducing hypotensive effects and expanding the vascular tree of the lower third of the body.
2. Insertion of an epidural catheter at the L_3/L_4 vertebrae. Blood pressure, pulse rate and fetal heart rate should be carefully monitored, and the infusion of local anaesthesia should be altered by posture to achieve the desired analgesic effects.

Other forms of vaginal anaesthesia – Spinal anaesthesia is rarely used in the management of normal labour because it is not superior to epidural analgesia and it carries greater risk of complications.

Paracervical and pudendal blockade involve infiltration of the paracervical region or infiltration around the pudendal nerve as it leaves the pudendal canal (Fig. 13.8). These procedures are most commonly used for pain relief during operative vaginal delivery and are therefore introduced in the second stage of labour.

Complications of regional analgesia are minimal but include:

1. Toxic symptoms or convulsions with intravenous injection of local anaesthesia.
2. Spinal tap with spinal anaesthesia. Leakage of cerebrospinal fluid may result in persistent headache. Total spinal analgesia may result in respiratory paralysis.

3. Hypotension, which is treated by changing the patient to the left lateral position and infusing 500–1000 ml of Hartman's solution.

Regional anaesthesia

- Epidural catheter inserted at L_3/L_4
- Need to expand plasma volume
- Complications are spinal tap, hypotension and intravenous injection of anaesthetic

---

Posture in labour

Some women prefer to remain ambulant or to sit in a chair during the first stage of labour. However, most women prefer to lie down as labour advances, and should be encouraged to lie in the lateral supine position. Women who wish to have epidural analgesia need to remain supine as the procedure inevitably produces some temporary motor impairment of the legs.

Water births

Immersion of the mother in a water bath is now a common option for pain relief in labour on the basis that flotation improves support of the pregnant uterus. However, delivery should not occur in the bath as it may result in inhalation of the bath water during the first fetal breath and may result in fetal drowning.

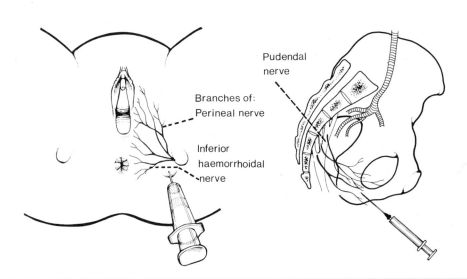

Fig. 13.8 Pudendal nerve blockade is achieved by injection of local anaesthetic around the pudendal nerve at the level of the ischial spine. Additional infiltration is used to block branches of the inferior haemorrhoidal and perineal nerves.

Nutrition in labour

No patient should be fed by mouth during labour, although occasional small sips of clear fluid are permissible. Delayed gastric emptying may result in vomiting and inhalation of vomitus if general anaesthesia is required. Intravenous therapy should be started where the labour persists for more than 6 hours and delivery is not imminent. The major cause of acidosis in labour is dehydration and not starvation, and therefore Hartman's solution and not 5% dextrose should be used at a rate of 1–1.5 litres/8 hours.

Fetal monitoring

Fetal distress (asphyxia) is associated with alterations in the fetal heart rate, the passage of meconium-stained liquor and excessive fetal movements. Diminution and cessation of fetal movements may indicate incipient placental failure and fetal demise.

During labour, the fetal heart rate can be monitored every 15 minutes using a Pinard fetal stethoscope, and contractions are monitored by manual palpation. However, it is now common practice to use electronic monitors to provide continuous surveillance, particularly in high-risk pregnancies.

Fetal cardiotocography

The pressure changes in the uterus are recorded by using either internal or external pressure transducers, and the resultant pressure wave is recorded on a continuous graphical record (tocograph).

Pressure is recorded either with a pressure sensor applied externally over the anterior abdominal wall and uterus or by inserting a pressure-sensitive transducer into the amniotic sac or alternatively a fluid-filled catheter, which is then attached externally to a pressure transducer (Fig. 13.9).

The **fetal heart rate** is recorded externally by the application of Doppler ultrasound over the fetal heart, or by the direct application of a clip and electrical lead directed to the fetal presenting part, after rupturing the fetal membranes. This has the advantages of giving a much clearer tracing. The heart rate is displayed as a continuous linear trace.

Basal heart rate

The normal fetal heart rate varies between 110 and 150 beats/minute (Fig. 13.10). It exhibits short-term fluctuations known as beat-to-beat irregularity. The normal heart rate fluctuates between 10 and 25 beats/minute. A 'silent' fetal heart rate of less than 5 beats/minute indicates fetal distress and jeopardy.

A summary of the definitions of heart rate are shown in Table 13.1.

Transient episodes of bradycardia

Three types of fetal bradycardia have been described:

1. *Early decelerations (type I)* – deceleration of the heart rate which commences with the onset of a contraction and returns to normal on completion

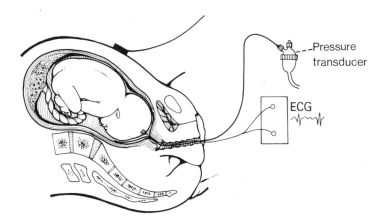

Fig. 13.9 Monitoring during labour – contractions are recorded by intra- and extra-uterine tocography; the fetal heart rate is recorded externally by Doppler ultrasonography or by direct application of an ECG electrode to the presenting part.

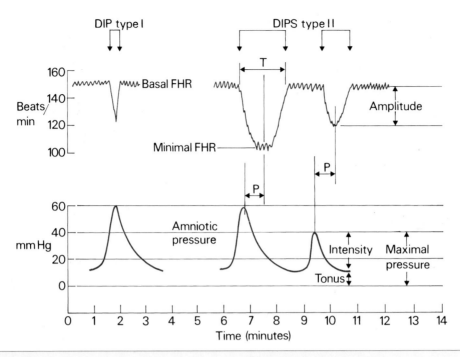

Fig. 13.10 Patterns of fetal heart rate change and amniotic pressure change in labour.

Table 13.1 Fetal heart rate definitions

Definition		Heart rate (beats/minute)
Baseline rate		
Normal		110–150
Tachycardia	– moderate	150–180
	– severe	>180
Bradycardia	– moderate	100–110
	– severe	<100
Variability		
Normal		>5
Reduced		3–5
Absent		<3

of the contraction. This is commonly innocuous and indicates head compression.

2. *Late decelerations (type II)* – deceleration occurs well after the contraction has started and does not return to normal until 20 seconds after completion of the contraction. This is generally considered to be pathological and to indicate fetal asphyxia and placental insufficiency – particularly when it is associated with a resting tachycardia.

3. *Variable deceleration* – this may occur at any time independent of contractions and is sometimes pathological. It may be associated with cord compression.

The fetal electrocardiogram

The fetal electrocardiogram (FECG) can be recorded from scalp electrodes but the signal is often difficult to interpret because of electrical noise. Techniques are now available using computer technology that allow isolation of the signal from background noise, and continuous real-time monitoring of all changes in time constants and the configuration of the FECG. In the presence of fetal hypoxia, the relationship between the PR interval and heart rate changes from negative to positive, the ST segment becomes depressed and the T wave height increases.

Fetal acid–base balance

Where abnormalities of the fetal heart rate occur in labour, the fetal acid–base status should be examined. Fetal blood can be obtained directly from the scalp through an amnioscope, which is inserted through the cervix and enables direct visualization of the presenting part. A scalp blood pH measurement is made. A pH of less than 7.25 indicates mild acidosis and necessitates repetition of measurement after 1 hour. A value of less than 7.20 indicates a significant degree of asphyxia and the need for delivery.

Fetal monitoring

- Normal basal fetal heart rate = 110–150 beats/minute
- Beat-to-beat variation should be > 5 beats/minute
- Decelerations are a fall in FHR of > 15 beats/minute for more than 30 seconds and are described by their relation to contractions
- Significant fetal hypoxia is indicated by a scalp pH of < 7.2
- Significant hypoxia is more likely in the presence of meconium-stained liquor

MANAGEMENT OF THE SECOND STAGE OF LABOUR

The onset of the second stage of labour is indicated by a desire to bear down and, often, to vomit. The diagnosis is confirmed by vaginal examination. This stage occupies less than 2 hours in the primigravida and 1 hour in the multiparous woman. The progress of the second stage is assessed by the degree of distension of the perineum. The desire to bear down may not be present if epidural anaesthesia is effective, and, in this situation, the onset of the second stage can be identified only by the recognition of full cervical dilatation.

Preparation for delivery

The attendant scrubs and puts on gown and gloves. The mother is commonly placed in the left lateral or supine position and may also be placed in the lithotomy position. Some women prefer to deliver in the squatting position. As the head is pushed down with each contraction, it distends the perineum and anus. The anus is covered with a pad, and the descent of the occiput controlled with the left hand, the head being kept well flexed until crowned when it is allowed to extend. This process minimizes perineal distension. The head then delivers, and the eyes and naso-pharynx are cleared.

If the perineum appears to be tearing, an episiotomy is performed, the incision is made in the medio-lateral direction from the midpoint of the posterior margin of the introitus (Fig. 13.11). With the next contraction, the head is gently pulled towards the perineum until the anterior shoulder is delivered under the subpubic angle and then pulled anteriorly to deliver the posterior shoulder and the remainder of the trunk.

The cord is clamped twice and cut between the clamps. The infant will normally cry immediately

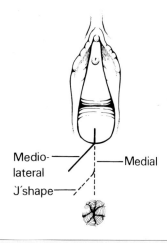

Fig. 13.11 Sites for episiotomy incisions: the object is to avoid extension of the incision or tear into the anal sphincter or rectum.

Table 13.2 Evaluation of the Apgar score

	0	1	2
Colour	White	Blue	Pink
Tone	Flaccid	Rigid	Normal
Pulse	Impalpable	<100 beats/ minute	>100 beats/ minute
Respiration	Absent	Irregular	Regular
Response	Absent	Poor	Normal

after birth, but, if the onset of respiration is delayed for more than 1 minute, the naso-pharynx should be aspirated and the baby's lungs inflated with oxygen. If the onset of respiration is further delayed, intubation will be necessary.

The condition of the baby is assessed at 1 and 5 minutes using the Apgar scoring system (Table 13.2).

MANAGEMENT OF THE THIRD STAGE

The mother is turned on to her back if she is not already in the supine position. A dish is placed under the cord and beneath the introitus and buttocks to collect any blood loss. The left hand is rested on the abdomen on the uterine fundus. An oxytocic drug such as Syntometrine, which contains both ergometrine and Syntocinon, is given by intramuscular injection with crowning of the head, and the uterus should contract firmly shortly after delivery of the fetus.

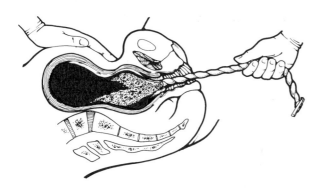

Fig. 13.12 Brandt–Andrews technique for assisted delivery of the placenta: the uterine fundus must be contracted before this technique is attempted.

As soon as the uterus is contracted, cord traction is applied with the right hand whilst monitoring fundal descent with the left hand against the uterine fundus (Fig. 13.12). Assisted delivery of the placenta is usually completed within 5 minutes of delivery.

The placenta and membranes are checked to see if any cotyledons are missing and whether the membranes are complete or incomplete. The blood loss is recorded.

Repair of perineal damage

If there is an episiotomy or tear, this is now repaired (Fig. 13.13). The episiotomy or tear may be first degree, second degree or third degree. First-degree tears involve vaginal and perineal skin only. Second-degree tears involve the underlying levator ani muscles. Third-degree tears involve the anal sphincter and, if gross, the rectal mucosa.

The perineal structures are sutured with size 0 or 1 chromic catgut, and the perineal skin may be sutured with non-absorbable or absorbable suture material. The former are removed 5 days later. There are many other satisfactory variants of this procedure. Many practitioners prefer to use absorbable suture materials throughout so that the sutures do not need to be removed. The use of subcuticular sutures results in an excellent scar but demands meticulous haemostasis. The use of synthetic absorbable suture materials which have greater strength and can be used at finer grades are now tending to replace traditional catgut.

Closure of the vaginal wound requires a clear view of the apex of the incision; a 'tagged' pack should be inserted into the vagina to keep the operative field clear of blood. After closure of the vaginal wound, the levator muscle and fascia should be approximated with interrupted sutures and the skin closed with careful haemostasis. If the superficial external sphincter is cut, then the ends should be identified and sutured together.

On completion of the procedure:

1. Remove the pack.
2. Ensure that the vagina is not constricted and admits two fingers easily.

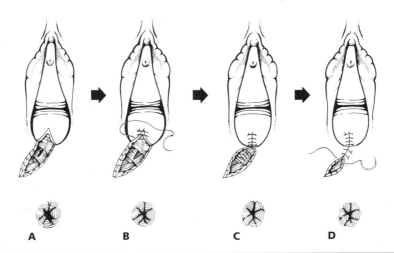

Fig. 13.13 Repair of the episiotomy: the posterior vaginal wall may be closed with continuous or interrupted sutures; apposition of the cut levator muscle ensures haemotasis before skin closure. **A** Episiotomy wound; **B** continuous suture of posterior vaginal wall; **C** interrupted sutures into the cut edges of the levator; **D** interrupted suture into the perineal skin.

3. Perform a rectal examination and make sure that none of the sutures have penetrated the rectal mucosa. If this occurs, the sutures must be removed.

BIBLIOGRAPHY

Baylan P 1987 Intrapartum fetal monitoring. Baillières Clinical Obstetrics and Gynecology 1(1)
Spencer J A D (ed) 1991 Fetal monitoring. Oxford University Press, Oxford
Studd J 1985 The management of labour. Blackwell, Oxford

14 Abnormal labour

PREMATURE LABOUR

The onset of labour before 37 weeks gestation is described as premature labour. Some 6–10% of all labours are premature. Because uterine contractions may occur at any stage during pregnancy, it is often difficult to identify the onset of labour. However, it must be remembered that the onset of labour is defined as the presence of regular, painful uterine contractions that produce progressive cervical dilatation.

Aetiology

The mechanism of the onset of labour remains uncertain; this also applies to the onset of premature labour. Nevertheless, it is known that there is an association between premature labour and social class, overdistension of the uterus, as with hydramnios and multiple pregnancy, premature rupture of the membranes, antepartum haemorrhage, and uterine abnormalities (Fig. 14.1). A woman has

a 30% chance of repeating the situation with her second pregnancy; if she has a second premature labour, there is a 60% chance of a third premature labour.

The danger of premature labour lies mainly in the risk to the fetus and not to the mother. Premature labour remains the most common cause of fetal and neonatal loss.

Management of preterm labour

Once the diagnosis is established, the management of preterm labour is dependent on the stage at which the mother presents and on the quality of available neonatal services. It may, for example, be preferable to allow a labour to proceed at 32 weeks gestation if the neonatal unit of a particular service

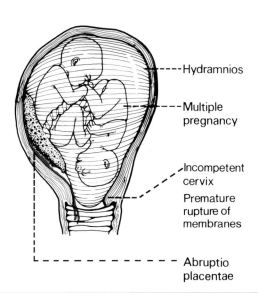

Fig. 14.1 Factors predisposing to premature labour.

- Hydramnios
- Multiple pregnancy
- Incompetent cervix
- Premature rupture of membranes
- Abruptio placentae

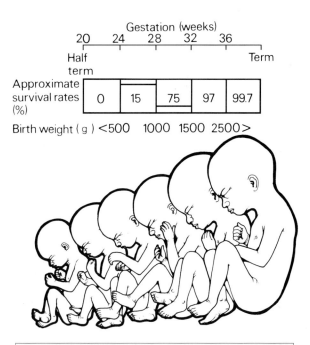

	Gestation (weeks)				
	20	24	28	32	36
	Half term				Term
Approximate survival rates (%)	0	15	75	97	99.7

Birth weight (g) <500   1000   1500   2500>

Fig. 14.2 Birth weight, gestational age and perinatal outcome.

provides a better opportunity of survival than can be achieved by attempting to suppress the labour (Fig. 14.2).

Those factors that indicate impaired prospects of conservative management of preterm labour include:

1. The presence of prematurely ruptured membranes
2. The occurrence of antepartum haemorrhage
3. Cervical dilatation in excess of 5 cm at the time of presentation.

Conservative management

If the cervix is less than 5 cm dilated and the membranes are intact, it is reasonable to attempt to stop labour. This is best effected using intravenous infusion of drugs which are sympathomimetic such as ritodrine, orciprenaline and isoxsuprine. These drugs inhibit uterine contractions when administered by intravenous infusion but they also have significant side effects such as tremor, tachycardia, hypotension, hypokalaemia, nausea and vomiting. Uterine activity can be effectively inhibited by the administration of prostaglandin synthetase inhibitors such as indomethacin, but these drugs also affect the ductus arteriosus and therefore may cause premature closure of the ductus in utero. Magnesium sulphate is also a potent inhibitor of uterine activity. Once labour is effectively inhibited, the drug can be administered orally until 36 weeks gestation after which it is doutful that any further advantage is gained by continuing the pregnancy. It is also important to realize that inhibiting labour after 36 weeks gestation will not improve perinatal outcome.

Prevention of respiratory distress syndrome

As long ago as 1972, Liggins and Howie demonstrated that the antepartum administration of glucocorticoids such as dexamethasone to mothers in preterm labour up to 34 weeks accelerated the production of surfactant in the fetal lung and therefore had a significant impact on fetal survival by reducing the incidence of respiratory distress syndrome and hence the need for neonatal ventilation. Administration of dexamethasone to the mother must precede delivery by 24 hours, and it is therefore necessary to inhibit uterine activity to allow the drug to improve fetal surfactant production. The effect of the drug will last for 7–10 days. Two doses of dexamethasone 12 mg are given by intramuscular injection 12 hours apart, or four doses of 6 mg given intramuscularly 12 hours apart.

Conservative management of preterm labour

Fifty to eighty per cent of threatened preterm labours will settle with no treatment. It is important to identify potentially treatable precipitating causes such as urinary tract infection. Tocolysis is probably only effective in delaying delivery by 48 hours. This is of clinical value in allowing time for in utero transfer to unite with advanced neonatal facilities if necessary and to allow time for glucocorticoid administration to take effect. Tocolysis is contraindicated in the presence of fetal death, chorioamnionitis and abruption and where there is an increased risk of maternal pulmonary oedema in diabetes, maternal cardiac disease and multiple pregnancy.

Method of delivery

When labour is established and there is no prospect of effectively inhibiting contractions, the labour should be allowed to proceed with appropriate pain relief. Shortening of the second stage by low forceps delivery and a generous episiotomy will serve to minimize the risk of intracranial haemorrhage.

The chances of survival are substantially enhanced with the availability of high quality neonatal services, and any woman in labour before 34 weeks gestation should be delivered in a hospital with appropriate facilities.

There is evidence that preterm labour with breech presentation is associated with a significant increase in perinatal loss and that survival is improved between 28 and 34 weeks gestation if the child is delivered by Caesarean section.

Perinatal mortality

The survival of infants weighing 1.5 kg or more is now in excess of 95%, and this percentage remains remarkably high even for birth weights down to 1 kg.

Premature labour

- Labour occurring before 36 weeks
- 6–10% of labours
- Associated with social class, 'uterine distension', antepartum haemorrhage and premature rupture of the membranes
- Tocolysis indicated if under 32 weeks, intact membranes and < 5 cm dilated

---

PREMATURE RUPTURE OF THE MEMBRANES

The time of spontaneous rupture of the membranes is determined by:

1. The tensile strength of the fetal membranes
2. The support of surrounding tissue, i.e. the degree of dilatation of the cervix
3. Intrauterine pressure.

Premature rupture of the membranes is defined as spontaneous rupture of the membranes before the onset of labour; it occurs in up to 10% of pregnancies.

Aetiology (Fig. 14.3)

The membranes may rupture prematurely as the result of:

1. *Weakened membranes* – This is associated with the presence of infection, and is the commonest explanation for premature membrane rupture.
2. *Cervical incompetence* – A dilated cervical canal will allow the membranes to bulge through the cervix and eventually rupture because of poor support.
3. *Abnormally raised intrauterine pressure* – This may be due to hydramnios, distension of the uterus by multiple pregnancy and sometimes abnormal external pressure.

Diagnosis

The mother usually observes that she has had a gush of fluid from the vagina or that she feels constantly wet. It may sometimes be very difficult to be certain whether the symptoms are related to vaginal discharge or to the passage of amniotic fluid. The diagnosis is confirmed by speculum examination and the direct observation of clear fluid in the vagina. The tests for protein in the vaginal discharge are not particularly helpful or reliable, and it can often be difficult to be certain if the membranes have ruptured. Sometimes the drainage of amniotic fluid may cease spontaneously, particularly if there is a high leakage rather than forewater rupture.

Management

It is advisable to admit the mother to hospital for observation.

The risks to the fetus and the mother are those of ascending infection, and in particular infection in the fetal lungs. Furthermore, prolonged drainage of amniotic fluid may lead to oligohydramnios and impaired fetal lung development.

On admission, the diagnosis must be established by direct speculum examination, and a high vaginal swab should be taken for culture. If negative, this should be repeated 1 week later and weekly thereafter. If the culture is positive or there are clinical signs of infection, then the appropriate antibiotic therapy should be given. After 36 weeks gestation, consideration should be given to induction, as the risks of prematurity will be minimal, whereas the risk of infection will continue.

If there are maternal signs of infection, such as maternal pyrexia, purulent vaginal discharge and uterine tenderness, then labour should be stimulated. If this is ineffective, as sometimes happens in these circumstances, then the child should be delivered by Caesarean section.

BREECH PRESENTATION

The fetus presents by the breech at delivery in about 3% of all pregnancies at term. The incidence of breech presentation is higher in early pregnancy, but in many cases the presentation spontaneously corrects itself.

Types of breech presentation

The breech may present in one of three ways (Fig. 14.4):

1. Frank breech – the legs lie extended along the body, and the buttocks present to the pelvic inlet (see Fig. 14.4). This is also described as a breech with extended legs.

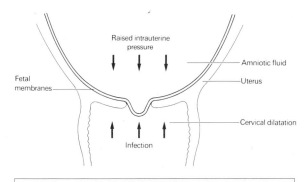

Fig. 14.3 Factors which determine the time of rupture of the fetal membranes.

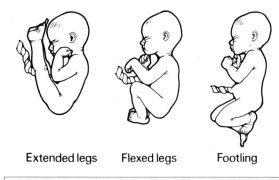

Extended legs   Flexed legs   Footling

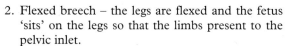

Fig. 14.4 Types of breech presentation.

2. Flexed breech – the legs are flexed and the fetus 'sits' on the legs so that the limbs present to the pelvic inlet.
3. Knee or footling presentation – one thigh is flexed and one is extended so that the foot or knee will descend first through the cervical os into the vagina.

The position of the fetus is described by using the sacrum as the denominator, rather than the occiput as with a vertex presentation.

Management

Antenatal

There are various conditions which predispose to breech presentation; these include multiple pregnancy, placenta praevia, congenital abnormalities of the uterus and fetal malformation. Increased muscle tone as found in primigravidae may also be a predisposing factor.

In the presence of any of these factors, it may be necessary to modify management accordingly.

Breech presentation is associated with an increased risk of perinatal loss associated with:

1. Asphyxia from cord compression during delivery
2. Intracranial haemorrhage and trauma to viscera during delivery.

It is therefore important to be certain that there will be no delay during delivery and that the pelvis is adequate and the fetus is not abnormally large.

External cephalic version

If the breech presentation persists after 34 weeks gestation, it may be appropriate to turn the fetus by manual manipulation to a vertex presentation. This

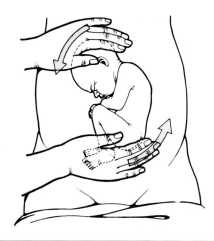

Fig. 14.5 External cephalic version: pressure is applied in the opposite direction to the two fetal poles.

process is known as **external cephalic version**. It is contraindicated if the ultimate intention is to deliver the child by Caesarean section, and if there has been a previous antepartum haemorrhage or placenta praevia.

The procedure is performed by applying pressure to both poles of the fetus after disimpacting the breech from the pelvis and rotating the fetus to a cephalic presentation (Fig. 14.5).

Complications include cord entanglement, fetal distress, premature rupture of the membranes and premature separation of the placenta. It is important to check the fetal heart before and during the procedure. If there are signs of fetal distress it may be necessary to return the fetus to its original presentation. If external cephalic version is not possible, then a decision must be made as to the method of delivery.

It may be difficult to define accurately the size of the fetus although modern ultrasound techniques have improved prenatal assessment. It is possible to examine the bony pelvis by clinical pelvimetry and radiological pelvimetry (Fig. 14.6). This should be performed at 36 weeks gestation.

Method of delivery

Caesarean section

If the pelvis is small or the fetus is large, then delivery should be by elective Caesarean section. A previous Caesarean section, pre-eclampsia or antepartum haemorrhage are also indications for delivery by

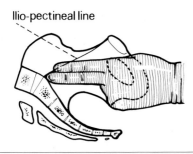

Ilio-pectineal line

Fig. 14.6 Clinical assessment of the pelvis and breech presentation.

elective Caesarean section. If the estimated birth weight is less than 1500 g, delivery by Caesarean section is associated with an improvement in both survival and morbidity.

Vaginal delivery

If all other factors are normal, vaginal delivery should be planned. The mother should be advised to present as soon as labour starts or the membranes rupture. Vaginal examination must be performed at the time of admission to exclude cord

presentation. The length of labour is the same as in a vertex presentation. Analgesia may be provided by epidural anaesthesia.

The presence of meconium-stained liquor carries the same significance of possible fetal hypoxia as with a vertex presentation.

Delivery technique (Fig. 14.7)

When the cervix is fully dilated, the mother is encouraged to bear down until the fetal buttocks and anus come into view (see Fig. 14.9). A wide episiotomy is performed and the mother is encouraged to expel the child to the level of the umbilicus. The legs are then lifted out of the vagina, and traction is applied to the legs downwards and backwards with the shoulders in the anteroposterior diameter. It should be possible to deliver the anterior arm by sliding the fingers over the shoulder and sweeping the arm downwards. The trunk is then moved laterally until the posterior arm can be delivered. The trunk is then allowed to hang for 30 seconds, and this helps to pull the head into the pelvis. The trunk is now swung upwards through 180° until the mouth comes on view. The mouth is cleared of fluid to allow respiration to

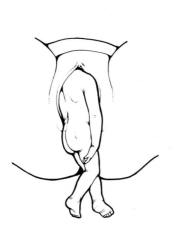

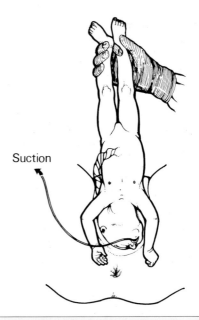

Suction

Fig. 14.7 Technique of breech delivery: initial delivery of the trunk allows descent of the head into the pelvis (left); subsequent anterior rotation of the trunk enables delivery of the fetal head with the application of forceps to safeguard the head from sudden compression and expansion (right).

start, and forceps are then applied to the aftercoming head to enable gradual delivery of the head and to protect against sudden expansion and expulsion. Syntometrine is given by intramuscular injection with delivery of the head. With proper selection and careful management, the perinatal mortality should be no greater than with vertex delivery.

Breech presentation

- 3% of term pregnancies
- Sacrum used as denominator
- Predisposing factors include multiple pregnancy, placenta praevia, and malformation of fetus or uterus
- Associated with increased perinatal morbidity and mortality
- Delivery by section is indicated if previous section, pregnancy-induced hypertension, antepartum haemorrhage or disproportion anticipated
- Length of labour should be normal
- Early deceleration more likely to indicate cord compression or fetal distress than in a vertex delivery
- Delivery of the after-coming head should be assisted

FACE PRESENTATION (Fig. 14.8)

This occurs in approximately 1 in 600 deliveries. The head is hyperextended so that the occiput rests on the cervical spine. It sometimes occurs as a continuing extension of a deflexed head in the occipito-posterior position. Occasionally the head is pushed back by a cervical tumour. The chin acts as the denominator.

Diagnosis

This can sometimes be made antenatally but it is usually recognized in labour. The head feels large on abdominal palpation and the nuchal groove can often be felt.

On vaginal examination, the fetal nose, eyes, mouth and chin can be felt but are sometimes obscured by considerable facial oedema. The diameter of engagement is the submento-bregmatic diameter, which is the same size as the sub-occipito–bregmatic diameter.

However, in a full-term fetus, delivery can occur vaginally only if the chin lies anteriorly.

Management

Vaginal delivery can be anticipated if the pelvis is normal and the chin rotates anteriorly. If progress is slow, it may be preferable to effect delivery by Caesarean section. The facial bruising and oedema are often gross but usually subside within a few days.

BROW PRESENTATION (Fig. 14.9)

Brow presentation is the cause of obstructed labour and occurs in about 1 in 3000 pregnancies. Unless the head is small or the pelvis very large, vaginal delivery is not possible.

Diagnosis

The head remains high and does not engage, and is therefore easily palpable. On vaginal examination, the brow is palpable between the bridge of the nose and supra-orbital ridges and the anterior fontanelle. The management is to deliver the child by Caesarean section.

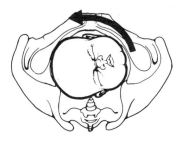

Left mento-transverse

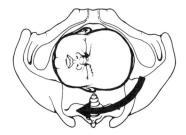

Right mento-transverse

Fig. 14.8 Position of the face presentation; the denomination is the chin.

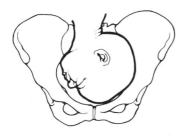

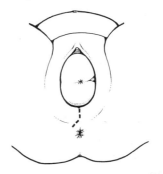

Brow presentation

Buttock presentation

Fig. 14.9 Brow and breech presentation at delivery.

UNSTABLE LIE, TRANSVERSE LIE AND SHOULDER PRESENTATION

An unstable lie is one which constantly changes. It is commonly associated with multiparity, placenta praevia, and uterine abnormalities such as a bicornuate uterus or uterine fibroids. Polyhydramnios may allow undue fetal mobility.

Complications

If the lie is unstable, there is a risk of prolapse of the cord and of obstructed labour from a malpresentation. Provided there is no evidence of placenta praevia, the lie should be corrected and the mother advised to come into hospital immediately labour begins. If the lie is still unstable at 38 weeks, it is safer to arrange hospital admission and await the spontaneous onset of labour. If induction of labour is indicated for other reasons, the lie should be corrected, the membranes, ruptured and labour stimulated with an oxytocin infusion.

TRANSVERSE LIE AND SHOULDER PRESENTATION

If labour starts when the lie is transverse, it is clear that vaginal delivery cannot occur unless the fetus is

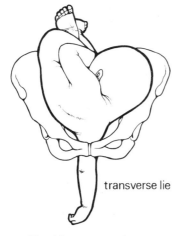

transverse lie

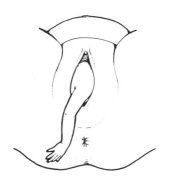

Shoulder presentation

Anterior arm presentation

Fig. 14.10 Prolapse of the arm into the vagina sometimes results in a shoulder presentation.

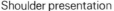

very small or macerated. The transverse lie may evolve into a shoulder presentation and as the cervix dilates, the arm may prolapse (Fig. 14.10).

Management

If the shoulder is presenting, no attempt should be made to replace or apply traction to the arm. Unless the lie can be corrected before the situation occurs, the only appropriate method of delivery is by Caesarean section. If the lie has been neglected, it may be necessary to perform a classical Caesarean section with a vertical incision in the upper segment.

CORD PRESENTATION AND PROLAPSE

Cord presentation occurs when any part of the cord lies alongside or in front of the presenting part. When the membranes rupture under these circumstances the cord will prolapse (Fig. 14.11).

Predisposing factors

Any condition that displaces the head or presenting part away from the cervix predisposes to cord prolapse. It is particularly likely to occur in the presence of malpresentations, cephalo-pelvic disproportion and polyhydramnios. If the membranes are ruptured artificially to induce labour, the cord may prolapse

but it is, in fact, no more likely to occur in this way than spontaneously.

Management

Cord prolapse is an obstetric emergency and delivery must be effected as quickly as possible. This means that unless the cervix is fully dilated and a forceps or ventouse delivery can be effected, Caesarean section is necessary.

As soon as the diagnosis is made, there is no point in trying to replace the cord, and indeed it should be handled as little as possible to avoid inducing arterial spasm. Pressure on the cord can be reduced by displacing the presenting part digitally per vaginam or by placing the woman in the knee–chest position (Fig. 14.11).

Despite the acute asphyxial insult inflicted on the fetus under these circumstance, fetal cerebral damage is surprisingly rare – probably because of the short-term nature of the asphyxia.

MALPOSITION OF THE FETAL HEAD

The occipito-posterior position (Fig. 14.12)

This is the commonest malposition of the fetal head, and is often associated with prolonged and painful labour with severe backache.

The head normally engages in the transverse diameter and the occiput rotates anteriorly as the head

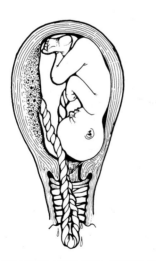
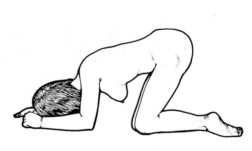

Knee-chest position

Fig. 14.11 Cord prolapse (left); pressure on the cord can be minimized by placing the mother in the knee–chest position (right).

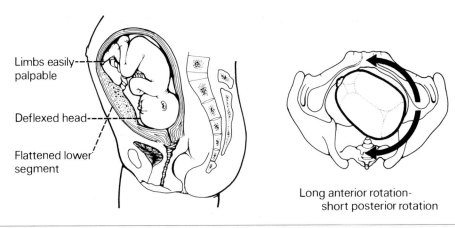

Limbs easily palpable

Deflexed head

Flattened lower segment

Long anterior rotation-
short posterior rotation

Fig. 14.12 Clinical findings in the occipito-posterior position (left); the head may rotate anteriorly or posteriorly or may arrest in the occipito-posterior position (right).

presses onto the pelvic floor. The head occupies the occipito-posterior position in 10% of vertex presentations. The head is deflexed and the presenting diameter – the occipito–frontal – is 11 cm, and therefore produces some degree of cephalo-pelvic disproportion.

Diagnosis

The occipito-posterior position can be diagnosed by both abdominal and vaginal palpation. The anterior abdominal wall looks flattened below the umbilicus as compared with the convexity of the normal presentation and position. The fetal limbs lie anteriorly and are easily palpable. The head engages late and tends to remain high. The occipito-posterior position is the commonest cause of non-engagement of the fetal head in the primigravida at term.

On vaginal examination, the posterior fontanelle lies behind the transverse diameter of the pelvic inlet. During labour, the cervix often dilates asymmetrically so that the anterior lip becomes thickened and oedematous whilst the posterior rim dilates normally.

Management

The essential features of management are to ensure that pain relief is adequate and that fluid replacement is maintained to prevent dehydration.

The head may rotate anteriorly and the labour progress normally (see Fig. 14.12) or it may rotate posteriorly and adopt a direct occipito-posterior position. The latter is particularly likely to occur in an anthropoid pelvis. It may remain in the occipito-posterior position but, when full cervical dilatation

occurs, the head must be rotated either manually or with Kielland's forceps and delivered by forceps extraction.

If the head occupies the occipito-posterior position and is low on the pelvic floor, it may be delivered as a direct occipito-posterior position. This can cause severe damage to the perineum because of the over-distension of the pelvic floor, and may result in a third degree tear.

Deep transverse arrest

Although the head usually engages in the transverse diameter, it normally rotates anteriorly. If this rotation does not occur, the head arrests at the level of the ischial spines. If the pelvis is android in shape, vaginal delivery may be impossible.

If the pelvis is normal, delivery is effected by either manual or forceps rotation. Deep transverse arrest results in a prolonged second stage of labour. This term should not be applied when forceps rotation is required for some other complication before the head has had the chance to rotate normally.

Other presentations

- Face presentation; 1 in 600 births, can be delivered if chin anterior
- Brow; 1 in 3000 births, usually requires Caesarean section
- Unstable lie; associated with multiparity, placenta praevia, polyhydramnios and uterine distortion
- Occipito-posterior position; 10% of births, commonest cause of non-engagement in primigravidae at term

ABNORMALITIES OF UTERINE ACTION

Labour may be prolonged because of abnormalities of uterine action. The degree to which these abnormalities contribute to dystocia has been a subject of considerable debate. Progress in normal labour depends on uterine polarity associated with fundal dominance and the progressive dilatation of the cervix.

Thus, lack of progress may result from either normal polarity and week contractions – **hypotonic uterine inertia** – or abnormal polarity and strong contractions – **hypertonic uterine inertia** (Fig. 14.13). In hypertonic uterine contractions, the contraction wave starts in the lower uterine segment and is often prolonged and painful. Contraction waves may also be asymmetrical resulting in a double peak in the uterine contraction wave.

Management

Abnormalities of uterine action are generally recognized by the failure of progress in labour. It is essential to exclude cephalo-pelvic disproportion by careful clinical assessment. Further management should include:

1. Adequate pain relief with epidural anaesthesia
2. Adequate fluid replacement by intravenous infusion
3. Stimulation of coordinate labour using a dilute solution of oxytocin.

Case study
Primary dysfunctional labour

A 22-year-old primigravid was admitted in labour with regular, painful contractions. The cervix was found to be 2.5 cm dilated. Four hours later, the cervix was 4 cm dilated and the rate of dilatation was significantly delayed (Fig. 14.14). The membranes were artificially ruptured, and clear amniotic fluid released. Progress in labour continued to be slow, and 3 hours later a dilute syntocinon infusion was commenced. This resulted in rapid progress to full cervical dilatation and delivery vaginally some 2 hours later.

Other disorders of uterine action

Constriction ring dystocia

This is a rare complication of uterine action where one part of the uterus constricts in a ring around the fetus. It commonly results from intra-uterine manipulations such as attempted internal podalic version or from the use of oxytocic agents where there is an abnormal fetal lie.

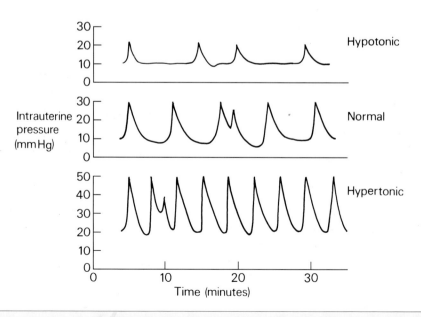

Fig. 14.13 Abnormalities of uterine action which commonly result in prolonged labour.

Case history: primary dysfunctional labour

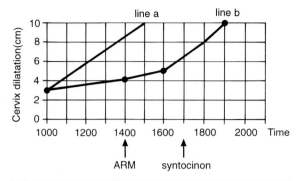

Fig. 14.14 Slow progress in the first stage of labour. The action time is line a, and line b is the actual cervical dilatation.

It is now a rare complication and can generally be reversed only with ether or halothane anaesthesia. It should not be confused with a retraction ring, which occurs as a ridge at the junction of the upper and lower uterine segments and is associated with obstructed labour.

Cervical dystocia

This rare cause of prolonged and obstructed labour is associated with various pathological conditions of the cervix. Factors that cause intensive scarring of the cervix, such as previous cautery or cone biopsy, may lead to a condition where the cervix will not dilate, despite intense uterine activity and, occasionally, this will result in spontaneous annular detachment of the cervix. However, when the condition is recognized, the labour should be terminated by Caesarean section.

TRIAL OF LABOUR AND CEPHALO-PELVIC DISPROPORTION

Every labour in a primigravida is, in a sense, a trial of labour. However, this term is reserved for the conduct of labour where borderline cephalo-pelvic disproportion is suspected. In many women, the only way in which the adequacy of the pelvis can be assessed is to allow the mother to labour and to carefully assess her progress.

Assessment of progress

This is achieved by assessing the rate of progress of cervical dilatation in relation to the normal cervico-gram or the nature of the uterine contractions, and the rate of descent of the fetal head. Uterine action is often ineffective in the presence of borderline cephalo-pelvic disproportion and it may be justifiable to employ a dilute oxytocin infusion to stimulate uterine activity.

The mother should be given intravenous fluids and no fluid or food orally. It is also important to ensure that there is adequate pain relief, which is best achieved with epidural anaesthesia. If cervical dilatation remains unchanged over a period of 6 hours, then the trial of labour should be concluded. Likewise, the trial of labour should also be terminated in the presence of fetal or maternal distress.

Case study
Secondary arrest (Fig. 14.15)

A 38-year-old multigravid woman was admitted in labour at term. After good initial progress in labour, significant arrest occurred at 8 cm dilatation. Vaginal examination confirmed the presence of the occipito-posterior position associated with relative cephalo-pelvic disproportion. The cervix eventually became fully dilated, and the fetal head was rotated and delivered with forceps. Delay in progress in a multi-parous patient should always be treated with caution as it is likely to be associated with malposition or cephalo-pelvic disproportion and there is a greater risk of uterine rupture with the injudicious use of oxytocic agents.

Case history: secondary arrest

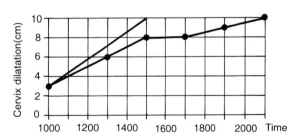

Fig. 14.15 Secondary arrest of cervical dilatation at 8 cm associated with the occipito-posterior position.

Causes of failure to progress

- Weak or incoordinate uterine activity
- Cervical dystocia
- Cephalo-pelvic disproportion
- Abnormal position

ABNORMALITIES OF THE THIRD STAGE OF LABOUR

The third stage of labour starts immediately after the delivery of the infant and ends with expulsion of the placenta. This is normally accomplished within 10–15 minutes and should be complete within 30 minutes.

Postpartum haemorrhage

Primary postpartum haemorrhage consists of blood loss from the vagina in excess of 500 ml and occurring within 24 hours of delivery (Fig. 14.16).

Secondary postpartum haemorrhage

This consists of excessive vaginal blood loss occurring at any subsequent time in the puerperium up to 6 weeks after delivery. Haemorrhage may occur from any part of the genital tract, but most commonly from the placental site as a result of (Fig. 14.17):

1. Uterine atony – if the uterus does not contract, then the decussation of myometrial fibres does not exert the usual haemostatic compression of the uterine vessels
2. Retention of the placenta or placental fragments.

A contracted empty uterus never bleeds.

> **Case study**
> **Primary post-partum haemorrhage**
>
> *A 37-year-old woman, para 5, was noted to have heavy bleeding following a normal delivery. The uterus was palpable abdominally above the umbilicus and was noted to be poorly contracted. On vaginal examination, 300 ml of clot was removed from the cervix and vagina, and uterine activity stimulated by rubbing the uterus and starting a Syntocinon infusion, after which the bleeding settled.*

Traumatic uterine haemorrhage

This may occur from cervical laceration, which commonly occurs at '3 o'clock' or '9 o'clock' positions, not anteriorly or posteriorly. It may also arise from uterine rupture and in particular, from rupture of a previous Caesarean scar.

Vaginal lacerations

Haemorrhage occurs from vaginal and perineal lacer-ations and this bleeding may be profuse – particularly when it involves vaginal or vulval varicosities.

> **Case study**
> **Postpartum haemorrhage from vaginal lacerations**
>
> *A 21-year-old woman delivered by rotational forceps was found to have steady, heavy vaginal bleeding following repair of her episiotomy. The uterus was felt to be well contracted and the bleeding did not respond to intravenous Syntocinon. Further bleeding required transfusion, and the patient was taken to theatre for examination under anaesthesia, when a laceration at the left vaginal fornix was repaired.*

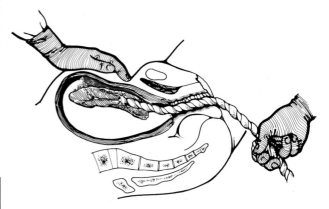

Fig. 14.16 Primary postpartum haemorrhage may occur in the presence of a retained placenta.

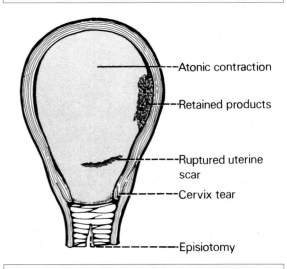

Atonic contraction

Retained products

Ruptured uterine scar

Cervix tear

Episiotomy

Fig. 14.17 Causes of postpartum haemorrhage.

Predisposing factors

Various factors predispose to postpartum haemorrhage, and these include:

1. Overdistension of the uterus, e.g. in multiple pregnancy, hydramnios
2. Uterine hypotonia associated with prolonged labour
3. Antepartum haemorrhage – placenta praevia
4. Multiple fibroids
5. Grand multiparity
6. General anaesthesia where agents such as halothane are employed.

Low implantation of the placenta appears to be associated with difficulties in efficient constriction of uterine blood vessels at the site of the implantation. Placental abruption is associated with an increased incidence of postpartum haemorrhage, partly because blood entrapped behind the placenta is expelled during the third stage but also because there may be difficulty with contractility in myometrium damaged by an antepartum haemorrhage. Occasionally haemorrhage may occur because of coagulation disorders.

Management

Postpartum bleeding may be sudden and profound and may rapidly lead to cardiovascular collapse. Treatment is directed towards controlling the bleeding and replacing the blood loss.

Controlling the haemorrhage – A brief visual inspection will suffice to ascertain:

1. The amount of blood loss
2. Whether the placenta has been expelled.

If the placenta has been expelled, the following actions are taken:

1. Palpate the uterine fundus. If the uterus is soft, then massage of the uterus will immediately stimulate a contraction and expel any retained clot.
2. Inject ergometrine maleate 0.5 mg intravenously and start an oxytocin infusion consisting of 10 units of Syntocinon in 500 ml of Hartman's solution. Although ergometrine has become less popular because of induced vomiting and raised blood pressure, it is still the most potent oxytocic agent available and should therefore be used as first choice in this situation.
3. Check that the placenta and membranes are complete. If they are not, then manual exploration of the uterine cavity is indicated.
4. If the bleeding continues despite the presence of a well-contracted uterus, the vagina and cervix

should be examined with a speculum under good illumination and any laceration sutured to ensure haemostasis.

If the placenta is retained:

1. Massage the uterus to ensure it is well contracted.
2. Apply cord traction and counter pressure against the uterine fundus. The placenta is partially separated and will often deliver with gentle but sustained cord traction as it may be trapped in the cervix.
3. If this manoeuvre fails, then proceed to manual removal of the placenta – with either regional or general anaesthesia.

If bleeding continues after deliver of the placenta and uterine exploration, and the uterus continues to be hypotonic despite physical and pharmacological measures to arrest the bleeding, it may be necessary to apply bimanual compression to the uterus as a first-aid measure. If this fails, it is necessary to proceed to hysterectomy.

There is no place for uterine packing – a technique that has been used in the past but is singularly ineffective.

Recently, the infusion of a solution of prostaglandin E_2 into the uterine cavity has been found to be an effective method of stimulating uterine contractions.

Replacement of blood loss and resuscitation – Although the healthy pregnant woman withstands sudden blood loss remarkably well, adequate replacement by transfusion is essential. Blood substitutes such as Haemacel can be safely used to replace up to 1500 ml blood loss, but thereafter a blood transfusion should be given.

Vaginal wall haematomas

Profuse haemorrhage does, at times, occur from vaginal and perineal lacerations and it is important to control this bleeding as soon as possible by suturing. Venous bleeding can be controlled by compression but arterial bleeding necessitates ligation of the vessel. If this is not achieved, then formation of haematomas will occur. These may be (Fig. 14.18):

1. Superficial – the perineum will be seen to bulge and distend and will be acutely painful. The sutures must be removed, the haematoma drained and haemostasis secured before closing the wound again with drainage.
2. Deep – blood loss may occur above the insertion of the levator ani and a large lateral vaginal wall

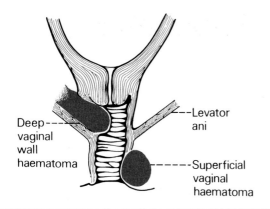

Fig. 14.18 The sites of vaginal wall haematomas.

Amniotic fluid embolism

This condition occurs around the time of delivery and results in cardiovascular and respiratory collapse. It is a rare condition occurring about once in 80 000 pregnancies but has a high mortality rate. Amniotic fluid enters the maternal circulation and causes sudden intravascular coagulation resulting in pulmonary insufficiency and a haemorrhagic diathesis.

The patient suddenly collapses with dyspnoea, cynanosis and hypotension. Treatment requires immediate oxygenation, monitoring of central venous pressure and adequate restoration of the circulating blood volume. Fresh frozen plasma is given if the fibrinogen level is low.

BIBLIOGRAPHY

Liggins G C, Howie R N 1972 A controlled trial of antepartum glucocoricoid treatment for prevention of respiratory distress syndrome in premature infants. Pediatrics 50: 515
Myerscough P R 1987 Munro Kerr's operative obstetrics. Baillière Tindall, London
Turnbull A, Chamberlain G V P 1989 Obstetrics. Churchill Livingstone, Edinburgh
Yu V Y H, Wood E C 1987 Prematurity. Churchill Livingstone, Edinburgh

haematoma may develop. This will not be visible externally but presents with continuing pelvic pain, unexplained anaemia and retention of urine. It can be readily recognized by pelvic examination, and must be drained by incision over the haematoma. It is usually very difficult to identify the bleeding point at this stage because extensive tissue damage occurs, but haemostasis should be attempted.

A large corrugated drain is inserted into the cavity and the vagina is packed. A catheter should be left indwelling and adequate blood transfusion and antibiotic therapy instituted.

Bleeding usually arises from a branch of the pudendal artery and may occur spontaneously after a normal vaginal delivery.

Postpartum haemorrhage

- May be primary or secondary
- Common causes are uterine atony, retained products, cervical or vaginal lacerations
- More likely in multiple gestation, prolonged labour, after antepartum haemorrhage (especially placenta praevia) and in grand multiparity
- Management consists of replacing loss, ensuring an empty well-contracted uterus, repair of lacerations and correction of abnormal clotting

---

15 Instrumental and operative delivery

Labour is induced when the risk to the mother or child of continuing the pregnancy exceeds the risks of inducing labour. The incidence of induction varies widely according to the practice of the obstetrician.

Indications

The major indications for induction of labour are:

1. Pre-eclampsia
2. Prolonged pregnancy (in excess of 42 weeks gestation)
3. Placental insufficiency and intra-uterine growth retardation
4. Antepartum haemorrhage – placental abruption and antepartum haemorrhage of uncertain origin
5. Rhesus isoimmunization
6. Diabetes mellitus
7. Chronic renal disease.

Prolonged pregnancy is defined as pregnancy exceeding 294 days from the first day of the last menstrual period in a woman with a 28 day menstrual cycle. The perinatal mortality rate doubles after 42 weeks and trebles after 43 weeks compared with 40 weeks gestation. However, routine induction of labour has minimal effect on the perinatal mortality rate. Conservative management of prolonged pregnancy involves frequent monitoring of the fetus with ultrasound assessment of liquor volume and induction if there is evidence of feto-placental compromise. However, many women request induction of labour on the basis of physical discomfort of the continuing pregnancy.

Methods of induction

The commonest method of inducing labour is by surgical rupture of fetal membranes.

Forewater rupture

Rupture of the membranes should be performed

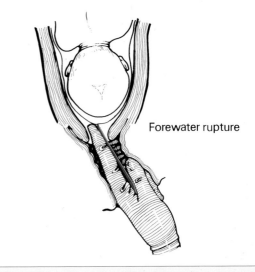

Forewater rupture

Fig. 15.1 Induction of labour by forewater rupture.

under conditions of full asepsis in the delivery suite. Under ideal circumstances, the cervix should be soft, effaced and at least 2 cm dilated. The head should be presenting by the vertex and should be engaged in the pelvis. In practice, these conditions are often not fulfilled, and the degree to which they are adhered depends on the urgency of the need to start labour. The mother is placed in the lithotomy position and, after swabbing and draping the vulva, a finger is introduced through the cervix, and the fetal membranes are separated from the lower segment – a process known as 'stripping the membranes'. The bulging membranes are then ruptured with Kocher's forceps, Gelder forewater amniotomy forceps or an amniotomy hook (Fig. 15.1). The amniotic fluid is released slowly, and care is taken to exclude presentation or prolapse of the cord. For purposes of monitoring the uterine activity and fetal heart rate, an intra-uterine catheter is inserted and a scalp electrode is attached.

Hindwater rupture

An alternative method of surgical induction involves

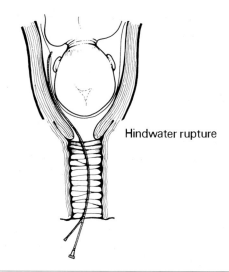

Fig. 15.2 Induction of labour by hindwater rupture.

rupture of the membranes behind the presenting part. This is known as hindwater rupture. A sigmoid-shaped metal cannula known as the Drewe–Smythe catheter is introduced through the cervix and penetrates the membranes behind the presenting part (Fig. 15.2). The theoretical advantage of this technique is that it reduces the risk of prolapsed cord. In reality, the risk is even lower with forewater rupture than with spontaneous rupture of the membranes and the technique of hindwater rupture is now rarely used.

Medical induction of labour

Various pharmacological agents can be used to stimulate uterine activity.

Oxytocin infusion – It is common practice to combine surgical induction with a Syntocinon infusion. A suitable regimen would begin at 1 mU/min and increase by 3 mU/min every 15 minutes until adequate contractions become established.

The hazards of induction

The principal hazards of combined surgical and medical induction of labour are:

1. *Hyperstimulation* – Excessive and prolonged uterine contractions reduce uterine blood flow and result in fetal asphyxia. Thus, contractions should not occur more frequently than every 2 minutes and should not last in excess of 1 minute. The Syntocinon infusion should be discontinued if

excessive uterine activity occurs or if there are signs of fetal distress.
2. *Prolapse of the cord* – This should be excluded by examination at the time of forewater rupture or subsequently if signs of fetal distress occur.
3. *Infection* – Prolonged induction–delivery intervals increase the risk of infection in the amniotic sac with consequent risks to both infant and mother. If the liquor becomes offensive and maternal pyrexia occurs, then the labour should be terminated and the infant delivered.

Cervical assessment

Clinical assessment of the cervix enables prediction of the likely outcome of induction of labour. The most commonly used method of assessment is the Bishop score (Table 15.1). This score involves clinical examination of the cervix.

A score of over 6 is strongly predictive of vaginal delivery following induction. A score of below 5 indicates the need for cervical ripening.

Medical induction of labour and cervical ripening

Medical induction is indicated where the cervix is unsuitable for surgical induction. The two most commonly used forms of medical induction are:

1. Syntocinon infusion
2. Administration of prostaglandins by various routes.

Syntocinon infusion – This induces uterine contractions but is a relatively ineffective method of inducing labour unless combined with surgical induction.

Prostaglandins – The most widely used form is prostaglandin E_2 (Prostin). This is used to ripen the cervix and may be administered:

1. Orally – tablets of 0.5 mg taken orally are increased to 2 mg/h until contractions are produced.
2. As an extra-amniotic infusion of prostaglandin E_2 – introduced via a catheter into the extra-amniotic

Table 15.1 Bishop's score			
Score	*0*	*1*	*2*
Consistency	Firm	Medium	Soft
Position	Posterior	Mid	Anterior
Dilatation	0	1–2 cm	3–4 cm
Length	3 cm	2 cm	–
Station	<–3	<–2	–1

space at a dose of 1 mg/min increasing to 4 mg/min until contractions are established. The advantage of this technique is that it produces minimal side effects of vomiting and diarrhoea.

3. As an intravenous infusion – this is now rarely used because of the severity of side effects and because it often causes thrombophlebitis at the injection site.

Cervical ripening can be achieved using vaginal pessaries of prostaglandin E$_2$ or by a xylose gel suspension in the vagina.

Induction of labour

- Common indications are pre-eclampsia, postmaturity, intra-uterine growth retardation, antepartum haemorrhage, rhesus disease and diabetes
- Can be performed by rupture of membranes, oxytocin infusion or vaginal prostaglandins
- Hazards are hypertonus, cord prolapse and infection

INSTRUMENTAL DELIVERY

Obstetric forceps were first introduced in the 17th century by the Chamberlain family, and have been modified and adapted in various forms. Forceps consist of a pair of fenestrated blades with a handle connected to the blades by a shank (Fig. 15.3). The blades normally exhibit both a pelvic and cephalic curve so that they can adapt both to the fetal skull and to the maternal sacral curve. The instruments are designed for application only to the fetal head and not to the buttocks.

Indications

The common indications for forceps delivery are:

1. Delay in the second stage of labour. This occurs most frequently as a result of pelvic floor resistance and a tight perineum. It may, however, also be caused by:
   a. Poor maternal expulsive efforts
   b. Cephalo-pelvic disproportion
   c. Malposition or malpresentation of the head
   d. Removal of the urge to bear down during epidural anaesthesia.
2. Fetal distress.
3. Maternal distress and maternal conditions necessitating minimal expulsive effort from the mother.
4. Forceps are applied to the after-coming head in a breech presentation and may also be used to extract the fetal head at Caesarean section.

Prerequisites to forceps delivery

When there is an indication for forceps delivery, the mother should be placed in the lithotomy position, and the thighs and perineum cleaned and draped. It is then important to check:

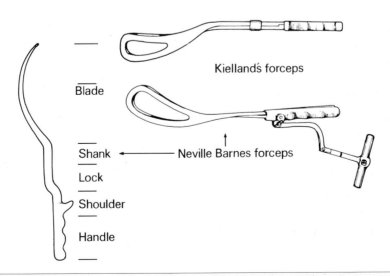

Fig. 15.3 Forceps parts (left) and commonly used forceps (right); the absence of the pelvic curve in Kielland's forceps enables rotation of the fetal head.

1. That the cervix is fully dilated.
2. That the bladder is not overdistended and requiring catheterization.
3. The position, presentation and status of the fetal head; it must be engaged and not palpable in the abdominal cavity.

Anaesthesia

This is commonly achieved with regional anaesthesia – epidural, spinal, sacral block or pudendal nerve block. On some occasions, general anaesthesia may be indicated.

Method of delivery

Low forceps (outlet forceps)

If the head is direct occipito-anterior in position, below the level of the ischial spine, and resting on the pelvic floor, low forceps delivery is performed (Fig. 15.4).

The forceps used where no rotation of the head is required are:

1. **Neville Barnes forceps** – this has an axis traction handle, which allows considerable force to be applied. This attachment is now rarely used.
2. **Simpson's forceps** – this is similar to the Neville Barnes forceps but with no axis traction handle.

Both these forceps have cephalic and pelvic curves.

The two blades of the forceps are designated according to the side of the pelvis to which they are applied. Thus, the left blade is applied to the left side

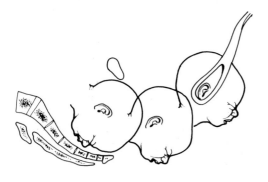

Low forceps delivery

Fig. 15.4 Low forceps delivery: traction is applied in line with the axis of the pelvis, and delivery is effected by lifting the head anteriorly once the occiput has passed beneath the subpubic arch.

of the pelvis. There is a fixed lock between the blades. Intermittent traction is applied in the direction of the pelvic canal until the occiput is on view and then the head is delivered by anterior extension. An episiotomy is usually, although not invariably, performed.

Mid-cavity forceps

Arrest of the head sometimes occurs in the mid-cavity when the presenting part reaches the level of the ischial spine. At this level, the position of the head is usually transverse or posterior.

The position of the head must first be corrected, by either manual rotation or forceps rotation, to a direct antero-posterior position before application of traction.

Kielland's forceps has a sliding lock and minimal pelvic curve so that rotation of the forceps will not lead to damage by the blades during the process of rotation.

High forceps

This type of delivery, where the head lies well above the level of the ischial spines, is very rarely performed. In fact, if the head can be palpated above the pelvic brim, this is a contraindication to vaginal delivery.

Trial of forceps

Occasionally, a situation arises where there is borderline disproportion, and this is an indication for a trial of forceps. This should be attempted only where there is a high expectation that vaginal delivery will be achieved without significant trauma to the mother or fetus.

A trial of forceps delivery should always be undertaken in an operating theatre with preparation made to proceed to Caesarean section.

Careful assessment of the pelvis and presenting part should be made before proceeding to apply the forceps blades. If firm traction does not produce steady descent of the head, then the blades should be removed and the child delivered by Caesarean section. It may be necessary to disimpact the head vaginally before section.

VACUUM EXTRACTION (VENTOUSE)

An alternative to forceps delivery is the application of a suction cup to the fetal scalp and extraction by

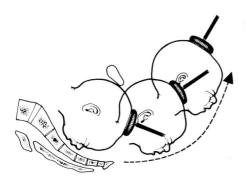

Ventouse extraction

Fig. 15.5 Ventouse extraction: the suction cup is attached by raising the 'chignon' on the fetal scalp.

traction (Fig. 15.5). The indications for vacuum extraction are the same as those for forceps delivery. The metal suction cups of the vacuum extractor are of three different sizes – 30, 40 and 50 mm. The vacuum inside the cup is slowly increased to $0.8 \, kg/cm^2$, and the scalp forms a 'chignon' inside the cup. Traction is applied with the contractions, and rotation of the head will generally occur as the head is pulled on to the pelvic floor.

Laceration of the scalp and caput or haematoma formation may occur with this procedure but the instrument rarely causes any maternal damage. Forceps, if incorrectly applied, may result in considerable maternal laceration, such as uterine and bladder or bowel damage. Fetal damage may involve facial bruising, facial nerve damage, skin abrasions and intracranial haemorrhage.

Instrumental delivery

- Common indications are delay in second stage, fetal distress, after-coming head in breech
- Prerequisites are full dilatation, empty bladder, head engaged and occipito-anterior position (for low forceps)
- Complications include laceration or bruising of scalp, facial nerve palsy and intracranial haemorrhage in fetus and vaginal laceration, fistula formation and uterine rupture in mother

---

CAESAREAN SECTION

This operation is the process whereby the child is removed from the uterus by direct incision through the abdominal wall and the uterus.

Lower segment Caesarean section

The most commonly performed procedure is the **lower segment Caesarean section**, where the bladder is reflected from the lower segment and a transverse incision is made (Fig. 15.6). The presenting part is then delivered through the lower segment. The wound is closed in two layers, taking care to exclude the decidua (Fig. 15.7).

The upper segment or classical Caesarean section

In this procedure, a vertical incision is made in the upper segment of the uterus, and the child is delivered through this incision (Fig. 15.8). This is not widely used because it has a much higher

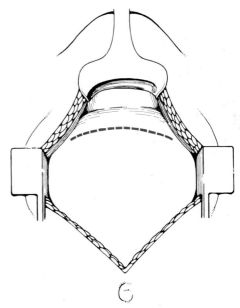

Lower segment incision

Fig. 15.6 Lower uterine segment Caesarean section: the bladder is reflected and a transverse incision is made in the lower segment.

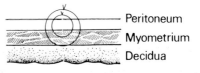

Peritoneum
Myometrium
Decidua

Fig. 15.7 Closure of the uterine wound in layers.

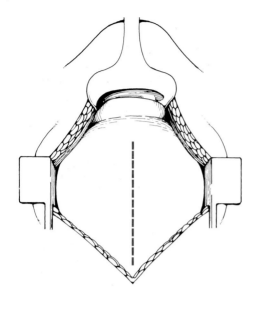

Upper segment incision

Fig. 15.8 'Classical' Caesarean section: a vertical incision is made in the upper uterine segment.

morbidity postoperatively, and a much higher incidence of subsequent rupture of the scar.

Caesarean hysterectomy

Caesarean section and hysterectomy are sometimes performed at the same time – where there is uterine rupture, uncontrollable postpartum haemorrhage and, occasionally, cervical malignant disease.

Indications for Caesarean section

It is not particularly helpful to state an incidence figure for Caesarean section because it varies widely from country to country. In the UK, it is about 15%, and the vast majority of the procedures are performed by the lower segment technique. The common indications for Caesarean section are:

1. Obstructed labour
2. Placenta praevia and antepartum haemorrhage
3. Fetal distress
4. Severe pre-eclampsia
5. Intra-uterine growth retardation and placental failure
6. Breech presentation and other malpresentations
7. Failed induction – prolonged labour

8. Diabetes mellitus
9. Prolapsed cord
10. Other rare indications such as cervical dystocia.

The rise in the Caesarean section rate over the last 20 years has led to a reassessment of the old dictum 'once a section always a section'. In those women with a non-recurrent indication for repeat Caesarean section, a vaginal delivery rate of 50–70% can be anticipated. The major concern is the risk of rupture of the uterine scar, although the risk is only 1%. The risk is higher where delivery has been effected by a classical upper uterine segment incision, and the rupture tends to occur before the onset of labour.

The decision to allow labour to proceed after a previous Caesarean section must take into account the indication for the original Caesarean section, the presentation and size of the present baby and the wishes of the mother. It is important that any woman who has a uterine scar should be delivered where there is ready access to an operating theatre. Blood should be taken for cross-matching, and all labours should be monitored. Signs of impending or actual scar dehiscence or rupture include pain over the scar, maternal tachycardia, fetal distress, incoordinate uterine activity, vaginal bleeding and collapse.

Complications

The immediate complications are those of haemorrhage, shock and the complications of anaesthesia. There may also be damage to the bladder or ureters. Rarely, the fetus may sustain lacerations during the incision of the uterus. Late complications include:

1. Secondary postpartum haemorrhage
2. Infection – uterine, vesical and wound
3. Pulmonary embolus
4. Deep vein thrombosis.

Caesarean section

- 15% of deliveries in UK
- Commonest indication is previous Caesarean section
- Usually transverse lower segment incision
- Complications include secondary postpartum haemorrhage, infection and thrombo-embolism

---

SHOULDER DYSTOCIA

Shoulder impaction occurs where there is a large infant or a small pelvis and particularly where the

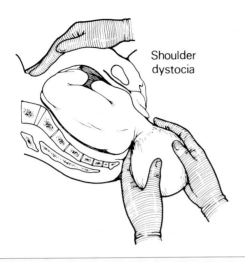

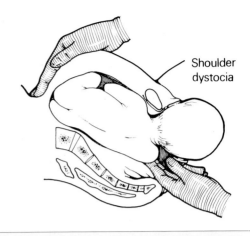

Fig. 15.10   Impacted shoulders: it is sometimes necessary to rotate the fetus to disimpact the posterior shoulder.

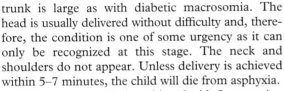

Fig. 15.9   Disimpaction of the anterior shoulder.

trunk is large as with diabetic macrosomia. The head is usually delivered without difficulty and, therefore, the condition is one of some urgency as it can only be recognized at this stage. The neck and shoulders do not appear. Unless delivery is achieved within 5–7 minutes, the child will die from asphyxia.

Delivery can usually be achieved with firm traction posteriorly to disimpact the anterior shoulder (Fig. 15.9) and then with traction anteriorly to deliver the posterior shoulder (Fig. 15.10). Firm downward pressure should be applied abdominally to the uterine fundus. The danger of this procedure is that excessive traction on the brachial plexus results in Erb's palsy.

Occasionally, the shoulders are disimpacted by rotation through 45° so that either the anterior or posterior shoulder may be disengaged.

Shoulder dystocia should be anticipated where the estimated fetal weight is over 5 kg, where there is evidence of macrosomia or where there is a history of previous dystocia. Such patients should be delivered where experienced obstetric and paediatric support is readily available.

BIBLIOGRAPHY

Bishop E H 1964 Pelvic scanning for elective induction. Obstetrics and Gynecology 24: 266–268
Pesso C 1994 Vaginal birth after Caesarean section. Current Opinion in Obstetrics and Gynecology 6: 417–425
Quilligan E J, Zuspan F P 1982 Douglas–Stromme operative obstetrics. Appleton-Century-Crofts, New York

16 The puerperium

The puerperium is defined as the 6 week period from the completion of the third stage of labour. During this time major physiological changes occur with the adaption of the mother to breast feeding and the return to the non-pregnant state of the various body systems.

PHYSIOLOGICAL CHANGES

Genital tract

The uterus undergoes rapid and massive change by a process of catabolism of muscle fibres. The fibres undergo autolysis and atrophy. Within 10 days, the uterus has involuted from a size where it is palpable at the umbilicus to one where it is no longer palpable as an abdominal organ (Fig. 16.1). By 6 weeks, the uterus has returned to the non-pregnant size. Where breast feeding is established, uterine involution may proceed to a level where the size is actually less than the usual non-pregnant

state. The endometrium regenerates within 6 weeks, and menstruation occurs within this time if lactation has ceased. If lactation continues, the return of menstruation may be deferred for 6 months or more.

Discharge from the uterus is known as **lochia**. At first this consists of blood, either fresh or altered, is called *lochia rubra*, and lasts from 2 to 14 days. It then changes to a serous discharge, *lochia serosa*, and finally becomes a slight white discharge, *lochia alba*. These changes may continue for up to 4–8 weeks after delivery. Abnormal persistence of lochia rubra may indicate retained placental tissue.

Cardiovascular system

Cardiac output and plasma volume return to normal within approximately 1 week. There is a fluid loss of 2 litres during the first week and a further loss of 1.5 litres over the next 5 weeks. This loss is associated with an apparent increase in haematocrit and haemoglobin concentration. There is an increase of serum sodium and plasma bicarbonate as well as plasma osmolality. An increase in clotting factors during the first 10 days after delivery is associated with a higher risk of deep vein thrombosis and pulmonary embolism. There is also a rise in platelet count and greater platelet adhesiveness. Fibrinogen levels decrease during labour, but increase in the puerperium.

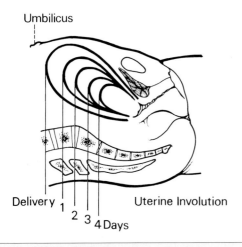

Umbilicus

Delivery
Uterine Involution
1 2 3 4 Days

Fig. 16.1 Uterine involution in the puerperium results in a rapid reduction in uterine size.

LACTATION AND BREAST FEEDING

Breast feeding is the preferred method of infant feeding because, in addition to fulfilling nutritional requirements, it also provides antibodies against infection and protection against various forms of gastro-enteritis associated with unhygienic preparation of artificial feeds. Women tend to avoid breast feeding for social and emotional reasons, and often for reasons of convenience. In a relatively small percentage of cases, there are physical reasons why lactation either is not possible or is inappropriate, such as inverted nipples, previous breast surgery, breast implants or cracked and painful nipples that do not respond to treatment.

Whilst breast feeding is desirable and women should be encouraged, it must be remembered that the majority of infants who are artificially fed also thrive. In other words, the enthusiasm of the attendants should not be allowed to override the mother's wishes. Encouragement and education in antenatal classes are important factors, but many women simply do not like the idea of breast feeding.

Breast preparation

The breasts and nipples should be washed regularly. The breasts should be comfortably supported and the nipples cleared of colostrum. Aqueous-based emollient creams may be used to soften the nipple and thus avoid cracking during suckling. Occasional expression of colostrum in the third trimester helps with subsequent milk secretion. Inverted nipples may present an insuperable barrier to breast feeding, and should be treated antenatally by the application of Waller's shields, which apply pressure to the areola and breast tissue surrounding the nipple (Fig. 16.2). These shields are worn inside the breast support for increasing lengths of time during the day.

Breast feeding

The child should be put to the breast as soon after delivery as possible. Suckling is initially limited to 2–3 minutes on each side, but subsequently this period may be increased. Once the mother

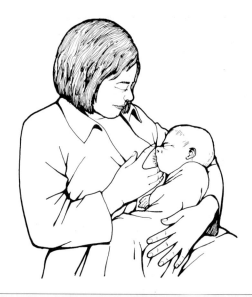

Fig. 16.3 The mother should be comfortable and the child placed well on to the breast to ensure adequate suckling.

is comfortably seated, the whole nipple is placed in the infant's mouth, taking care to maintain a clear airway (Fig. 16.3). After suckling, the child is held upright to enable swallowed air to be regurgitated.

Full milk flow supervenes by the third or fourth day after delivery, and may be accompanied by painful vascular engorgement.

Suppression of lactation

Many women elect not to breast feed. Firm support of the breasts, restriction of fluid intake, avoidance of expression of milk and analgesia may be sufficient to suppress lactation. The administration of oestrogens will effectively suppress lactation, but carries some risk of thrombo-embolic disease. It should, however, be noted that the original description of 'risk' was based on observation of doses of oestrogens far in excess of the quantities necessary to suppress lactation. There is, therefore, a case to be made for administering oral oestrogens to suppress lactation. Bromocriptine will inhibit prolactin release and hence suppress lactation, but the dosage necessary to produce this effect tends to create considerable side effects. It should, however, be emphasized that it is preferable to avoid all drug therapy if suppression can be achieved by conservative management.

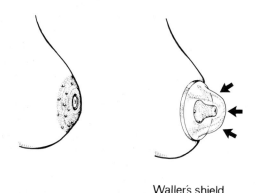

Waller's shield

Fig. 16.2 Inverted or flat nipples (left) may be enhanced by the application of Waller's shields (right).

> **Physiological changes in the puerperium**
>
> - Uterus involutes
> - Regeneration of endometrium
> - Reduced bladder sensitivity to over-distension
> - Increased coagulability
> - Fall in plasma volume

PSYCHOLOGICAL CHANGES AND DISORDERS IN THE PUERPERIUM

Mild degrees of depression and emotional liability are almost the 'norm' in the puerperium, but may become severe in some cases and require psychiatric support. Psychiatric illness may present as severe, incapacitating depression, but the more florid forms of puerperal psychosis involve confusion and delirium with disorientation in time and space, and a complete loss of interest in the child. In some women, frank mania may occur. Early recognition of these symptoms is important if danger to mother and child is to be avoided, and early psychiatric support must be sought. These problems are discussed in greater detail in a separate chapter.

COMPLICATIONS OF THE PUERPERIUM

Puerperal pyrexia

The commonest problem of the puerperium is the development of a pyrexia, i.e. a rise of temperature in excess of 38°C.

Aetiology

Puerperal pyrexia must be assumed to be due to infection until proved otherwise. A systematic investigation is undertaken to elucidate the cause and site of the infection (Fig. 16.4).

1. Genital tract infection – The genital tract is particularly vulnerable to infection. The commonest site is within the uterine cavity; infection may be introduced via external sources or arise from contamination from endogenous sources. Infection is particularly common following prolonged labour or prolonged rupture of the membranes.

The clinical signs include subinvolution of the uterus, which remains bulky and larger than would normally be anticipated. The uterus is often tender to palpation. The lochia may be offensive or puru-

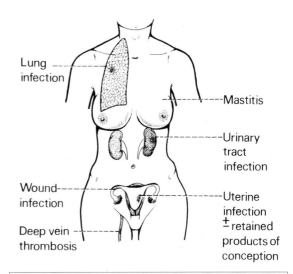

Fig. 16.4 The pathogenesis of puerperal pyrexia.

lent, but is often normal. Retained products of conception predispose to infection and will also result in excessive and persistent blood-stained lochia. A cervical swab should be taken for culture as a routine procedure in any women with puerperal pyrexia. The common organisms isolated from this site include *Escherichia coli*, *Staphylococcus pyogenes*, *Streptococcus faecalis* and *haemolytic streptococcus*.

Infection may also occur in episiotomy wounds of perineal tears, although these infections are relatively uncommon because the vascularity of the perineum provides a higher resistance to infection. The perineum becomes tender and reddened and may be seen to exude purulent discharge. Where genital tract infection is suspected, swabs should be taken for culture, and antibiotic therapy started before the culture results are available.

2. Urinary tract infection – The postpartum woman is particularly vulnerable to urinary tract infection. This is due to a combination of trauma to the bladder, incomplete emptying, particularly related to perineal pain, and the introduction of bacterial organisms by catheterization.

Urinary tract infection is often unaccompanied by any symptoms, with the exception of a low-grade pyrexia, but if ascending infection supervenes, then acute pyelonephritis may develop. This will produce bilateral loin pain, frequency of micturition and dysuria and lower abdominal pain after voiding. In cases of puerperal pyrexia, a midstream specimen of urine should be sent for culture.

3. Breast infection – Mastitis most often occurs in the second week after delivery and, therefore, may develop after discharge from hospital. Infection may be introduced through a cracked nipple, and often originates from the mother's skin or nasopharynx or from the infant's nasopharynx.

4. Other sites of infection – Following Caesarean section, infection may occur in the skin wound or in the peritoneal cavity. Where general anaesthesia is used, lung infection may occur although, with modern anaesthesia, this is an uncommon complication.

Signs and symptoms

The development of pyrexia is accompanied by pain and local tenderness. The breast develops a reddened, tender area and, if abscess formation occurs, the skin becomes oedematous and develops the classical 'peau d'orange' appearance.

Early recognition of infection enables early introduction of antibiotic therapy. If abscess formation occurs, then surgical drainage is necessary.

If the mother is still lactating, feeding is discontinued from the affected breast. In most cases, lactation should be suppressed unless there is strong motivation to continue.

Thrombo-embolic disease

Thrombophlebitis

This is the commonest form of thrombo-embolic disease and tends to arise within the first 3 or 4 days after delivery. Localized inflammation, tenderness and thickening occur in the superficial leg veins. Although the condition is painful and may spread along the leg veins, it rarely leads to serious embolic disease and does not require anticoagulant treatment. Anti-inflammatory drugs and local applications of glycerine and icthyol should be used.

Phlebothrombosis

Deep vein thrombosis is a much more serious complication which tends to arise 7–10 days after delivery, and is particularly likely to occur after operative delivery or prolonged immobilization. Clotting occurring in deep veins may be silent, and presents only when the clot breaks loose and lodges in the lung as a pulmonary embolus, with consequent chest pain and haemoptysis. Massive pulmonary embolus results in sudden death unless treated by prompt surgical management.

Management of phlebothrombosis – As soon as the diagnosis is established, anticoagulant treatment should be started with intravenous heparin. The limb should be rested until the anticoagulant therapy produces pain relief; then gradual mobilization may be introduced. When the acute process has been controlled, the anticoagulant therapy can be changed to warfarin and should be continued for 3 months. Specialized leg supports such as TED stockings are used to provide support for the affected leg.

Other complications of the puerperium

Urinary retention is a common problem in the immediate puerperium, and may result in overflow incontinence. The major cause of retention is pain from the perineum. Traditional methods of encouraging micturition include hot baths, relief of perineal pain by analgesic drugs and local applications of ice-packs. If these procedures fail, then the bladder should be catheterized on an intermittent basis until the residual urine is less than 50 ml.

True incontinence is a rare complication and is usually associated with a vesico-vaginal fistula resulting from pressure necrosis during obstructed labour, or following direct injury to the bladder. Injection of a coloured dye into the bladder will establish the diagnosis. A catheter is left indwelling until there is evidence of closure of the fistula or surgical repair is undertaken.

Faecal incontinence may occur following a third degree tear where a recto-vaginal fistula is present. Correct repair of the original tear with proper separation of tissue layers should avoid this complication. Surgical closure is necessary, but repair is delayed until the wound area is clear. Some faecal incontinence may occur where the external anal sphincter is damaged.

Complications of the puerperium

- Genital tract infections
- Urinary infection
- Wound infection
- Mastitis
- Thrombo-embolism
- Incontinence/urinary retention

BIBLIOGRAPHY

Ledward R, Cruikshank S H 1995 Drug treatment in obstetrics and gynaecology. ISIS
Ledward R S, Hawkins D F 1983 Drugs and breast feeding. In: Ledward R S, Hawkins D F (eds) Drug treatment in obstetrics. Chapman and Hall, London

17 Psychiatric disorders in childbirth

M. R. Oates

THE IMPORTANCE OF PSYCHIATRY IN OBSTETRICS

1. There is a substantial psychiatric morbidity associated with children

Childbirth contributes a substantial risk to the mental health of women. For women who were previously well, their risk of being admitted to a psychiatric hospital, being referred to a psychiatrist, of suffering from a psychotic illness or from a severe depressive illness in the year *following childbirth* is greatly elevated over their lifetime risk and much greater than for other women or men (Fig. 17.1). At least 10% of all women delivered will suffer from a depressive illness severe enough to meet the criteria for a major depressive illness. If less severe cases are included, then the incidence of postnatal depression is even higher, between 15 and 20% of all deliveries. Approximately 3–5% of all women delivered will meet the criteria for moderate to severe depressive illness (of a type that requires antidepressant medication). Just under 2% of all women delivered will be referred to a psychiatrist in the postpartum year. Four per 1000 deliveries will be admitted to a psychiatric hospital, of whom half (2 per 1000) will be suffering from a psychotic illness. Over 80% of these women will be suffering from their first ever psychiatric illness, but 20% will have had a previous postpartum illness or a non-childbirth-related psychiatric disorder. For women with an existing psychiatric disorder, childbirth poses a predictable risk of relapse for those with chronic disability or concerns about their ability to care for their child.

Importance of psychiatry

- Substantial morbidity
- Effective treatment
- Adverse consequences
- Predict risk
- Regular medical contact
- Prevention

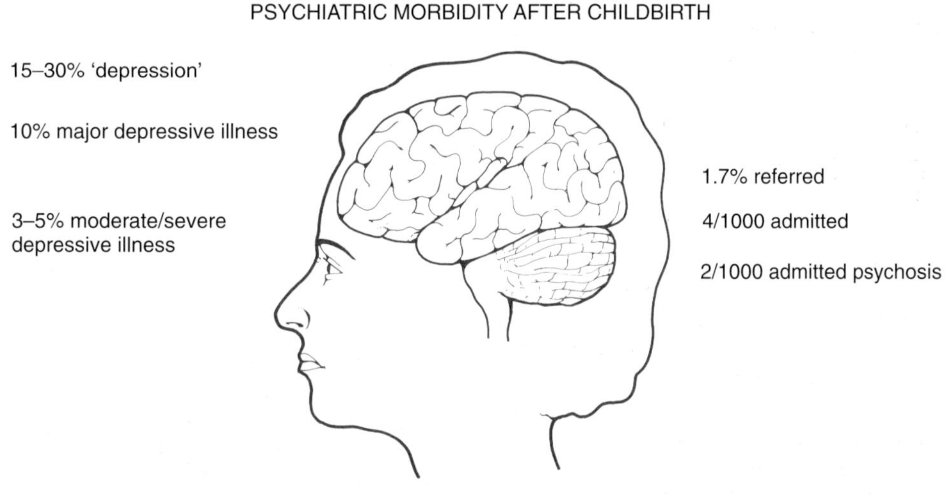

PSYCHIATRIC MORBIDITY AFTER CHILDBIRTH

15–30% 'depression'

10% major depressive illness

3–5% moderate/severe depressive illness

1.7% referred

4/1000 admitted

2/1000 admitted psychosis

Fig. 17.1 The incidence of psychiatric morbidity after childbirth.

In contrast to the increased risk of serious psychiatric disorder following childbirth, a woman is less likely to be seriously mentally ill, to be referred to a psychiatrist, to take an overdose, commit suicide or be admitted to a psychiatric hospital *during pregnancy*. However, a significant *minority* of women do become mentally ill during pregnancy (15% in the first trimester, 8% in the second and 5% in the third). The majority of these conditions are not serious and will resolve as the pregnancy progresses; and some will not have implications for the mental health of those women after delivery. Women may also present at the booking clinic currently well but who have past histories of psychiatric disorder and are concerned about the effect that childbirth might have upon their mental health. The obstetrician will also be required to manage women who have become pregnant whilst suffering from a mental illness and receiving treatment. Thus, a substantial minority of patients seen by obstetricians and the maternity services (between 15 and 20% of all patients) will have mental health problems which have to be taken into account in their management.

2. Treatment is effective

For those mothers becoming ill for the first time following childbirth, the diagnosis is likely to be that of a variant of an affective disorder. These range in severity from the most severe and rarest *puerperal psychosis* (a form of manic depressive or bipolar disorder) through *severe depressive illness* to less severe and milder forms of *depression*. Effective treatments are available for all of these conditions. There is evidence to suggest that postpartum affective disorder is particularly sensitive to treatment, has a shorter illness duration and better lifetime prognosis. Approximately half of these women will become ill following a subsequent childbirth.

3. Untreated there can be major adverse sequelae

Although the majority of these illnesses are self-limiting and will recover by 6 months postpartum, 30% of women are still ill at 1 year postpartum and over 10% at 2 year postpartum. Long-standing postnatal depressive illness affects mother–infant attachment and relationships and interferes with the social and cognitive development of children. Such adverse effects can be detected beyond the resolution of the mother's illness up to the age of 5 to 7 years old. These effects are particularly marked in boys

and when combined with social and marital adversity. Prolonged postnatal mental illness may also lead to the breakdown of marriages. These adverse consequences of postnatal mental illness underline the importance of early detection and vigorous treatment. Psychiatric morbidity and hazard to mother and infant may be reduced to a minimum by speedy diagnosis and referral for treatment by obstetricians, midwives and general practitioners.

Adverse sequelae of postnatal depression

- Immediate:
  - Physical morbidity
  - Suicide/infanticide
  - Prolonged psychiatric morbidity
  - Social attachments mother–infant
  - Emotional development
- Later:
  - Social–cognitive affects child
  - Psychiatric morbidity child
  - Marital breakdown

---

4. It is sometimes possible to predict risk

It is now known that well women with a *family history* of serious affective disorder are at a 1 in 3 risk of developing such an illness following childbirth. Women with a *previous history* of postnatal depression or puerperal psychosis are at a 1 in 2 risk of developing such a condition following every subsequent childbirth. The illness is likely to present at about the same time as before, thus allowing the woman's medical attendants and family to be aware of the necessary period of vigilance. Women with a previous history of non-postpartum affective disorder are also at increased risk of becoming ill following childbirth. If the illness was manic–depressive (bipolar) the risk is also 1 in 2. If the illness was a non-psychotic depressive illness or other neurotic condition the risk is also elevated, and is thought to lie between 1 in 5 and 1 in 3. Women with chronic schizophrenia may not be at a particularly elevated risk of relapse, either during pregnancy or during the early postpartum period, but may face later problems with the stresses of child-rearing.

Risk factors for serious mental illness

- Primiparity
- Past psychiatric history
- Family psychiatric history

Some of the risk factors for a primiparous woman developing a mild postnatal depressive illness are also known. However, they are less specific or useful in predicting individuals at risk, more for identifying a vulnerable population. They include such factors as previous psychiatric history, youth, being single, prior social services involvement, antenatal admission for non-obstetric reasons and ambivalence about the pregnancy.

Risk factors for mild postnatal depression

- Single
- Young
- Short interval
- Early deprivation
- Chronic life difficulties
- Society adversity trend
- Lack of confidante
- Past psychiatric history
- Question TOP index pregnancy
- Antenatal admission, non-serious conditions
- Life events
- Prior social services involvement

---

5. Structured contact with maternity and primary health care services

Pregnant and postpartum women are in frequent and regular contact with medical services. With a little modification these contact points could be modified so that risk factors for developing illnesses could be identified at the booking clinic and during the pregnancy. The postnatal check at 6 weeks could be modified to include screening for all women for postnatal depression, early identification and prompt treatment.

6. Prevention

For the small minority of women with predictable risk factors, particularly those who have had a previous postpartum illness or serious mental illness, an exciting opportunity exists for prevention, both psychological and pharmacological interventions. Secondary prevention is a reality now in screening, early detection and prompt treatment. Primary prevention is also a possibility.

CLINICAL SYNDROMES

The majority of women who have become mentally ill following childbirth will have been well previously ('a new episode'). Most of these women will be suffering from their first ever mental illness ('lifetime first episode'). However, some women have had previous postpartum illness or an illness at another time in their life and have recovered from it. The overwhelming majority of these 'new' illnesses are affective or mood disorders which vary in severity from the mildest, minor postnatal depression through to moderate to severe postnatal depression to the most severe form, puerperal psychosis – a variant of manic–depressive or bipolar disorder.

The problems faced by women with enduring mental health problems who become pregnant can usually be identified before conception or during the pregnancy, and require a special approach. These are considered later in the chapter.

The risk of developing a new episode of mental illness (usually affective disorder) following childbirth is substantial and is elevated over lifetime risk. Women run a 16-fold increased risk of being admitted to a psychiatric hospital suffering from puerperal psychosis, a 10-fold increase in risk suffering from a severe depressive illness, a fivefold increase of risk of suffering from non-psychotic postnatal depression and of being referred to a psychiatrist.

Postpartum (puerperal) psychosis
(Fig. 17.2)

This is a severe form of affective psychosis (manic–depressive or bipolar illness). Up to one-third of these patients are manic, and two-thirds are suffering from a depressive psychosis. The onset is very abrupt, rarely before the third postpartum day, the most common day of onset being day 5. They therefore need to be carefully distinguished from the 'blues', which will be experienced by over half of all women. The 'blues' will settle, usually within 24 hours. Postpartum psychoses will rapidly deteriorate. The majority of postpartum psychoses will have presented before the 16th postpartum day. In the first few days these abrupt onset psychoses take the form of an acute undifferentiated illness, hallmarked by restless agitation, perplexity, confusion, fear and suspicion, insomnia, not eating or drinking and rapidly forming delusional ideas about themselves and their babies. After 3–5 days, the illness becomes more clearly that of a manic or depressive psychosis. However, many of these women will also experience first-rank symptoms of schizophrenia with frightening hallucinations and delusions, so that the diagnosis is often that of a schizo-affective psychosis. Despite this, and the fact that they are very seriously disturbed, it is important to

PUERPERAL PSYCHOSIS

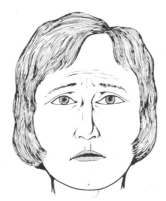

Risk factors:
  family/personal history
  Caesarean section

Abrupt onset 80% 3–14 days

Rapidly changing clinical picture

Delire triste

99% manic depressive/
  schizo-affective

Good prognosis

Treatment issues:
  admission with baby

Vigorous treatment

Risk 1:2 next baby

Fig. 17.2 Risk factors, presentation and treatment in puerperal psychosis.

remember that the treatment and prognosis is that of an affective psychosis and that the majority of these patients will recover quickly and fully, although the risk after subsequent childbirth is 1 in 2.

Management

The patient should be referred urgently to a psychiatrist, and will usually require admission to a psychiatric unit. If possible, this should take place in a specialized setting where the mother and her infant can be managed together – a psychiatric mother and baby unit. The immediate priority will be to sedate the patient with neuroleptic medication to a level that allows her to be safely contained within her environment. Such medication will also reduce the perplexity, fear and distress, and over a period of 48 hours should begin to make some impact on hallucinations and delusions. Patients with first-onset postpartum psychoses or those with postpartum-only psychoses are often effectively treated with smaller doses of neuroleptics than would be usual for non-postpartum conditions. A suggested initial regime would be 50 mg of chlorpromazine three times daily or its equivalent of haloperidol 5 mg twice a day or trifluoperazine 5 mg twice a day. The dose can be titrated up or down to an equivalent of 150 mg of chlorpromazine three or four times a day. These medications are also available as intra-muscular injections or syrups which may aid compliance in a highly disturbed state. These drugs commonly induce extra-pyramidal side effects, particularly in postpartum women, both Parkinsonism and acute dystonias.

These can be prevented or treated by using an anti-Parkinsonian agent such as procyclidine 10 mg twice a day. Lithium carbonate can also be used to treat acute episodes of mania, as well as its more familiar use as a prophylactic against recurrence of manic depressive illness. For severe depressive psychoses, electroconvulsive therapy (ECT) is the treatment of choice. Antidepressants, because they take between 10–14 days to begin their effect, are rarely appropriate as a first-line treatment for a severely disturbed, depressive psychosis. Puerperal psychosis usually responds very quickly to treatment. There should be substantial improvement within days, with recovery taking place within 2 weeks for mania and 4–6 weeks for the depressive psychoses. In the latter, antidepressants will need to be started to maintain recovery after the cessation of ECT.

Risk of relapse

Early onset puerperal psychoses, although responding to treatment very well, frequently relapse after recovery. Continuation of medication is, therefore, very important for 6 months following recovery. A patient who has presented with a manic psychosis may relapse with a depressive psychosis or a further episode of mania. If this happens on more than one occasion, the clinician may well think of using lithium carbonate in order to stabilize the mood for up to 6 months to 1 year postpartum. If the patient has suffered from a previous episode of non-postpartum manic depressive illness, prophylaxis should be continued for 2 years following delivery.

Risk of recurrence

The risk is now estimated to be 1 in 2 following any subsequent childbirth. The risk is likely to be highest if she has a baby within 2 years of recovery from her illness. Such patients should therefore be advised to delay their next pregnancy until they have been well for at least 2 years.

Severe major postnatal depression
(Fig. 17.3)

This affects between 3 and 5% of all women delivered. It too develops in the early weeks following delivery but does not show the abrupt onset of the puerperal psychosis, developing more slowly. A third of the patients present within the first 3 weeks after delivery and they are the most severely disturbed. However, two-thirds present later, between 10 and 12 weeks postpartum. Most of these women would have been diagnosable at the 6 week postnatal check. This latter group are often missed and go untreated. Women with severe postnatal depression have classical biological syndrome of early morning wakening, a mood which is worse in the morning, impaired appetite, concentration and interests. They are often indecisive, and find it uncharacteristically difficult to cope with everyday life. Their mood is profoundly lowered. They feel flat, empty and weary, there is a loss of zest and interest in life and a loss of the ability to feel pleasure or enjoyment (anhedonia). They feel guilty and incompetent, and about one-third have intrusive obsessional thoughts of harm coming to their children. They are often frightened that they are bad mothers.

Treatment – management

Anti-depressants – The biological syndrome and the severity of the depressed mood predict a response to antidepressants. Tricyclic antidepressants are usually the treatment of choice, unless there is a contra-indication or a previous response to another class of antidepressant. A suggested initial regime would be dothiepin, starting at 75 mg at night increasing over a few days to 150 mg at night. Improvement can be expected within 2 weeks, and resolution of the illness between 4 and 6 weeks. Antidepressants will need to be continued for 6 months following recovery before gradually reducing the dose.

Hormones – Progesterone therapy, both as prophylaxis and treatment, as suggested by Katerina Dalton, has much popular support. However, neither its scientific basis nor the efficiency or treatment have been replicated by others. Research on the use of transdermal *oestrogens* to treat postnatal depression is underway, and the early results are encouraging. However, this too remains to be replicated by others.

Risk of relapse – Providing medication is continued for 6 months, the majority of women can expect to fully recover. However, some will need to continue their medication for longer. The risk following future pregnancies is 1 in 2 for those women who have postpartum-only illnesses. The risk of recurrence outside of childbirth is low. However, for those

MAJOR DEPRESSIVE ILLNESS

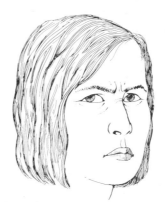

Onset in first 2 weeks
  postpartum more gradual

2 peaks presentation:
  2–4 weeks
  10–14 weeks

Early presentation:
  often missed because atypical

Overt-guilt/worthlessness
  anomie
  ruminative worry
  anxiety

Treatment:
  antidepressants/counselling

good prognosis

Risk 1:2 next baby

Fig. 17.3 Risk factors, presentation and management of major depressive illness in the puerperium

women who have had episodes outside of childbirth, the risk following subsequent births is lower than this, but the risk of non-postpartum episodes is increased.

Mild postnatal depression (Fig. 17.4)

This is the most common condition following childbirth. At least 7% of women will reach the criteria for mild major depressive illness, and many more would meet the criteria for minor depressive illness. This form of depression tends to affect a vulnerable population, and usually presents later in the postpartum year, often via the health visitor, with problems coping, particularly with the infant. The symptoms are variable, and the patient is often tearful, having difficulty in coping, complaints of irritability and lack of satisfaction with motherhood. Symptoms of anxiety, initial insomnia and a sense of loneliness and isolation are common. The patient is often distractible and better in company. She frequently has social and marital problems. The full biological syndrome of major depressive illness is absent.

Management

Psychological treatments are as effective as antidepressant and more effective than standard care for this group of patients. Six-weekly sessions of specific counselling by a trained health visitor are effective treatment, as is a similar course of cognitive psychotherapy. The latter form of treatment would appear to be particularly popular with patients, and confers some benefit to those patients who are suffering from depression only within the context of childbirth and to their children. Social support and practical help from a female confidante improves the mental health and wellbeing of the mother and the child both as a preventative and treatment strategy. This form of common depression, often associated with social adversity and marital conflict, may become chronic and have adverse effects on the child. Social and psychological interventions are particularly important but are likely to take place in primary care. Preventative strategies, using modified antenatal classes, could possibly reduce morbidity in this group in their next pregnancy.

AETIOLOGY OF POSTPARTUM MOOD DISORDERS

It is generally assumed that biological factors are the most important aetiological factors for the severe illnesses, i.e. postpartum psychosis and severe depressive illness, and psychosocial factors the most important for mild postnatal depressive illness.

Neuro-endocrine factors

The constancy of incidence across cultures and over time, the close temporal relationship of the onset to childbirth and the more recent findings of a high risk of subsequent postpartum illness and a lowered risk of non-postpartum episodes would tend to suggest a neuro-endocrine basis for the

MILD POSTNATAL DEPRESSION

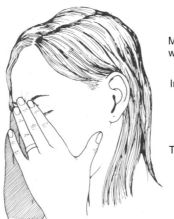

Vulnerable 'at risk'

Insidious onset in 1st week

Present 3 months to 1 year

'Understandable'

All unhappy and tearful
i.e. depressed

Most express problems
with mothering

In addition symptoms of:
anxiety
phobias

Treatment:
counselling
social support

Fig. 17.4   Risk factors, presentation and management of mild postnatal depression.

severe condition. Changes in cortisol, oxytocin, endorphins, thyroxine, progesterone and oestrogen have all been implicated in the causation of this condition. Comparable dramatic changes in steroidal hormones, outside the postpartum period, have a well-known association with affective psychoses and mood disorders. A plausible recent theory is that the sudden fall in oestrogen triggers a hypersensitivity of E_2 receptors in a predisposed group of women and may be responsible for the very severe mood disturbance that follows. The occurrence and severity of the postnatal 'blues' has been shown to be related to both the absolute level of progesterone and to the relative drop from a prepartum level. However, there is no known association between the postpartum 'blues' and affective psychoses and no evidence as yet to implicate progesterone in the aetiology of these conditions.

Obstetric factors

Caesarean section has been shown to be associated with postpartum psychosis in first-time mothers. Previous obstetric loss has been associated with severe postnatal depressive illness, as has infertility and an adverse experience of childbirth. However, there is no direct evidence to suggest that other obstetric complications predispose to severe psychiatric illness.

Social factors

Severe postpartum illness can affect women with much-wanted babies from happy and stable marriages, who live in comfortable economic circumstances. Apart from a family history and personal history of psychiatric disorder, there is little to distinguish women suffering from severe mental illness from other postpartum women.

However, women suffering from minor postnatal depression do show significant differences when compared to well women and to women suffering from severe postnatal depression or puerperal psychoses. The risk factors for mild postnatal depression appear to be predominately psychosocial. They include being young, either single or with a short marriage, lack of a female confidante, chronic social adversity, marital discord, previous psychiatric history, prior social services involvement and antenatal admission in the last trimester of pregnancy. They are significantly more likely than other women to have been admitted on multiple occasions, but for non-serious conditions, usually abdominal pain

with no explanation or unfounded concerns about retarded uterine growth.

BREAST FEEDING AND MEDICATION

Many women who present with mental illness early in the puerperium are breast feeding, and its continuation is usually very important to them. Depressed women are often advised to stop breast feeding, partly because it is commonly believed that psychotropic medication adversely affects the infant and partly because it is commonly believed that the mother's mood will improve. There is no evidence that stopping breast feeding in itself improves the mother's mental state. In reality it often adds to the burden of guilt they feel. Continuing breast feeding, particularly when depressed, often helps to maintain a relationship with the baby and a feeling of usefulness and may protect the infant from the effects of maternal depression. Continuing breast feeding requires a great deal of skill on the part of the psychiatric nurse when women are so very disturbed. Totally breast feeding the infant may not be possible in the first few days of a severe puerperal psychosis. Nonetheless, it should be possible to maintain lactation with a combination of expressing the milk and frequent suckling of the infant. When it is clearly important to continue breast feeding, the choice of psychotropic medication becomes very important (Fig. 17.5). Lithium should probably not be given to breast feeding women. The available evidence suggests that tricyclic antidepressants in full dosage are safe for breast feeding. They are present in only very small amounts in breast milk, and significant quantities are not detectable in the infant's serum. The use of neuroleptics is more contentious. Phenothiazines, such as chlorpromazine in a single dosage of 50 mg and not more than 200 mg a day or trifluoperazine in a single dosage of 5 mg and not more than 15 mg a day, are also probably safe for breast feeding mothers. However, the long-term effects on the developing child and adult are unknown. The infant should be closely monitored, and the breast feeding suspended if the baby is drowsy, does not wake and cry for its feeds or does not suckle strongly. If the severity of the mental state requires the use of parenteral medication or a single dosage of more than the equivalent of 100 mg of chlorpromazine, it is probably safer to suspend breast feeding for a period of 12–24 hours and express the milk. Paediatric advice should be sought if the baby is premature, or of low birth weight or jaundiced.

DRUGS AND BREAST FEEDING

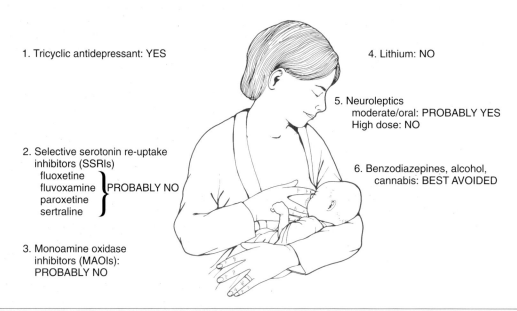

Fig. 17.5 Drug secretion in breast milk.

Summary

Although few psychotropic drugs are known to be teratogenic or to have adverse effects on the developing fetus or neonate, no psychotropic drug is of proven safety. It is therefore very important that psychotropic medication should not be prescribed lightly during pregnancy or lactation and that such drugs should be prescribed only where there are positive indications for their use. Close collaboration between the obstetrician and psychiatrist is recommended before treatment of a mental illness with psychotropic medication. Breast feeding should not routinely be suspended in mothers who require psychotropic medication. There is an adequate range of psychotropic drugs available to safely treat the mentally ill pregnant or lactating woman.

MENTAL ILLNESS IN PREGNANCY

There is probably a slightly increased risk of minor (neurotic) mental illness during the first trimester of pregnancy, with about 15% of pregnant women suffering from such conditions having been previously well prior to conception. These illnesses usually resolve spontaneously as the pregnancy progresses. The incidence of psychiatric disorder in the second trimester of pregnancy is 8%, and in the third 5%. Women who develop a minor illness (usually anxiety or reactive depression) in the first trimester of pregnancy are not thought to be at increased risk of developing postnatal depression after delivery. However, those very few women who develop such an illness in the last trimester of pregnancy may be at increased risk of postnatal depression, and should be followed up. Psychotropic medication is not usually required for women who develop minor mental illness in pregnancy. Counselling and improving social support is the preferred and effective treatment.

The risk of developing a new episode of major mental illness (manic–depressive illness or schizophrenia) is low during pregnancy and probably lower than at other times in a woman's life. This is in contrast to the dramatic increase in risk following childbirth. Similarly, women with a past history of major psychiatric disorders are probably not at increased risk of relapsing during pregnancy. However, on the rare occasion that they do, or when such an illness develops for the first time in pregnancy, it will require treatment. For severe depressive illnesses, tricyclic antidepressants, e.g. dothiepin 150 mg daily, can be used, but they will need to be reduced by 25 mg per 2 weeks so that the mother is receiving less than 75 mg or, preferably, has stopped the antidepressant before delivery. This is because there have been some reports of babies born to mothers receiving a full therapeutic dose of tricyclic antidepressants suffering from neonatal jitteriness and anti-cholinergic side effects. Once delivered, the anti-depressant can be gradually increased back to a therapeutic level. This is to mitigate the substantial risk of the mother developing a postpartum relapse. Very rarely, a new episode of mania can occur during pregnancy. This can be treated, as is usual, with chlorpromazine or another neuroleptic in the smallest possible dose that effects resolution of the symptoms. Again, this will need to be reduced to a minimum possible dose before delivery. There have been some reports of mothers suffering from hypotensive episodes following delivery on large doses of neuroleptics. There have also been reports of babies suffering from hypotonia and extra-pyramidal side effects. Once delivered, the neuroleptic should be increased again to mitigate the substantial risk of a manic relapse follow-ing delivery. Lithium should not be used in preg-nancy as it is teratogenic in the first trimester and may cause cardiac defects, and in the last trimester has been associated with fetal hypothyroidism. However, if the mother is not breast feeding, lithium may be reintroduced after delivery, aiming at a therapeutic serum level by day 5. This has been shown in non-randomized clinical studies to be very effective at preventing a postpartum manic relapse.

The risk to the fetus from receiving psychotropic medication in utero has to be balanced against the risk posed by maternal disturbance.

Chronic mental illness and pregnancy

With the exception of anorexia nervosa, no psychiatric condition is associated with a reduction in biological fertility. Therefore, all forms of psychiatric disorder may present associated with pregnancy. A particular problem for the psychiatrist and obstetrician is posed by those women whose stability of mental health and social functioning depends upon taking regular medication.

Manic–depressive illness

If a woman has a history of multiple episodes of manic–depressive illness, she may be receiving a combination of one or more of the following group of drugs: antidepressants, neuroleptics and lithium. She may often be given the advice to stop these drugs before conceiving, and may face, therefore, not only a dramatic increase in the risk of relapsing following delivery (1 in 2) but also a risk of relapsing during pregnancy in the weeks following cessation of medication. If at all possible, such women should discuss with their psychiatrist before conception the likely effects of stopping their medication and of childbirth on their mental health. If the patient, family and psychiatrist have every reason to believe that, given a stable mental state, she can meet the needs of the developing child, then she will need assistance to manage her condition. She should be advised to gradually reduce her lithium before con-ception. If necessary, her mental state will need to be stabilized with antidepressants, if she becomes depressed, or with a small dose of neuroleptic if she becomes hypomanic. Her mental health should then improve as the pregnancy progresses. Once delivered, she should be restarted on her normal regime. If she wishes to breast feed, this should include a neuroleptic. If she does not wish to breast feed, then lithium can be started on the first postpartum day.

Chronic schizophrenia

These women will usually be maintained either on an oral neuroleptic or, commonly, an intramuscular depot injection of a neuroleptic such as fluphenazine decanoate (Modecate) or flupenthixol (Depixol). If this medication is stopped they run a substantial risk of having a relapse in their schizophrenic illness within 3 months. Again, ideally these women should discuss with their psychiatrist their capacity to parent as well as the effects of pregnancy and the postpartum period on their mental health. If, when well and stable even on medication, they have the resources to effectively parent a child then they should be advised not to stop their medication in order to conceive or during pregnancy. However, as they approach delivery their medication should be reduced to the minimum possible level compatible with mental health and then increased on the day of delivery to the normal regime. Women with chronic schizophrenia may benefit from a period of in-patient admission to a mother and baby unit to help them get off to the best possible start with their infant and provide an opportunity to assess their capacity to care for their infant. Providing medi-cation is continued, the risk of relapse in the immediate postpartum period is not high. However, such women may remain vulnerable to the stresses and strains of child-rearing for some months and years to come.

PREVENTION

Secondary prevention

The identification of vulnerable women and those at high risk, vigilance in the first 2 weeks, early detection and vigorous treatment will reduce maternal morbidity and adverse affects on the child. The inclusion of routine questions designed to detect postnatal depression or the use of a simple screening schedule such as the Edinburgh Postnatal Depression Scale would allow for the detection of the 10% of women suffering from major depressive illness and their treatment with either anti-depressant or psychological therapies as indicated.

Primary prevention

Hormonal strategies have yet to be confirmed by clinical trials. For those women at high risk of a bipolar illness by virtue of a previous postpartum episode or past psychiatric history, the use of lithium carbonate has been shown in non-randomized clinical studies to be effective. Such a strategy will involve a high degree of cooperation between the psychiatrist and obstetrician. Lithium should be started at 400 mg at night on the first postpartum day, increasing to a dose which produces a thera-peutic level (0.6–0.8 mmol/l) by the third to fifth postpartum day. Breast feeding is not possible on this regime. For those women who wish to breast feed, a small dose of a neutroleptic such as 1.5 mg of haloperidol at night may be equally effective. Women with a past history of severe depressive illness may wish to start antidepressant on the day of delivery. They should start their previously effective antidepressant at half-dosage on the day of delivery (e.g. 75 mg of dothiepin) and gradually increase the antidepressant by 25 mg every 3–4 days until they are taking a therapeutic dose (150 mg of dothiepin) by 2 weeks postpartum.

Psycho-social interventions

Mothers with chronic life difficulties, poor marriages, lack of a female confidante and a past history of maternal deprivation and previous depressive epi-sodes are at risk of developing mild postnatal depression following delivery. However, just as important is the risk that they will not enjoy their children. Providing specially modified antenatal classes for this vulnerable group with an emphasis on social support and anticipatory learning of the likely difficulties that face new mothers has been shown to be effective in reducing the rates of postnatal difficulties that face new mothers. Also effective is the providing of a social confidante, practical assistance and advice-giving through link-ing such women with an experienced volunteer mother.

Prevention of mental illness

- Counsel women with chronic severe mental illness about pregnancy
- Manic–depressive illness: consider restarting treatment after delivery
- Maintain chronic schizophrenic medication throughout pregnancy
- Previous history of puerperal psychosis/severe postnatal depression: close contact first week
- Consider prophylaxis after delivery
- Assess all women at 6 weeks postnatal check for postnatal depression

---

THE 'BLUES'

The majority of women experience some alteration in their emotional state between the third and 10th day postpartum. This is known as the 'baby blues'. The most common day of onset is day 5. The 'blues' is probably associated with both the absolute level of progesterone and the relative drop of progesterone from the predelivery to postpartum level. However, despite its likely hormonal basis, it should be remembered that bouts of low mood and tearfulness are very common 3–5 days after an exciting event and also after many surgical events. The 'blues' is characterized by a low, tearful and labile mood, irritability, insomnia and a tendency to be over-sensitive to criticism and transient bouts of despair and catastrophizing – 'blowing things out of proportion'. The severity of the 'blues' varies from being relatively mild to quite distressing, but it is an essentially normal and probably inevitable con-sequence of childbirth and should not be confused with mental illness. Unlike mental illness it usually only lasts 48 hours, it responds to kindness and reassurance and does not deteriorate over the fol-lowing days as postnatal depression does. However, tearful and anxious episodes may occur on occasion for a number of weeks following childbirth, parti-cularly when tired or when the baby is difficult to settle. It is important that all professionals involved with the care of newly delivered mothers know of the timing, characteristics and essentially benign nature of the 'blues'. It is also important that women

Table 17.1 Psychiatry and obstetrics

Booking clinic	Take family and personal history Psychiatric disorder Refer to past history	Severe postnatal depression Puerperal psychosis Previous serious psychiatric disorder
Antenatal care	Vigilance	Previous baby, previous loss, infertility Multiple antenatal admissions High anxiety
Delivery	Vigilance	Caesarean section Maternal danger
Postnatal	Vigilance	SCBU Maternal readmission Early maternal disturbance
Postnatal examination	6 weeks	Screen for postnatal depression

themselves and their partners are made aware of this phenomenon during antenatal classes.

Postpartum mood disorder of all severities is a common complication of childbirth. In many cases it is predictable and perhaps avoidable. In all cases awareness by the obstetrician of risk factors and the clinical syndromes will allow for early detection, prompt treatment and a reduction in morbidity with subsequent benefits to the woman, her infant and her family (Table 17.1).

BIBLIOGRAPHY

Cox J L, Holden J M, Sagovshy R 1987 Detection of postnatal depression: development of the 10-item Edinburgh postnatal depression scale (EPDS). British Journal of Psychiatry 150: 782–786

Holden J M, Sagovsky R, Cox J L 1989 Counselling in a general practice setting: a controlled study of health visitors; intervention in treatment of postnatal depression. British Medical Journal 298: 223–226

Oates M (ed) 1989 Baillières Clinical Obstetrics and Gynaecology. Baillière Tindall, London, vol 3

Ruben P C 1987 Prescribing in pregnancy. British Medical Association, London

Stewart D E, Klompenhouwer J L, Kendell R E, van Hulst A M 1991 Prophylactic lithium in puerperal psychosis: the experience of three centres. British Journal of Psychiatry 158: 393–397

Wieck A, Kumar R, Hirst A D et al 1991 Increased sensitivity of dopamine receptors and recurrence of affective psychosis after childbirth. British Medical Journal 303: 613–616

18 Perinatal mortality

DEFINITIONS

The definition of perinatal death is linked to the concept of viability and, as the likelihood of survival of a low birth weight infant has increased progressively over recent decades, current UK definitions are not satisfactory. The present World Health Organization definitions are:

- Stillbirth – the term 'stillborn' is used when there are no signs of life in a child born after the 22nd week of gestation or 500 g. The stillbirth rate is the number of stillbirths per 1000 total births per year.
- Neonatal death – this is defined as death of a liveborn infant within 28 days of birth. The neonatal death rate is the number of infants dying within 28 days after birth per 1000 live births per year.
- Perinatal death rate – this is the total number of stillbirths and first-week deaths per 1000 total births per year.

INCIDENCE

Perinatal mortality rates vary widely – both between different countries and within different regions of the same country. For example, in 1995 the highest rate occurred in Somalia and the lowest in Japan (Table 18.1). In Western European countries, perinatal mortality has fallen markedly over the last 20 years; these trends are clearly demonstrated in the figures for England and Wales (Fig. 18.1). The causes for this improvement include:

1. Improved antenatal and intrapartum care
2. Improved socio-economic conditions
3. Reduction in parity
4. An active screening programme for common congenital abnormalities such as Down's syndrome and abnormalities of the central nervous system such as anencephaly and spina bifida.

Table 18.1 International comparison of perinatal mortality rates in 1995 (per 1000 total births)

Country	Rate/1000 births
Somalia	120
Mozambique	105
Bangladesh	85
Nepal	75
China	45
Greece	15
UK	10
USA	10
Germany	5
Sweden	5
Japan	5

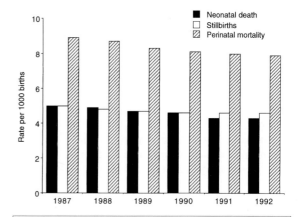

Fig. 18.1 Perinatal mortality in England and Wales.

Factors which are known to affect perinatal mortality in England and Wales include social class, country of birth of the mother, maternal age and parity and marital status. Smoking also has a significant adverse effect on birth weight and perinatal mortality.

Many developing nations in Sub-Saharan Africa and Asia do not collect routine statistics, and the data available are collected by governmental and other agencies. Among the poorest countries in terms of their GNP (gross national product), such as Mozambique, Tanzania, Bangladesh and Nepal, the perinatal mortality rate is above 75 per 1000 total births. A comparison of the role of obstetric care in perinatal mortality must take account of the incidence of congenital abnormalities and low birth weight.

AETIOLOGY

The commonest causes of stillbirth are those related to:

1. Major congenital abnormalities incompatible with life, such as heart disease and abnormalities of the central nervous system and renal agenesis.
2. Asphyxia – a final diagnosis of intra-uterine asphyxia may represent the end product of a variety of different pathological processes including:
   a. Placental abruption
   b. Pre-eclampsia and eclampsia
   c. Placental dysfunction associated with intra-uterine growth retardation
   d. Cord entanglement or prolapse
   e. Abnormal uterine activity and cephalo-pelvic disproportion.
3. Traumatic cerebral haemorrhage and intracranial damage from difficult labour and delivery.
4. Blood group incompatibility – this is now a rare cause of intra-uterine death associated with severe rhesus iso-immunization and hydrops fetalis.

The common causes of neonatal death are those related to:

1. Major congenital abnormalities incompatible with life.
2. Prematurity – the most important single factor in causing neonatal death associated with:
   a. Respiratory distress syndrome and hyaline membrane disease
   b. Pneumonia
   c. Intracranial haemorrhage and cerebral damage sustained either during labour and delivery or in the early neonatal period
   d. Necrotizing enterocolitis.

SOCIAL FACTORS AND PERINATAL MORTALITY

Maternal age

Maternal age at both extremes is associated with an increase in perinatal mortality. The death rate in the under 16 years age group is twice as high as at any other age.

Parity

There seems to be little doubt that the introduction of the 1967 Abortion Act has been a major factor in the reduction of perinatal mortality. High parity is associated with high fetal and neonatal loss.

Social class

Each country tends to exhibit in microcosm the international differences that are dependent on economic status. The impact of socio-economic class on perinatal mortality means that women of social classes 4 and 5 have a higher perinatal mortality rate.

Many countries do not collect annual routine statistics and in those countries where figures are published, there are often difficulties in interpreting the data because of inaccuracies in the data collection. However, the more gross discrepancies generally do say something about social indices in a country and the quality of medical care.

The figures published for 1995 show a remarkable 24-fold difference between those countries with the highest and lowest perinatal mortality rates (Table 18.1). Although perinatal mortality rates have tended to fall over the last 10 years in most countries, there are still marked differences between countries. The magnitude of these differences is tending, if anything, to increase.

Perinatal mortality

- Major causes are congenital abnormalities, asphyxia and prematurity
- Predisposing factors are maternal age, high parity, low social class

---

THE IMPACT OF LOW BIRTH WEIGHT ON NEONATAL MORTALITY

Low birth weight is defined as a live birth of less than 2500 g. The rate varies from 4% in Sweden to an estimated 25% in Bangladesh. The overall figure in Britain is 6.7% of all live births. The mortality rate in relation to birth weight is shown in Figure 14.2. The figures shown are national figures and tend to vary substantially in relation to the quality of special intensive care units.

MATERNAL MORTALITY

Maternal mortality rate is the number of maternal deaths per million maternities in 1 year. A maternal death is defined as death occurring within 1 year of delivery. Death may be directly due to pregnancy and childbirth including abortion, or may simply occur within a year of childbirth, but be unrelated to the process.

The statistics in Figures 18.2 and 18.3 are based on the triennial reports from the Department of Health in England and Wales. The report for 1988–1990 showed a direct death rate of 61/million maternities (Fig. 18.2) and an 'indirect' death rate of 39.4/million maternities (Fig. 18.3). The rates in Britain vary according to the region – as with the perinatal mortality rate.

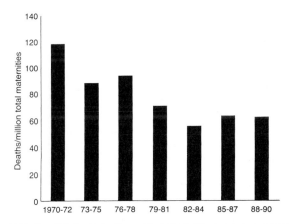

Fig. 18.2 Deaths due to direct maternal causes per million maternities.

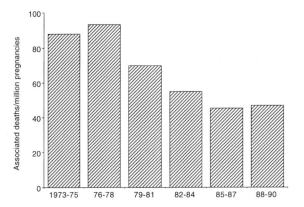

Fig. 18.3 Maternal deaths associated with pregnancy.

The major causes of maternal death in order of importance are as follows:

1. Thrombo-embolism
2. Hypertensive diseases of pregnancy
3. Ectopic pregnancy/abortion
4. Uterine haemorrhage
5. Amniotic fluid embolism
6. Sepsis excluding abortion
7. Anaesthesia
8. Genital tract trauma.

The system of confidential enquiries into maternal death

The system of confidential enquiry was introduced in England and Wales in 1952, and triennial reports have been published since that time. Ninety-nine per cent of all deaths are now documented in the reports. Information gathered by the area or, now, district medical officers, based on reports of all those staff involved in management of the pregnant woman, together with the results of the postmortem are passed to regional obstetric assessors and finally to central assessors who are the Department of Health advisers in obstetrics and gynaecology. Strict confidentiality is maintained throughout this procedure, and the name of the patient is removed from the public record. An attempt is made to classify deaths into avoidable and unavoidable groups.

Maternal mortality

- Deaths within 1 year postpartum.
- 103 per million
- Major causes include pulmonary embolism, pregnancy-induced hypertension, anaesthetic, haemorrhage

---

BIBLIOGRAPHY

Antonov A 1947 Children born during the siege of Leningrad in 1942. Journal of Paediatrics 30: 250–259

BMJ 1980 Quality, not quantity, in babies. British Medical Journal 1: 347–348

Department of Health 1996 Report on confidential enquiries into maternal deaths in England and Wales 1991–1993. HMSO, London

Field D J, Hopkin I, Milner A D, Madeley R J 1985 Changing overall workload in neonatal units. British Medical Journal 290: 1539–1542

HMSO 1994 Health and personal social service statistics for England 1994. HMSO London

OPCS Monitors Series DH3

Pharoah P O D, Alberman E D 1981 Mortality of low birthweight infants in England and Wales 1953 to 1979. Archives of Disease in Childhood 56: 86–89

World Bank 1993 World development report. Oxford University Press, New York

19 Imaging techniques in obstetrics and gynaecology

The major techniques used in imaging the fetus and the pelvic organs are:

1. Radiological imaging
2. Ultrasonography
3. Magnetic resonance imaging
4. Immunoscintigraphy.

The last two new methods are important but are not yet widely used.

RADIOGRAPHY IN OBSTETRICS AND GYNAECOLOGY

Radiological imaging in pregnancy has now largely been replaced by ultrasound imaging because of risk factors. Nevertheless, there are specific examples where it is still used, although magnetic resonance imaging and ultrasound imaging have largely superseded most of these functions.

Indications for radiography in pregnancy

X-ray pelvimetry

Assessment of the bony pelvis remains the commonest indication for the use of radiography in pregnancy. The erect lateral views of the pelvis are the most valuable because they enable assessment of the true conjugate diameter and the shape of the sacrum. Pelvic inlet views are used for assessment of the transverse diameter of the inlet and also for measurement of the narrowest diameter of the pelvic cavity – the interspinous diameter. Outlet views are less important because the pelvic outlet is amenable to clinical assessment.

Radiological diagnosis in gynaecology

Plain radiography of the abdomen has a role to play in the diagnosis of pelvic tumours. Dermoid cysts often contain radio-opaque material such as teeth and bone, which can be seen in the pelvis. Uterine fibroids are not visible radiologically but can be detected if there is calcification in the fibroid.

Hysterosalpingography (Fig. 19.1)

The injection of a radio-opaque water-soluble dye through the cervix into the uterine cavity is used to visualize the cavity of the uterus, the cervical canal and the Fallopian tubes. This procedure is performed by injecting the dye through a Leech–Wilkinson or Ruben's cannula, having first filled the instrument with dye to exclude air bubbles. The cavity of the uterus is filled with 2–3 ml of dye, and the presence of filling defects caused by polyps or submucous fibroids can be demonstrated. These defects usually show a rounded margin. Intra-uterine synechiae have a sharp demarcation but an irregular edge. Abnormalities of

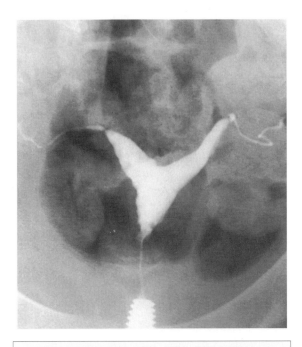

Fig. 19.1 Hysterosalpingogram of a subseptate uterus; the Fallopian tubes can also be clearly defined.

the uterine cavity such as uterus bicornis bicollis and septate uteri can also be demonstrated.

Tubal obstruction associated with fimbrial confluence shows up as a retort-shaped structure. If dye leaks through the tube, it can be seen smeared over the surface of the bowel. If it becomes loculated around the end of the tube, it may indicate the presence of peritubal adhesions.

The site of tubal obstruction can also be demonstrated. It is important to be gentle in performing the procedure. Rough manipulation of the uterus may result in utero-tubal spasms and thereby give a false indication of organic tubal obstruction.

Radiography

- Obstetrics – assessment of bony pelvis, gestational age, skeletal malformations, multiple pregnancy
- Risk of leukaemia in child
- Gynaecology – dermoids, hysterosalpingography and lost IUCD

ULTRASONOGRAPHY IN OBSTETRICS AND GYNAECOLOGY

The principle of ultrasound usage in medical diagnosis is based on the transmission of sound frequencies of the order of 2–20 MHz into human tissues and the subsequent measurement of returning echoes from interfaces of differing densities. Ultrasound will not penetrate a gaseous medium and has therefore not been particularly useful in the diagnosis of disorders of the bowel and lung.

Ultrasound is produced by excitation of a piezo-electric crystal, which vibrates at a predetermined frequency. The transmitting phase is short, and the crystal reverts to a receiving phase. Scanners are divided into static and real-time machines.

Real-time scanners

There are three forms of real-time scanners: linear array, mechanical array and phased array. Only linear and phased array methods are now commonly used. These techniques enable positive identification of moving or pulsating parts, particularly fetal movements and fetal heart beats. Transvaginal probes of a higher frequency are now widely used as they give better imaging of the pelvis.

Estimation of gestational age

In the first 90 days of pregnancy, the most accurate measurement for estimation of gestational age is the

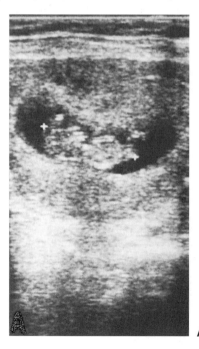

A

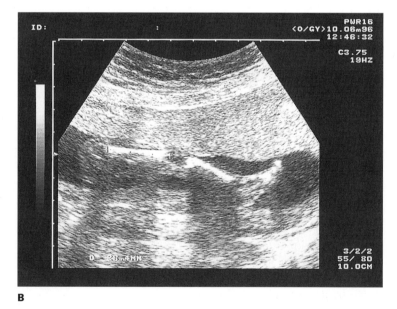

B

Fig. 19.2 **A** Crown–rump length in an 8 week fetus; **B** the measurement of femur length may enhance the accuracy of the assessment of gestational age and fetal growth.

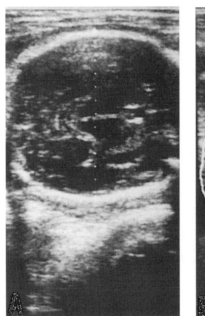 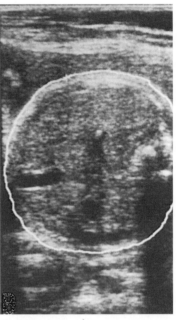

Fig. 19.3 **A** Biparietal diameter as measured by ultrasound; the midline shadow of the falx cerebri can be clearly identified. **B** Abdominal circumference measured at the level of the umbilical vessels.

measurement of crown–rump length (Fig. 19.2). This is best performed with real-time apparatus as it is possible to measure the maximum longitudinal axis.

In the second trimester, gestational age can be estimated by measurement of biparietal diameter (Fig. 19.3). The scatter around the mean increases with gestational age, and the most accurate estimate of gestational age can be obtained between 16 and 20 weeks gestation.

Images of the normal fetus

Modern ultrasound real-time techniques have increasingly high resolution and enable high-quality images of the general structures of the fetus to be obtained. Figure 19.4 for example shows a sagittal view of the face and brain in a normal fetus in a low-power section (A) and in a high-power section (B).

Ultrasound assessment of blood velocity profiles in the fetus

The assessment of the velocity of blood flow in blood vessels can be calculated using the principle of Doppler shift. Ultrasound waves reflected from a moving target such as red blood cells in a vessel produce a frequency change which is proportional to the velocity of the target. The y-axis records the height of the Doppler shift and the x-axis reflects the time (Fig. 19.5). A typical waveform in the fetal umbilical artery is shown in Figure 19.5A. Figure 19.5B shows a cross-sectional image of the umbilical vessels. All profiles in this section should be considered to provide an index of blood velocity. The peak of the waveform is known as the A wave and the trough of the wave is known as the B wave. The AB ratio therefore represents the ratio of peak systole to end diastole.

The resistance index is the ratio of peak systole minus end diastole over peak systole. In general terms, fetal growth retardation is associated with an increase in the AB ratio, suggesting an increase in resistance to flow in the placenta. An increase in the resistance index also suggests a deterioration in the condition of the placenta. These tests are being used increasingly in the assessment of placental function.

Abnormalities in early pregnancy

Ectopic pregnancy

Direct identification of an ectopic pregnancy by ultrasound is difficult (see Fig. 19.6) but the com-

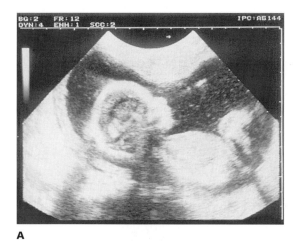
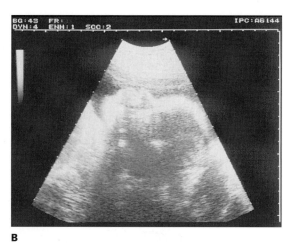

A **B**

Fig. 19.4 **A** Ultrasound image of the fetal face and brain; **B** the same view with greater magnification.

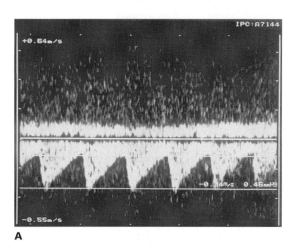
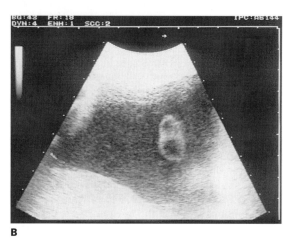

A **B**

Fig. 19.5 **A** The velocity profile of the umbilical artery measured from insonation of the fetal umbilical artery; **B** cross-sectional image of the vessels.

bination of:

1. The absence of a gestation sac in the uterus
2. An adnexal mass with or without a fetal pole
3. Fluid in the pouch of Douglas
4. A positive pregnancy test

is highly specific for an ectopic pregnancy.

Early embryonic demise

In this condition, the fetus can be clearly identified, and usually grows at a normal rate until death occurs, and the fetal heartbeat can no longer be seen. One of the difficulties created by routine scans in early

pregnancy is that the diagnosis of early embryonic demise may be established before there is any indication that the pregnancy is abnormal. It is sometimes preferable to repeat the scan a week later rather than proceed to immediate uterine evacuation, to enable the mother to come to terms with the diagnosis.

Anembryonic pregnancy

The absence of fetal development results in the presence of a gestational sac which does not contain a fetus (Fig. 19.7). This can be readily identified but as with early embryonic demise, it is advisable to repeat the scan after at least 1 week.

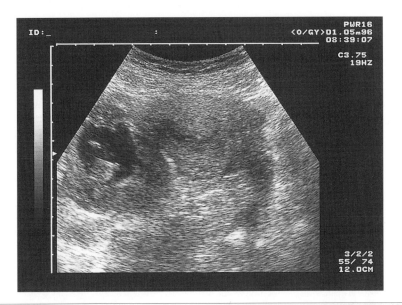

Fig. 19.6 The uterus and the endometrial cavity can be seen centrally. A fetal pole can be seen in the cavity to the left of the uterus.

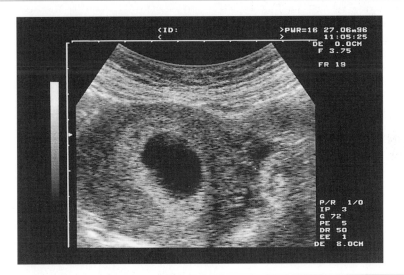

Fig. 19.7 The empty gestation sac in a blighted ovum.

Hydatidiform mole

The classic appearance of a molar pregnancy makes this condition easy to recognize. The uterus is filled with echoes, which give it a snowstorm appearance. There is usually no evidence of a fetus, but this is not invariably the case. The presence of haemorrhage within the molar tissue may lead to some confusion with the possibility of a missed abortion and fetal resorption.

Detection of fetal malformations

Ultrasound is widely used for the diagnosis of congenital abnormalities. Real-time scanning enables imaging in both longitudinal and transverse sections and is particularly useful in the diagnosis of abnormalities of the central nervous system.

Spina bifida

The entire length of the fetal spine can be demonstrated by real-time imaging with both longitudinal and transverse scans (Fig. 19.8). The normal spine appears as a complete bony ring, but with spina bifida the posterior aspect of the ring is open, with a bulging meningo-myelocoele, and the neural elements can be seen outside the spinal canal. The most difficult area to visualize is the lower lumbar and sacral spine.

Anencephaly

Ultrasound diagnosis of anencephaly is relatively easy but also less important than the diagnosis of spina bifida, because the anencephalic fetus does not survive.

Hydrocephaly can be diagnosed by the abnormal enlargement of the biparietal diameter and lateral ventricles. In the detection of microcephaly, the head circumference must be compared with trunk measurements in order to obtain a sure diagnosis.

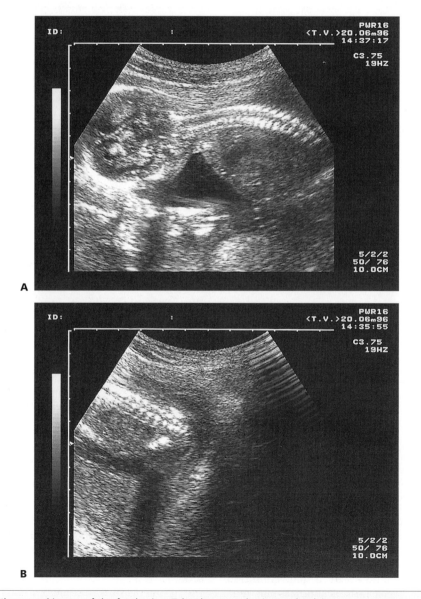

Fig. 19.8   **A** Ultrasound image of the fetal spine; **B** lumbar–sacral spine and pelvis.

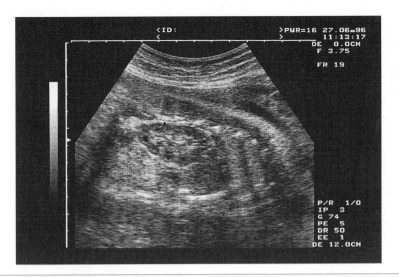

Fig. 19.9 An image of a normal fetal kidney.

Renal tract anomalies

The bladder can be visualized after 14 weeks gestation but may vary considerably in size according to the voiding cycle of the fetus. Renal agenesis can be recognized by the absence of kidneys and of urine in the bladder. Other anomalies that can be diagnosed by ultrasound include isolated renal cysts, multicystic dysplasia, infantile polycystic kidneys and obstructive uropathy.

An image of a normal fetal kidney is shown in Figure 19.9.

Abnormalities of the gastrointestinal tract

Oesophageal atresia can be identified by the absence of a stomach bubble and the presence of polyhydramnios. Duodenal atresia is associated with a double bubble, and diaphragmatic hernia is suggested by deviation of the heart and a fluid-filled space in the chest. It is also feasible to establish a diagnosis of omphalocoele and gastroschisis. Foreign bodies can also be identified in the uterus (Fig. 19.10).

Chromosomal defects

Structural abnormalities of the heart, gut and neck can be identified in about 50% of infants with trisomy 21. Findings include the 'double bubble' sign of duodenal atresia, cardiac abnormalities such as ventricular septal defect, and echogenic foci in the wall of the ventricle. An increase in the thickness and translucency of the skin over the neck (nuchal translucency) is more specific for Down's syndrome and can be detected in the first trimester. Although not specific for trisomy, the presence of these markers, especially where more than one sign can be identified or where the mother is aged over 35 years may indicate the need for karyotyping the fetus.

Ultrasound imaging of the placenta

The placenta can be easily identified on ultrasound scan but is often difficult to localize in relation to the lower uterine segment and the cervix. The reflection of the bladder from the uterus facilitates the demarcation of the lower uterine segment anteriorly, but it is difficult to identify the cervix with ultrasound and localization of the posterior placenta with any great degree of accuracy is not possible. Apparent placental migration is due to the changing shape of the uterine musculature with advancing gestational age. Although the placental site will be identified as low in up to 30% of pregnancies at 20 weeks gestation, less than 3% of these cases will ultimately have a placenta praevia. However, location of the cervix has now improved, and hence location of the posterior placenta praevia has improved.

The role of ultrasound in the diagnosis of placental abruption is limited because it is difficult to differentiate between normal intravascular blood and retroplacental clot. A diagnosis of abruption should be made only where the state of the blood collection is non-physiological.

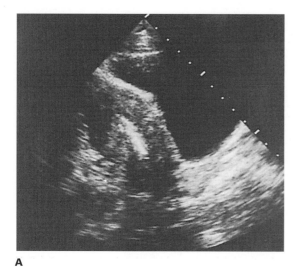

A

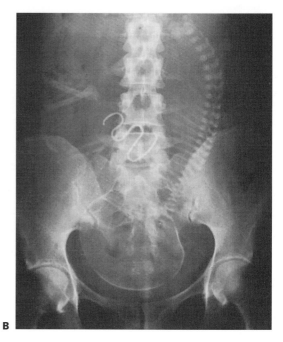

B

Fig. 19.10 **A** Ultrasound diagnosis of a plastic intra-uterine contraceptive device; **B** radiography of the abdomen showing a Lippes loop and a full-term pregnancy.

Assessment of fetal growth

The assessment of fetal growth is dependent on serial measurement of various parts of the fetus, and no valid estimate can be obtained from an isolated measurement. **Cephalometry** involves the measurement of the fetal biparietal diameter. These measurements can be misleading in breech presentation because of the dolico-cephalic shape of the head; in this instance it is necessary to measure the occipito-frontal diameter as well, to establish a ratio between the two measurements.

Abdominal measurements

The size of the fetal abdomen provides a sensitive indication of fetal growth. Measurements are aimed at the lower edge of the liver and are expressed in terms of either abdominal circumference or abdominal area. Abdominal size in relation to head size gives a sensitive indication of intrauterine growth retardation. Late onset of placental insufficiency gives rise to a 'head-sparing' effect and asymmetrical growth retardation. Symmetrical growth retardation may be associated with fetal abnormality or infection, and intra-uterine growth retardation of early onset. Various nomograms have been devised for growth of the long bones of the limbs. In particular, measurements of the femur in relation to abdominal girth are useful in the assessment of fetal growth.

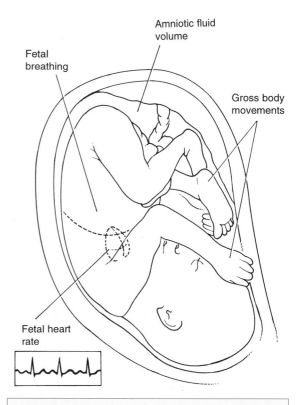

Fig. 19.11 Components of the biophysical profile assessment.

Assessment of fetal welfare

Biophysical profile

The assessment of fetal wellbeing is now commonly performed by using a composite measurement of five indices that indicate fetal health. These include observations on fetal breathing, body movements, fetal tone, reactive fetal heart rate and amniotic fluid volume. (Fig. 19.11) The scoring system is shown in Table 19.1. Interpretation and management of the findings is shown in Table 19.2. The decision concerning management will also take account of the clinical situation. In other words, the use of this type of assessment as with all forms of antenatal fetal assessment must take account of the maternal medical history, previous obstetric history and the history of events and complications during the current pregnancy.

Fetal imaging of the normal fetus

In scanning of the fetus at various gestational ages, it is now possible to obtain high-quality images of the face and lips (Fig. 19.12) and of the cerebral ventricle (Fig. 19.13). In addition, the thickness of the nuchal fold can be measured as an indicator of Down's syndrome (Fig. 19.14). The fetal appendages – the hands and feet – can be clearly identified, particularly in relation to fetal movement (Fig. 19.15). Four-chamber views of the fetal heart allow detection of fetal cardiac anomalies (Fig. 19.16).

Detection of pelvic pathology

Ultrasound is now used extensively for the detection of pelvic pathology. It can be used to measure the size of various pelvic tumours such as ovarian cysts, be they benign or malignant, and the presence of minor cysts in the ovary as with polycystic ovarian syndrome (Fig. 19.17).

Ultrasound

- Uses frequencies of 2–20 MHz
- Most valuable in estimation of gestational age, missed abortion, mole, fetal central nervous system and renal tract malformations, fetal growth, anterior placenta praevia
- Less useful in ectopics, posterior placenta praevia, abruption

---

Table 19.1   Biophysical profile: assessment over 30 minutes

	Biophysical variable	Normal (2)	Abnormal (0)
1	Fetal breathing movements	> 1 episode of 30 seconds duration	No episode in 30 minutes
2	Gross body movements	At least 3 discrete body/limb movements in 30 minutes	≤ 2 movements
3	Fetal tone	At least 1 episode of active extension and flexion of limbs. Opening and closing of hand	Absent fetal movement. Slow extension, partial flexion
4	Reactive fetal heart rate	≥ 2 accelerations of ≥ 15 beats/minute lasting 15 seconds associated with fetal movements	< 2 accelerations in 30 minutes
5	Qualitative amniotic fluid volume	At least 1 pocket of amniotic fluid at least 1 cm in two perpendicular planes	No amniotic fluid pockets > 1 cm

Table 19.2   Management based on biophysical profile

Total score results	Interpretation	Recommended management
10	Normal	Conservative management. Repeat in 1 week or in 3 days if diabetic or postmature
8	Normal	If oligohydramnios present, review for delivery. If oligohydramnios and postmature, deliver
6	Equivocal	Repeat within 24 hours. If normal, proceed as for a score of 8 or 10. If the score is 6 or less, evaluate for delivery
≤ 4	Abnormal	Deliver unless ≤ 26 weeks

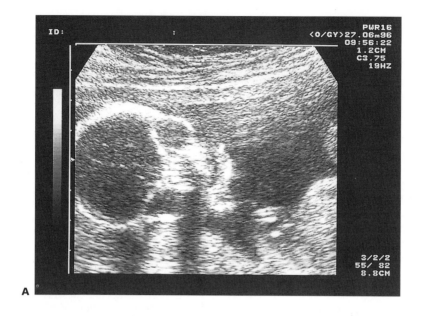

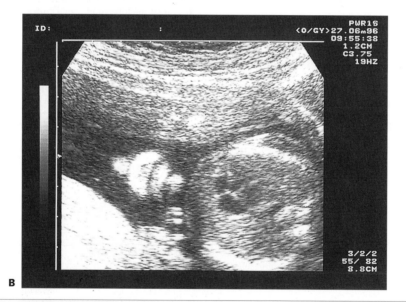

Fig. 19.12 **A** Lateral view of the fetal face and cranium; **B** ultrasound image of the fetal face and lips.

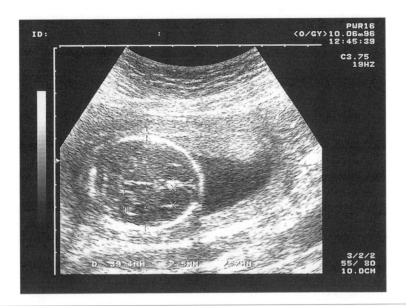

Fig. 19.13 Ultrasound view of the anterior and posterior horns of the ventricles in the brain.

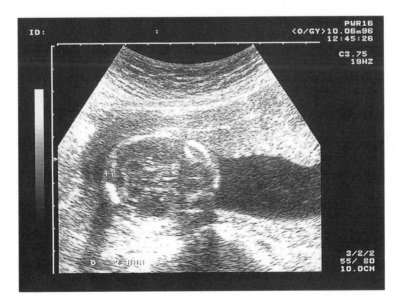

Fig. 19.14 Measurement of the nuchal fold thickness and the appearance of the cerebellum dumbbell-shaped ventricles.

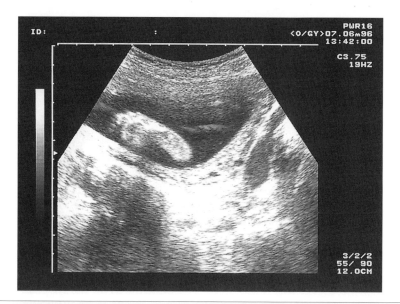

Fig. 19.15 Ultrasound image of a fetal foot.

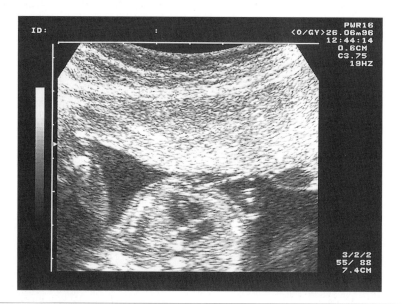

Fig. 19.16 Four-chamber view of the fetal heart.

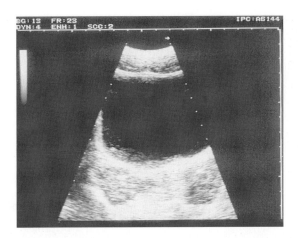

Fig. 19.17   Bilateral polycystic ovarian disease showing the mottled appearance in both ovaries characteristic of multiple small cysts.

Ultrasound is now used extensively to assess follicular growth and rupture (Fig. 19.18) during normal follicular maturation and to assess hyperstimulation of the ovaries (Fig. 19.19). Finally, detection of pelvic tumours such as uterine fibroids (Fig. 19.20) are readily identifiable by ultrasound.

MAGNETIC RESONANCE IMAGING
(Figs 19.21–19.24)

Magnetic resonance imaging (MRI) or tomography is a new technique of imaging. Soft tissue definition is at a premium with this method and it has the advantage that images can be obtained in any plane. Furthermore, the technique is not dependent on

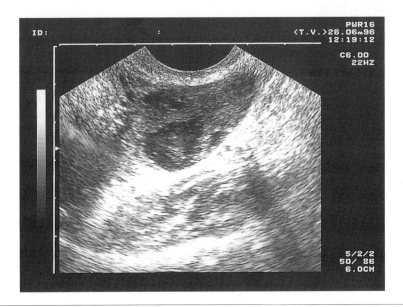

Fig. 19.18   Ultrasound image of a collapsing ovarian follicle.

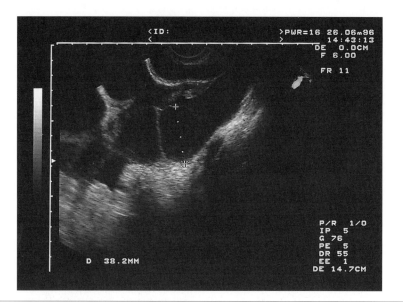

Fig. 19.19   Ovarian hyperstimulation with multiple follicles.

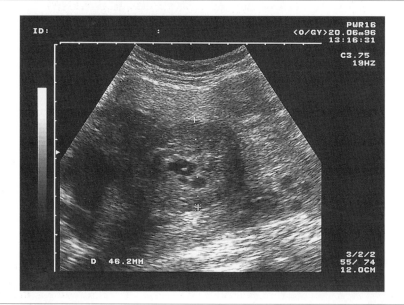

Fig. 19.20   Ultrasound image of a uterine fibroid.

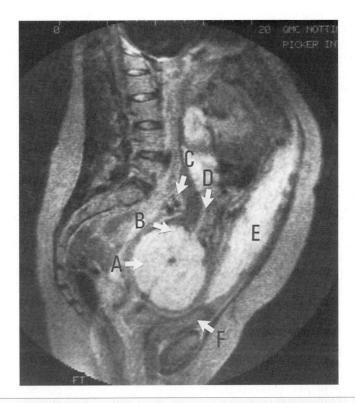

Fig. 19.21 Magnetic resonance imaging; a sagittal section of a mature fetus. A, cerebral cortex; B, cerebellum; C, umbilical cord vessels; D, spinal cord; E, anterior placement of the placenta; F, bladder.

ionizing radiation, and at the present time does not appear to be associated with any hazard. The nucleus of the hydrogen atom contains a single spinning proton which generates a small magnetic field. The application of a powerful external magnetic field polarizes the hydrogen-ion-containing sample and aligns the hydrogen ions. When radio-waves of the appropriate frequency are passed through the tissue, the protons are displaced and, in returning to their basal state, energy is emitted as a radio frequency. Images are created from a series of measurements in the time domain. The use of this technique in obstetrics is now under investigation. It enables very accurate localization of the placental site because the cervix can be identified with considerable clarity. The fetal brain can also be imaged in late pregnancy (Fig. 19.21), but it is difficult to image the fetus in early pregnancy using existing techniques because of fetal movement.

MRI is particularly useful in the diagnosis of pelvic tumours (Fig. 19.23). Endometrial carcinoma can be clearly identified, and the depth of invasion into the myometrium accurately measured. Tumour invasion for cervical, uterine and ovarian carcinomas can be seen in transverse, sagittal and coronal sections.

The technique promises considerable advances in morphological and biochemical imaging.

Three-dimensional MRI

The introduction of post echo-planar imaging removes fetal movement artifacts, and using multiple slices reconstruction allows computer-enhanced images of the total fetal body and of individual organs. A computer reconstruction of a fetal brain in a mature fetus is shown in Figure 19.24. This technology enables accurate estimates of fetal volume/weight and therefore enables differentiation between normal and abnormal fetal growth. This technology is rapidly advancing, and should be particularly valuable in 'weighing' the macrosomic fetus. The Nottingham MRI programme has demonstrated that brain growth is spared in asymmetrical fetal growth retardation, but liver size and hence the brain/liver volume ratio is significantly different in infants with intra-uterine growth retardation.

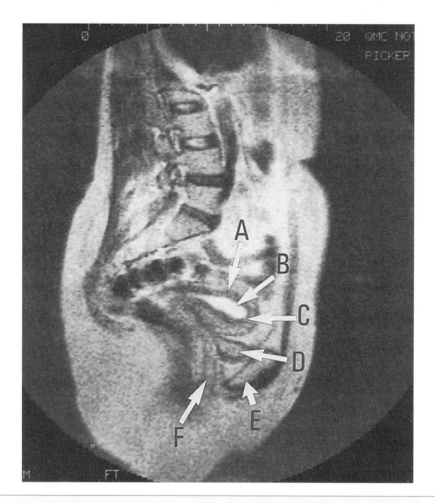

Fig. 19.22 Sagittal section of the normal non-pregnant female pelvis with magnetic resonance imaging. A, outer layers of the myometrium; B, endometrium; C, low-resonance band of the myometrium; D, bladder; E, pubic symphysis; F, vagina.

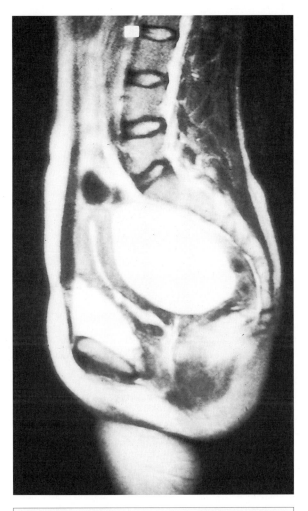

Fig. 19.23 Magnetic resonance imaging of a large ovarian cyst; the tumour can be seen distending the uterus and elongating the endometrium.

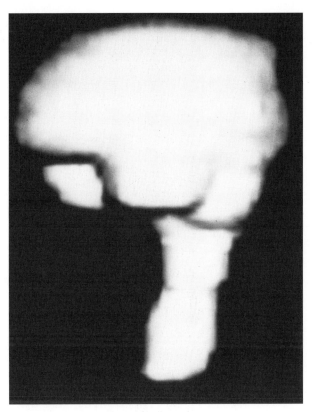

Fig. 19.24 Reconstructed image of the fetal brain using echoplanar imaging and multiple brain sections. (By courtesy of Professor I. R. Johnson.)

been principally used in studies on ovarian tumours to identify recurrent disease. Perhaps its greatest potential lies in the prospect of using the target antibody to carry cell toxins to the tumour cells.

IMMUNOSCINTIGRAPHY

This technique involves the injection of specific monoclonal antibodies to tumours into the circulation for the purpose of targeting radioactive isotopes on to tumour deposits. Remote metastases can be identified, and so far the technique has

BIBLIOGRAPHY

Chervenak F A, Isaacson G C, Campbell S 1993 Ultrasound in obstetrics and gynecology. Little Brown, Chicago, vols 1 and 2
Powell M C, Worthington B S, Symonds E M 1993 Magnetic resonance imaging in obstetrics and gynaecology. Butterworth/Heinemann, London

20 Contraception and sterilization

The ability to control fertility by reliable artifical methods has transformed both social and epidemiological aspects of human reproduction. Family size is determined by a number of factors including social and religous customs, economic aspirations, knowledge of contraception and the availability of reliable methods to regulate fertility.

The most fertile phase of the menstrual cycle occurs at the time of ovulation. In a 28 day cycle, this occurs between day 12 and day 14 of the cycle. Thus, natural methods of family planning include:

1. The **rhythm method** – avoiding intercourse midcycle and for 3–4 days either side of midcycle. The efficacy of this method depends on the ability to predict the time of ovulation.
2. **Coitus interruptus** – a traditional and still widely used method of contraception which relies on penile withdrawal before ejaculation. It is not a particularly reliable method of contraception.

Artificial methods of contraception act by the following pathways:

1. Inhibition of ovulation
2. Prevention of implantation of the fertilized ovum
3. Barrier methods of contraception whereby the spermatozoa are physically prevented from gaining access to the cervix.

Efficacy – The effectiveness of any method of contraception is measured by the number of unwanted pregnancies that occur during 100 women years of exposure, i.e. during 1 year of 100 women who are normally fertile and having regular coitus. This is known as the '**Pearl index**'.

BARRIER METHODS OF CONTRACEPTION

These techniques involve a physical barrier which prevents spermatozoa from reaching the female upper genital tract.

Condoms

The basic condom consists of a thin, stretchable latex film which is moulded into a sheath, lubricated and packed in a foil wrapper. The sheath has a teat end to collect the ejaculate. The disadvantages of sheaths are that they need to be applied before intercourse and that they reduce the level of sensation for the male partner. The advantages are that they are readily available, that they are without side effects for the female partner, and that they provide a degree of protection against infection. The failure rate is variable, but averages around 3.9 pregnancies per 100 women years.

Diaphragms

The female equivalent of the sheath is the diaphragm. The modern diaphragm consists of a thin latex rubber dome attached to a circular metal spring. These diaphragms vary in size from 45 to 100 mm in diameter. The size of the diaphragm required is ascertained by examination of the woman. The size and position of the uterus are determined by vaginal examination, and the distance from the posterior vaginal fornix to the pubic symphysis is noted. The appropriate measuring ring is inserted. This usually varies between 70 and 80 mm and, when correctly in position, the anterior edge of the ring or diaphragm should lie behind the pubic symphysis and the lower posterior edge should lie comfortably in the posterior fornix (Fig. 20.1).

The woman should be advised to insert the diaphragm either in the dorsal position or in the kneeling position whilst bending forwards. The diaphragm can be removed by simply hooking an index finger under the diaphragm rim from below and pulling it out. The diaphragm should be smeared on both sides with a contraceptive cream, and it is usually advised that the diaphragm be inserted dome down. However, some women prefer to insert the diaphragm with the dome upwards.

The diaphragm must be inserted prior to intercourse and should not be removed until at least

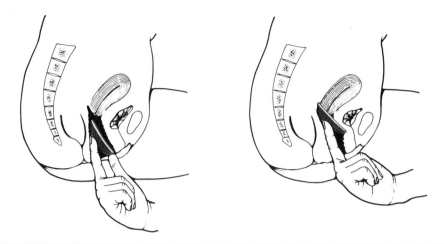

Fig. 20.1 Insertion of the vaginal diaphragm to cover the cervix and anterior vaginal wall.

6 hours later. The main advantage of this technique is that it is free of side effects to the woman, apart from occasional reaction to the contraceptive cream. The main disadvantages are that the diaphragm must be inserted before intercourse and that there is a failure rate of 7.2 per 100 women years. There are a variety of vault and cervical caps which are of much smaller diameter than the diaphragm. These are suitable for women with a long cervix or with some degree of prolapse, but otherwise have no particular advantage over the diaphragm.

Spermicides

Spermicides in general are only effective if used in conjunction with a mechancial barrier.

Pessaries or suppositories have a water-soluble or wax base and contain a spermicide. They must be inserted approximately 15 minutes before intercourse. Common spermicides are nonoxynol-9 and benzalkonium.

Creams consist of an emulsified fat base and tend not to spread. Care in insertion is essential so that the cervix is covered.

Jellies or pastes have a water-soluble base which spreads rapidly at body temperature. They therefore have an advantage over creams as they spread throughout the vagina.

Foam tablets and foam aerosols contain bicarbonate of soda so that carbon dioxide is released on contact with water. The foam spreads the spermicide throughout the vagina. Pregnancy rates vary with different agents, but average around 9–10 per 100 women years.

Sponges consist of polyurethane foam impregnated with nonoxynol-9. The failure rate is between 10 and 25%, and their use is not recommended as an isolated method.

Barrier contraception

- Condom: 3.9 pregnancies/100 women years but also some protection against infection
- Diaphragm: 7.2/100
- Spermicides: 10/100 (need to be used with other barrier)

INTRA-UTERINE CONTRACEPTIVE DEVICES (IUDs)

A wide variety of devices have been designed for insertion into the uterine cavity (Fig. 20.2). These devices have the advantage that, once inserted, they are retained without the need to take alternative contraceptive precautions. It seems likely that they act by preventing implantation of the fertilized oocyte, although some produce changes in cervical mucus which interfere with the ability of spermatozoa to penetrate into the uterine cavity.

The first device to be widely used was the Grafenberg ring, and was made of a silver–copper alloy. Introduced in the 1930s, it ran into considerable difficulties with haemorrhage, infection, abortions and uterine perforations. With the development of plastic devices in the 1960s, IUDs entered a new phase of acceptance, and are now in common usage.

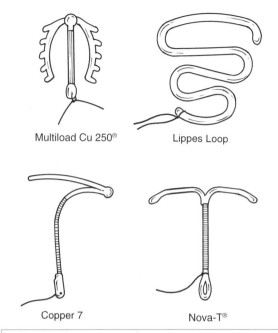

Multiload Cu 250®

Lippes Loop

Copper 7

Nova-T®

Fig. 20.2 Some intra-uterine contraceptive devices.

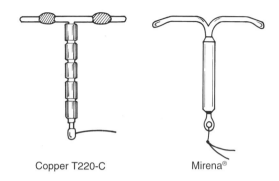

Copper T220-C

Mirena®

Fig. 20.3 Recent developments in copper and hormonal systems: the levonorgestrel intra-uterine system of delivery in the Mirena IUD.

Types of device

The devices are either inert or pharmacologically active.

Inert devices

Lippes loops, Saf-T-coils and Margulis spirals are plastic or plastic-coated devices. They have a thread attached which protrudes through the cervix and allows the woman to check that the device is still in place. Inert devices tend to be relatively large.

Pharmacologically active devices

The addition of copper to contraceptive devices produces a direct effect on the endometrium by interfering with endometrial oestrogen-binding sites and depressing uptake of thymidine into DNA. It also impairs glycogen storage in the endometrium. Examples of such devices are Copper-T or Copper-7 (first generation) or combined Multiload Copper-250.

Devices containing progestogen

Some devices such as the Mirena® contain 52 mg of levonorgestrel (Fig. 20.3). This provides protection against pregnancy for 5 years with a failure rate of 0.3–1.1%.

The levonorgestrel-containing device also suppresses the normal build up of the endometrium so that, unlike most IUDs, it causes a fall in menstrual blood loss. However, there is a high incidence of irregular scanty bleeding in the first 3 months after insertion of the device. Unlike previous progesterone- containing devices it does not appear to be associated with a higher risk of ectopic pregnancy.

Selection of patients

IUDs are best reserved for older parous women where there are difficulties with other methods of contraception, or where the motivation to remember to use methods which involve action before intercourse is deficient. These devices are not really suitable for nulliparous women under the age of 20 years, as the infection rate can be up to 18%. There are often difficulties with insertion of the device and expulsion rates are high. Menorrhagia, dysmenorrhoea and dyspareunia are common.

Insertion of devices

The optimal time for insertion of the device is in the first half of the menstrual cycle. With postpartum women, the optimal time is 4–6 weeks after delivery. Insertion at the time of therapeutic abortion is safe and can be performed when motivation is strong. It is unwise to insert IUDs following spontaneous abortion because of the risk of infection. Devices may be inserted within a few days of delivery, but there is a high expulsion rate. Ideally, the woman should be placed in the lithotomy position. A cervical smear should be taken, and a swab taken

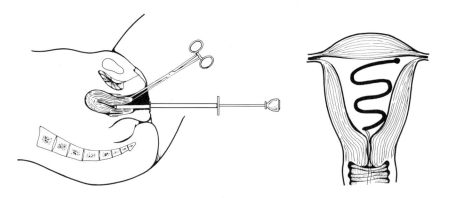

Fig. 20.4 Insertion of the IUD.

for culture if there is any sign of infection. The uterus is examined bimanually, and the size, shape and position ascertained. The cervix is swabbed with an antiseptic solution and a vulsellum can be applied to the anterior lip of the cervix, although this is not essential and may cause discomfort. The passage of a uterine sound will indicate the depth and direction of the uterine cavity, and the dimensions of the cavity may be assessed by devices known as cavimeters, which measures its length and breadth. Many IUDs are available in different sizes, and cavimeters help to choose the appropriate IUD. Insertion devices vary in construction, but generally consist of a stoppered plastic tube containing a plunger to extrude the device, which may be linear or folded (Fig. 20.4). The device is inserted in the plane of the uterine lumen and care is taken not to push it through the uterine fundus.

Attempts at insertion of a device where the cervical canal is tight may result in vagal syncope. Acute pain following insertion may indicate perforation of the uterus.

The woman should be instructed to check the loop strings regularly and to notify her doctor immediately if the strings are not palpable. Copper devices generally require replacement every 3–5 years, but other devices may be left in situ for longer periods.

Complications (Fig. 20.5)

Pregnancy rates

Pregnancy rates vary according to the type of device used, from 2–6/100 women years for non-medicated IUDs and 0.5–2/100 for early generation copper devices to less than 0.3/100 women years for third-generation copper and levonorgestrel IUDs. If the

device or its strings are easily grasped, it is sensible to remove it to reduce the incidence of a septic abortion, there being a high incidence of spontaneous abortion in such pregnancies. If it is not accessible, it should be left and removed at the time of delivery. The risk of failure of the IUD diminishes with each year after insertion.

Perforation of the uterus

About 0.1–1% of devices perforate the uterus. In many cases, partial perforation occurs at the time of insertion, and later migration completes the perforation. If the woman notices that the tail of the device is missing, then it must be assumed that one of the following has occurred:

1. The device has been expelled
2. The device has turned in the uterine cavity and drawn up the strings
3. The device has perforated the uterus and lies either partly or completely in the peritoneal cavity.

If there is no evidence of pregnancy, an ultrasound examination of the uterus should be performed. If the device is located within the uterine cavity, then it is removed and, unless part of the loop or strings is visible, it will generally be necessary to remove the device with formal dilatation of the cervix under general or local anaesthesia. If the device is not found in the uterus, a radiograph of the abdomen will reveal the site in the peritoneal cavity. It is advisable to remove all extra-uterine devices by either laparoscopy or laparotomy. Inert devices can probably be left with impunity, but copper devices promote considerable peritoneal irritation and should certainly be removed.

COMPLICATIONS OF IUCD

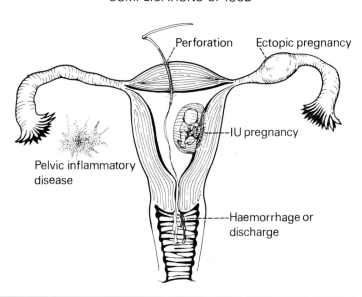

Fig. 20.5 Complications of IUDs.

Pelvic inflammatory disease

Acute pelvic inflammatory disease occurs in 1–2% of high-income patients and 8–10% of indigent populations. Pre-existent pelvic inflammatory disease is a contraindication to this method of contraception.

If pelvic inflammatory disease does occur, then the device should be removed immediately and antibiotic therapy commenced. If the infection is severe, it is preferable to complete 24 hours antibiotic therapy before removing the device.

Abnormal uterine bleeding

Increased menstrual loss occurs in most women with an IUD, but can be tolerated by the majority. However, in 15% of such women it is sufficiently severe to necessitate removal of the device. It can be controlled by drugs such as dicynene, amino-caproic acid or danazol. Intermenstrual bleeding may also occur, but if the loss is slight it does not constitute a reason for removal.

Pelvic pain

Pain occurs either in a chronic low-grade form or as severe dysmenorrhoea. The incidence is widely variable, with up to 50% of women suffering some pain. However, the pain may be acceptable if it is not severe, and this is a decision that has to be made by the patient in relation to the convenience of the method.

Vaginal discharge

Vaginal discharge may be due to infection, but most women with an IUD develop a slight watery or mucoid discharge.

Ectopic pregnancy

Compared with women having unprotected intercourse, the incidence of pregnancy is lower in women with an IUD in situ (2.5/100 women years). However, should pregnancy occur, there is a higher risk (3–4%) of the pregnancy being extra-uterine. It is therefore essential to think of this diagnosis in any woman presenting with abdominal pain and irregular vaginal bleeding and who has an intrauterine device in situ.

IUDs

- Prevent implantation
- Inert or pharmacologically active
- Best for older multiparous women
- Can be inserted at TOP
- Replace after 3–5 years
- 2 failures per 100 women years
- Complications: perforation, pelvic inflammatory disease, abnormal bleeding, ectopic pregnancy

---

HORMONAL CONTRACEPTION

Oral contraception is given as a combination of oestrogen or progestogen, either as a combined pill or triphasic pill, or as progesterone only.

Combined pill

These preparations contain oestrogen and a progestogen in a variety of combinations. The oestrogen used is either oestradiol or mestranol, and is given in a dosage between 20 and 50 µg daily. The progestogens used are derived from 17-hydroxyprogesterone or 19-norsteroids.

The only derivative of 17-hydroxyprogesterone commonly used is medroxyprogesterone acetate in the form of Depo-provera. The 19-norsteroids used include:

1. Norethisterone
2. Ethynodiol
3. Norgestrel
4. Levonorgestrel
5. Norethisterone acetate
6. Lynestrenol.

Triphasic pill

These pills have a variable dose of progestrogen and oestrogen components and are used to reduce the side effects from the progestogen.

Progesterone-only pill

Progesterone-only pills contain either norethisterone or ethynodiol diacetate and are taken continuously on the basis of one tablet daily. Because of the low dose, they should be taken at the same time every day.

Injectable compounds

Medroxyprogesterone acetate is administered as a depot preparation given in a single injection which lasts for 3 months. This compound has been criticized because of its side effects, which include irregular vaginal bleeding, loss of hair and skin eruptions.

Norplant contains 36 mg of levonorgestrel, impregnated into a silicone rubber rod, and implanted subcutaneously in the arm. The effects last from 3 to 5 years, and it requires surgical removal.

Mode of action

Combined and triphasic pills act by suppressing gonadotrophin secretion and, in particular, the luteinizing hormone peak. The endometrium becomes unsuitable for nidation and the cervical mucus becomes hostile. Progesterone-only pills alter the endometrial maturation and affect cervical mucus. Ovulation is suppressed in only 40% of women.

Contraindications

There are various contraindications to the pill, some being more absolute than others.

The absolute contraindications include pregnancy, pulmonary embolism, deep vein thrombosis, sickle cell disease, porphyria, liver disease and jaundice – particularly where it is associated with a previous pregnancy or carcinoma of the breast. It is necessary to maintain a high level of vigilance in women with varicose veins, diabetes, hypertension, renal disease, chronic heart failure and oligomenorrhoea, but none of these conditions constitutes an absolute contraindication, and, in some cases, the adverse effects of a pregnancy may substantially outweigh any hazard from the pill. Women who smoke and those over the age of 35 years have a significantly increased risk of thromboembolic disease.

The occurrence of migraine for the first time, severe headaches or visual disturbances, or transient neurological changes are indications for immediate cessation of the pill. There are a series of minor side effects which may sometimes be used to advantage or may be offset by using a pill with a different combination of steroids.

Oestrogenic effects	*Progestogenic effects*
Fluid retention and oedema	Premenstrual depression
	Dry vagina
Premenstrual tension, and irritability	Acne, greasy hair
Increase in weight	Increased appetite with weight gain
Nausea and vomiting	Breast discomfort
Headache	Cramps of the legs and abdomen
Mucorrhoea, cervical erosion	Decreased libido
Menorrhagia	
Excessive tiredness	
Vein complaints	
Breakthrough bleeding	

Therapeutic uses other than contraception include the treatment of menorrhagia, premenstrual syndrome, endometriosis and dysmenorrhoea.

Major side effects

The mortality rate from thrombo-embolic disease is

1.3 per 100 000 below 34 years of age and 3.4 per 100 000 above 35 years. Cardiovascular problems are increased, and this appears to be associated with increased levels of low-density lipoproteins or reduced levels of high-density lipoproteins. Prolonged amenorrhoea may occur in women coming off the pill, but the direct relationship remains unclear. Smoking increases the risks of thrombo-embolic disease two- to threefold.

Beneficial effects

In addition to the prevention of unwanted pregnancy, the use of the pill is associated with a 50% reduction in blood loss at menstruation, a lower incidence of ectopic pregnancy (0.4/1000) and some protection against pelvic inflammatory disease and benign ovarian cysts. Pill users also have a reduced risk of both endometrial and ovarian cancer of up to 50% depending on the length of use.

Counselling

It is important to obtain a complete general history and examination before prescribing the pill, and also to perform annual check-ups and cervical cytology. There are a large number of compounds commercially available, and some pills marketed by different companies contain the same compounds at the same concentrations.

Interaction between drugs and contraceptive steroids

Many drugs affect the contraceptive efficacy of the pill, and therefore additional precautions should be taken (Table 20.1). Vomiting and diarrhoea also result in loss of the pill and hence the return of fertility – particularly with the low-dose pills now widely in use. Progesterone-only pills must be taken every day if they are to be effective.

Failure rates

The failure rate of combined pills is 0.5 per 100 women years. The failure rate for progesterone-only preparations is higher and varies between 0.9 and 4.3 per 100 women years.

The pill and surgery

The pill increases the risk of deep vein thrombosis and should therefore be stopped at least 6 weeks before surgery. It should not be stopped before minor

procedures – particularly before laparoscopic sterilization procedures. The risk of an unwanted pregnancy occurring before admission is substantially greater than the risk of thrombo-embolus.

The pill and lactation

Combined preparations tend to inhibit lactation and are therefore best avoided. The pill of choice at this time is the progesterone-only pill as it has minimal effect on lactation and may, indeed, promote it.

Postcoital pill

Following unanticipated intercourse around mid-cycle, there is sometimes a need for emergency measures to prevent conception.

The regime recommended by the Committee of Safety in Medicines as an emergency measure is that of a combined oestrogen–progestogen pill. The preparation of choices should contain 50 μg of ethinyloestradial and 250 μg of levonorgestrel. Two pills of this combination should be given within 72 hours of exposure and then repeated 12 hours later. If one dose is lost through vomiting, the complete course should be repeated.

Combined oral contraceptive pill

- Suppress gonadotrophins
- Oestradiol and progestogen
- Pregnancy, thrombo-embolism and liver disease contraindicate
- 1.3/100 000 mortality
- 0.5/100 women years failure rate

STERILIZATION

Contraceptive techniques have the major advantage that they are easily reversible and provide a high level of protection against pregnancy. They have the disadvantage that they require a conscious act on behalf of the individual before intercourse. When family size is complete or there is a specific medical contraindication to continuing fertility, then sterilization becomes the contraceptive method of choice.

Counselling

It is essential to counsel both partners about the nature of the procedures and their implications and to discuss whether it is better for the male or female

Table 20.1 Interaction of various drugs with oral contraceptives

Interacting drug	Effects of interaction
Analgesics	
Amidopyrine	Breakthrough bleeding
Phenazone	
Pethidine	Possible increased sensitivity to pethidine
Anti-inflammatory agents	
Phenylbutazone	Possible decrease in contraceptive reliability
Oxyphenbutazone	
Anticoagulants	
Dicoumarol	Possible reduction of effect of anticoagulant. An increased dosage of anticoagulant may be necessary
Anticonvulsants	
Hydantoins:	
Ethotoin	
Methoin	
Phenytoin	Possible decrease in contraceptive reliability
Methylphenobarbitone	Careful observation is necessary for signs of fluid retention
Phenobarbitone	
Primidone	
Ethosuximide	
Carbamazepine	
Tricyclic antidepressants	
Imipramine	
Clomipramine	Reduced antidepressant response; increase in antidepressant toxicity
Amitriptyline	
Antihistamines	
Antihistamines	Possible decrease in contraceptive reliability
Anti-infective agents	
Ampicillin	
Chloramphenicol	
Neomycin	Possible decrease in contraceptive reliability
Nitrofurantoin	Possibility of breakthrough bleeding
Penicillin V	This is most likely with rifampicin
Rifampicin	
Sulphamethoxypyridazine	
Antimigraine agents	
Dihydroergotamine	Possible decrease in contraceptive reliability
Barbiturates	
Phenobarbitone	Probable decrease in contraceptive reliability
Methylphenobarbitone	
Hypoglycaemic agents	
Insulin	Control of diabetes may be reduced
Oral hypoglycaemics	
Anti-asthmatics	
Anti-asthmatics	Asthmatic condition may be exacerbated by concomitant oral contraceptive ingestion
Sedatives and tranquilizers	
Chlordiazepoxide	
Chlorpromazine	Possible decrease in contraceptive reliability
Diazepam	Possibility of breakthrough bleeding
Meprobamate	
Systemic corticosteroids	
Systemic corticosteroids	Increased dosage of steroids may be necessary as plasma corticoid-binding protein increases

partner to be sterilized. In many cases, only one partner will be seeking sterilization, in which case only one point of view needs to be considered.

Counselling should include reference to the failure rates and to the question of reversibility. With the improvements brought about by microsurgery, it is no longer acceptable to say that sterilization is irreversible and the patient should be counselled according to the technique to be used. The partner to be sterilized will be a matter of choice and motivation. If one partner has a reduced life expectancy from chronic illness, then that partner should be sterilized.

Timing of sterilization

The operation is best performed in the first half of the menstrual cycle. If this is not possible, then it is important to ascertain that the woman is not pregnant. Sterilization at the time of abortion or delivery is generally unwise because of the high failure rate and relatively high 'regret' rate. It is preferable to perform sterilization as an 'interval' procedure some 3 months after delivery.

Techniques

Female sterilization

The majority of procedures involve interruption of the Fallopian tubes, but may vary from the application of clips on the tubes to total hysterectomy. In general terms, the more radical the procedure, the less likely there is to be a failure. However, very low failure rates can now be achieved using methods with high reversibility prospects and these should be the methods of choice.

Tubal ligation (Fig. 20.6) – The common technique involves simple ligation of a loop of tube using a 'mini'-laparotomy procedure. This is known as the **Madlener procedure**.

The **Pomeroy technique** is the same, but the loop of tube is excised and absorbable suture material used for the ligation. There are several variations to this technique, including the separation of the cut ends of the tubes on contralateral sides of the broad ligament.

Failure rates vary with the technique but may be as high as 3.7% with the Madlener operation, and as low as 0.6% for the Pomeroy technique. This type of procedure may also be performed by the vaginal route, either through the pouch of Douglas or through the utero-vesical fold of peritoneum. The failure rates tend to be higher than those achieved via abdominal incision.

Laparoscopic sterilization – The use of the laparoscope for sterilization procedures has substantially reduced the duration of hospital stay.

1. Tubal coagulation and division – Sterilization is effected by either unipolar or bipolar diathermy of the tubes in two sites 1–2 cm from the utero-tubal junction. A considerable amount of tube can be destroyed with this technique. Division of the diathermied tube is said to reduce the risk of ectopic pregnancy. The failure rate with this procedure is about 0.7%. The major complication of the procedure is the danger of burning bowel with subsequent leakage and faecal peritonitis.

2. Tubal clips – The application of clips or rings through the laparoscope has become popular because it avoids the risk of diathermy damage. The clips are made of plastic and inert metals and are locked on to the tube (Fig. 20.7). They have the advantage of causing minimal damage to the tube, but their disadvantage is a higher failure rate.

   The **Hulka–Clemens clip** has been reported as having a failure rate of up to 2.6%. Failures may be due to application on the wrong structure or extrusion of the tube from the clip, recanalization, or fracture of the clip so that it falls off the tube.

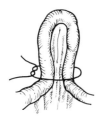
Madlener

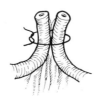
Pomeroy

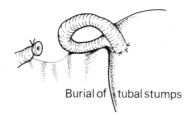
Burial of tubal stumps

Fig. 20.6 Sterilization by tubal ligation and excision.

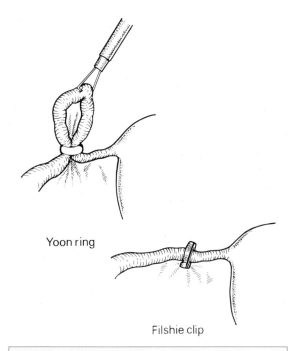

Fig. 20.7 Sterilization by clip occlusion.

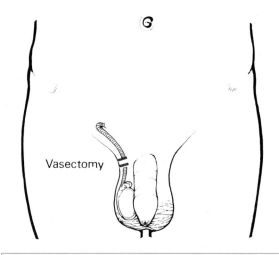

Fig. 20.8 Vasectomy involves excision of a segment of the vas deferens.

The **Filshie clip**, which has a titanium frame lined by silicone rubber, has a lower failure rate (0.2%) and is easier to apply.

Yoon rings are applied over a loop of tube and are similar to a Madlener procedure. This technique is associated with considerably greater abdominal pain postoperatively, and the failure rates vary between 0.3 and 4%. The rings are not suitable for application to the tubes in the puerperium where the tube is swollen and oedematous.

Complications – Apart from the complications of laparoscopy, the longer-term complications are those of tubal recanalization and pregnancy, ectopic pregnancy, menstrual irregularity and loss of libido.

Table 20.2	Comparative failure rates
Method	*Pregnancies (per 100 women years)*
Sheath	3.9
Diaphragm	7.2
Spermicides	10
Combined pill	0.5
Progesterone-only pill	0.9–4.3
IUD	0.3–3.0
Clip sterilization	0.2 (%)
Vasectomy	1–2/1000

Vasectomy

This procedure is generally performed under local anaesthesia. Two small incisions are made over the spermatic cord and 3–4 cm of the vas deferens are excised (Fig. 20.8).

The advantage of the technique is its simplicity. The disadvantages are that sterility is not immediate, and should not be assumed until all spermatozoa have disappeared from the ejaculate. On average, this takes about 14 ejaculations. The procedure is more difficult to reverse and, even when satisfactory re-anastomosis is achieved, only about 50% of patients will sire children, because of the production of sperm-immobilizing and sperm-agglutinating antibodies. Failures may follow spontaneous recanalization and excision of an inadequate length of vas deferens. The excised segments should always be examined histologically to confirm that the vas has been excised. Complications of the operation include haematoma formation, wound infection and epididymitis. Also a painful granuloma may form at the cut end of the vas due to a foreign body reaction induced by spermatozoa.

Sterilization

- Counsel re. irreversibility, failure rate and risks
- Laparoscopy/mini-laparotomy
- 0.2–4% failure rate
- Complictions: laparoscopic, ectopic pregnancy, menstrual irregularity

---

TERMINATION OF PREGNANCY

In the UK this is carried out in approved centres under the provision of the 1967 Abortion Act. This Act requires that two doctors agree that continuation of the pregnancy would either involve greater risk to the physical or mental health of the mother or her other children than termination, or that the fetus is at risk of an abnormality likely to result in it being seriously handicapped. The most recent amendment to the Act sets a limit for termination under the first of these categories at 24 weeks, although in practice the majority of terminations are carried out prior to 20 weeks. All terminations carried out in the UK must be notified. Approximately 200 000 legal terminations per year are carried out in the UK, and this number is still rising.

Indications for termination of pregnancy

- Pregnancy involves greater risk to the mother's life than termination
- To prevent grave permanent injury to the mother's health
- Pregnancy involves a greater risk to the mother's mental or physical health (under 24 weeks)
- Risk to the health of the existing children of the woman (under 24 weeks)
- Fetal abnormality likely to result in serious mental or physical handicap

---

Surgical termination of pregnancy

This is the method most commonly used in the first trimester. The cervix is dilated under general anaesthesia, and the conceptus removed using a suction curette. A variation involving piecemeal removal of the larger fetal parts with forceps (dilatation and evacuation) allows the method to be used for later second-trimester pregnancies. Cervical dilation can be made easier by administration of prostaglandin pessaries before the operation.

Medical termination of pregnancy

This is the method most commonly used for pregnancies after 14 weeks. Abortion is induced using prostaglandins administered either as vaginal pessaries or as an extra-amniotic infusion through a balloon catheter passed through the cervix. After delivery of the fetus, an examination under general anaesthetic may be necessary to remove the placenta. Medical termination can also be carried out in the first trimester using the oral progesterone antagonist mefipristone. A single oral dose induces complete abortion in 60–85% of cases when given alone and in up to 98% of cases when given with a vaginal prostaglandin pessary.

Complications of termination

Early complications include bleeding, uterine perforation (with possible damage to other pelvic viscera), cervical laceration, retained products and sepsis. All the procedures also have a small failure rate. Late complications include infertility, cervical incompetence, isoimmunization and psychiatric morbidity. Adequate counselling and explanation of the procedures and their risk are essential.

Contraception following termination

Referral for termination should also be an opportunity to discuss future contraception and to ensure that adequate provision is made for this after the termination. The procedure can be combined with sterilization. This has the advantage of preventing further terminations for the woman who is certain she has completed her family, but there is a slightly higher failure rate for some forms of sterilization carried out at this time and an increase in the 'regret rate'. IUD insertion can be carried out at the same time as termination and is not associated with an increased risk of perforation or failure. If the oral contraceptive is being used, this can be started on the same or following day.

BIBLIOGRAPHY

Department of Health 1990 Handbook of contraceptive practice. HMSO, London
Loudon N 1991 Handbook of family planning, 2nd edn. Churchill Livingstone, Edinburgh
Szarciwski A, Guillebaud J 1994 Contraception. Oxford University Press, Oxford

The changes of the menstrual cycle

The nature of the menstrual cycle has been described in a previous chapter. Menstruation is the periodic change occurring in primates which results in the flow of blood and endometrium from the uterine cavity, and which may be associated with various constitutional disturbances.

PUBERTY AND MENARCHE

Puberty is the process of sexual maturation beginning with the maturation of the hypothalamus. This results in an increased release of pituitary gonadotrophins and, hence, stimulation of the ovary with the production of sex hormones. Other trophic hormones such as adrenocorticotrophic hormone (ACTH), thyroid-stimulating hormone (TSH) and growth hormone also gradually increase over a period of 3–4 years. The sexual changes of puberty can be divided into three phases.

Thelarche

The first of the sexual changes to occur is the development of the breast (Fig. 21.1). Nipple enlargement begins between 9 and 11 years of age with thickening of the duct system as a result of increasing oestrogen production. At the same time, the vaginal epithelium increases in thickness and vaginal pH decreases.

Adrenarche

The growth of pubic hair occurs at about 11–12 years of age, and is followed by the development of axillary hair (Fig. 21.2). Both phenomena are dependent on adrenal development.

Menarche

The final manifestation of sexual maturity in the female is the onset of mestruation. The average age of the menarche in the UK is 13 years, and occurs in 95% of girls between the ages of 11 and 15 years. There has been a lowering of the age of the menarche

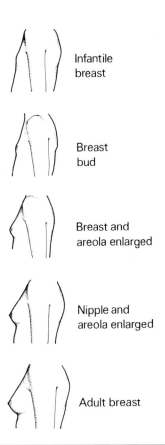

Infantile breast

Breast bud

Breast and areola enlarged

Nipple and areola enlarged

Adult breast

Fig. 21.1 Development of the female breast during the thelarche.

in Western Europe and there is some variation between different ethnic groups.

The menstrual cycle is often irregular in the first 2 years and may show intervals of 4–6 months between periods. The cycles are frequently anovulatory, and prolonged bleeding may occur.

The growth spurt

Throughout the period of sexual maturation, marked changes occur in growth (Fig. 21.3). A rapid increase

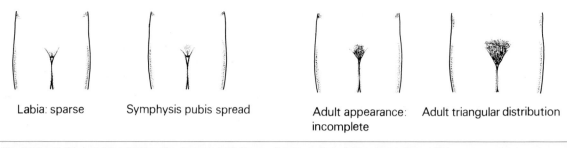

Labia: sparse   Symphysis pubis spread   Adult appearance: Adult triangular distribution
                                           incomplete

Fig. 21.2 Pubic hair distribution leading up to full sexual maturation during the adrenarche.

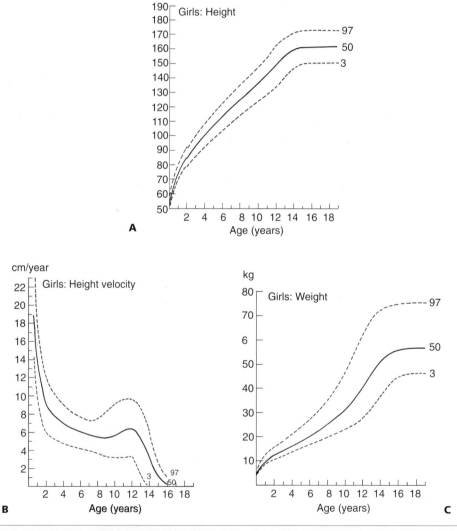

Fig. 21.3 **A** Centile change for height in the female; **B** height velocity indicates the slowing down of the rate of growth with a secondary acceleration around the time of puberty; **C** changes in weight show a wider scatter than with height.

in growth occurs between 11 and 14 years. The legs lengthen first, and this is followed by increases in shoulder breadth and in trunk length. The pelvis enlarges and changes in shape. Maximal height occurs between 17 and 18 years, and growth is terminated by the fusion of femoral epiphyses.

Puberty/Menarche

- Hypothalamic maturation
- Breast enlargement 9–11 years
- Pubic hair 11–12 years
- Menarche 11–15 years
- Growth spurt 11–14 years

Precocious puberty

The development of physical signs of sexual maturation before the age of 8 years and the onset of menstruation before the age of 10 years are indications of precocious puberty. The majority of cases carry no pathological connotation.

Aetiology

Precocious puberty may occur at any point in the hypothalamic–pituitary–ovarian axis or as a result of abnormalities in the adrenal or thyroid glands. Causes may be (Fig. 21.4):

- Constitutional
- Neurological – meningitis, encephalitis, polyostotic fibrosus, dysplasia, neurofibromatosis, cerebral tumours, hydrocephalus, cysts

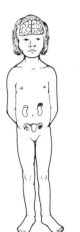

Constitutional

Neurological

Ovarian tumours

Adrenal tumours

Gonadotrophin secretory tumours

Others: hypothyroidism, exogenous oestrogens

Fig. 21.4 The aetiology of precocious puberty.

- Ovarian tumours
- Adrenal tumours
- Gonadotrophin-secreting tumours – chorio-epithelioma, hepatoblastoma
- Others – hypothyroidism, exogenous oestrogens.

The majority of cases of precocious puberty are constitutional in origin. It is, however, important to exclude other organic causes before classifying the problem as constitutional. There are a group of cases where the activity of the hypothalamic–pituitary axis is stimulated by intracranial lesions such as meningitis, encephalitis, ventricular hamatoma and pineal tumours. The **McCune–Albright syndrome** is a disorder of bone involving widespread polyostotic fibrous dysplasia with disturbed function of the hypothalamus and pituitary resulting in premature menstruation. There is also a skin disorder manifested by the development of skin pigmentation and cafe-au-lait spots. Of the ovarian lesions, the commonest are the granulosa cell tumours. These must be differentiated from follicular cysts, which may be associated with hypothalamic causes.

Investigation

All children exhibiting precocious sexual development must be investigated to exclude any underlying pathology. General and pelvic examination may reveal evidence of ovarian lesions. A skeletal survey should be undertaken for any bony abnormalities. Skull radiography and computerized axial tomography (CAT) scanning may reveal the presence of abnormalities of the sella turcica, suprasella calcification and lesions involving the floor of the fourth ventricle.

Ultrasound scanning of the pelvis should reveal any ovarian tumours.

Management

In children where there is a specific lesion causing precocious sexual maturation, the management depends on the treatment of the condition. In constitutional precocious puberty, management is concerned with the abnormal bone growth and the emotional and psychological problems contingent on early sexual maturation. Advanced bone growth results in the girl initially being much taller than her classmates, but the early fusion of epiphysis means that her ultimate stature is smaller than normal. It is sometimes possible to inhibit hypothalamic activity by the administration of medroxyprogesterone acetate 100–200 mg i.m. every 2–4 weeks or by giving the anti-androgenic agent cyproterone acetate by the oral route.

These children may need protection from sexual assault as they may conceive if coitus occurs. The youngest recorded pregnancy and confinement occurred in a 6-year-old child with precocious sexual development.

> **Precocious puberty**
> • Menarche before 10 years of age
> • Usually constitutional
> • Exclude intracranial/ovarian lesions
> • Investigations, ultrasound scanning of pelvis, radiography of pituitary fossa, skeletal survey

Delayed puberty

Delayed puberty commonly presents as primary amenorrhoea. This is defined as the failure to menstruate by the age of 16 years. However, delayed puberty is also revealed by failure in development of secondary sexual characteristics.

If the secondary sexual characteristics are normal apart from amenorrhoea, the diagnosis is likely to be (Fig. 21.5):

1. Hematocolpos – the retention of menstrual fluid because of an imperforate hymen
2. Vaginal agenesis – congenital absence of the vagina
3. Resistant ovary syndrome (see below)

4. Testicular feminization or other chromosomal abnormalities.

If the secondary sexual characteristics are poor, then the amenorrhoea may be due to (Fig. 21.6):

1. Constitutional delay in puberty
2. Gonadal dysgenesis – primitive streak ovaries or the congenital absence of ovarian tissue
3. Hypothalamic–pituitary failure.

If there are signs of virilization in the female, then the following diagnoses should be considered (Fig. 21.7):

1. Congenital adrenal hyperplasia
2. Virilizing adrenal tumours
3. Virilizing ovarian tumours
4. Cushing's syndrome
5. Chromosomal abnormalities such as the 46 XY female.

General examination should take account of the age, height, weight and arm span of the individual and also features of abnormal somatic structures such as neck webbing and short metatarsal bones. Pelvic examination will reveal whether there are any abnormalities of the genital tract.

The resistant ovary syndrome

This is a rare but important cause of primary amenorrhoea. Secondary sexual characteristics are usually normal. Follicle-stimulating hormone (FSH)

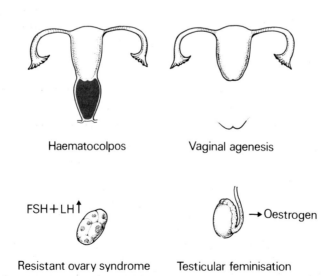

Haematocolpos Vaginal agenesis

Resistant ovary syndrome Testicular feminisation

Fig. 21.5 The aetiology of primary amenorrhea (FSH, follicle-stimulating hormone; luteinizing hormone).

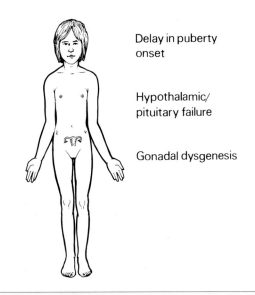

Fig. 21.6 Aetiology of delayed puberty with poor secondary sexual characteristics.

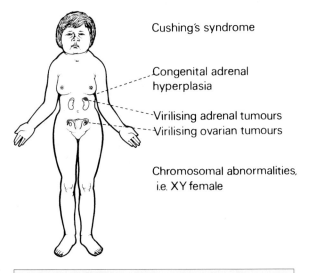

Fig. 21.7 Aetiology of virilization and hirsutism in the female.

and luteinizing hormone (LH) levels are raised to the menopausal range but, unlike true ovarian failure, the ovaries contain numerous ova. Stimulation with human menopausal gonadotrophin or with human chorionic gonadotrophin meets with little success. It must be remembered that these women are able˙ to conceive and may sometimes ovulate spontaneously. Prognosis for childbearing must be guarded, but, unlike true ovarian failure,

ovulation and spontaneous menstruation may occur.

Intersexuality

Ambiguous genital development is a rare, but disturbing problem and successful management at a physical and psychological level should be started as soon after birth as possible.

Causes of ambiguous genitalia may be:

1. Where the fetus has a Y chromosome and so is karyotypically male, the testes may not form, or they may function abnormally and produce oestrogens, as in testicular feminization. The failure of androgen production or androgen insensitivity at the target organ site will result in development of female external genitalia.
2. Virilization may occur in a karyotypic female with androgens being produced from some outside source such as in congenital adrenal hyperplasia.
3. Mosaicism – on occasions, true hermaphroditism does occur, and testicular and ovarian tissues form in the same fetus.

The appearance of the hermaphrodite, the undermasculinized male and the masculinized female are all similar. Differential diagnosis is dependent on establishing the karyotype, and measuring 17-oxosteroids and the intermediate products of cortisol metabolism as well as electrolyte levels.

Congenital adrenal hyperplasia needs early recognition if fetal and neonatal survival is to occur. Salt loss may be a major factor in this condition, and the infant should be treated with cortisone acetate and prednisone or bromohydrocortisone.

Sexual assignment is particularly important in all intersex cases and should be allocated on the basis of phenotypic sex.

Delayed puberty

• Primary amenorrhoea
• Poor secondary sex characteristics
• Consider chromosome disorders and adrenal tumours

THE MENOPAUSE

At the other end of the spectrum, the termination of menstrual life occurs, and is accompanied by a variety of different manifestations.

The **climacteric** is that part of the ageing process which embraces the transition from the reproductive

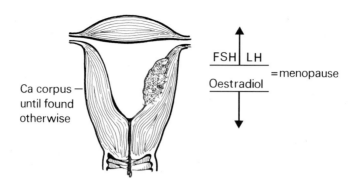

Fig. 21.8   Postmenopausal bleeding must always be assumed to result from corpus carcinoma until the diagnosis is excluded. The menopause can be confirmed by the presence of high FSH/LH levels and low oestradiol levels in the plasma.

to the non-reproductive phase of life. It is divided into the **premenopause, menopause** and **post-menopause**. The menopause marks the end of menstruation but, as with the menarche in relation to puberty, it reflects only one manifestation of a series of changes. The age of the physiological menopause varies with race and socio-economic conditions, but in Western Europe and the USA the average age of onset is between 49 and 50 years.

Spontaneous cessation of the periods before the age of 40 years is defined as premature menopause. The menopause may be physiological or artificial, when it is associated with removal of the ovaries or the uterus.

Hormonal and menstrual changes in the premenopause

The menstrual cycle shortens in women over the age of 40 years, and the change in the cycle length is related to shortening of the follicular phase. FSH levels are higher at all stages of the cycle than levels seen in younger women, whilst oestradiol levels are lower.

The transition from menstruation to amenorrhoea is often characterized by menstrual irregularity. Prolonged episodes of bleeding following a period of amenorrhoea may be associated with anovulatory cycles and with hyperplastic endometrium. Persistent irregular bleeding in the premenopausal phase should never be considered normal, because it may be associated with uterine neoplasms.

Vaginal bleeding which occurs more than 1 year after the menopause is known as postmenopausal bleeding. The possibility of carcinoma of the body of the uterus should be considered, and diagnostic curettage or endometrial aspiration performed in all cases (Fig. 21.8).

Other causes of postmenopausal bleeding include other benign and malignant tumours of the lower genital tract, stimulation of the endometrium by exogenous oestrogen (e.g. hormone replacement therapy and oestrogens from ovarian tumours), infection and senile atrophic vaginitis. Diagnostic curettage should be accompanied by direct inspection of the uterine cavity to minimize the risk of missing localized disease. Ultrasound measurement of endometrial thickness can also be used, as significant endometrial pathology is unlikely where this is less than 3 mm.

Hormone changes in the menopause

There is a marked reduction in ovarian production of oestrogen and, in particular, of oestradiol. Some oestrogen production occurs in the adrenal gland, but the major source of oestradiol appears to be the 'fat' organ with peripheral conversion of both oestrone and testosterone. Thus, heavy women have higher circulating oestradiol levels than slender women. There is considerable variation in the circulating levels of oestradiol in the menopause, and this may account for the variation in severity of menopausal symptoms. The absence of any significant oestrogen production results in excessive release of FSH and LH, with the major increases occurring in FSH. The levels of gonadotrophins continue to show random oscillations similar to the pattern seen in the premenopausal phase. Androgens produced in the ovary and adrenal gland are mainly androstenedione and testosterone and these levels fall in menopausal women. There is also a reduction in adrenal androgen secretion, including that of dehydroepiandrosterone (DHEA) and DHEA sulphate. Oestrogen production by the ovary is reduced, but the production of testosterone persists.

Symptoms and signs of the menopause

Vascular disturbances

The commonest symptom of the menopause is the development of hot flushes. These episodes consist of flushes and perspiration, occur in about 80% of the female population and may persist for up to 5 years after the menopause. The flushes are associated with an increase in skin temperature and conductance. They are also associated in some way with high gonadotrophin levels, but this relationships is not as clear as might at first appear. There are other women where oestrogen levels are low and gonadotrophin levels are high, but who do not develop hot flushes. There is no doubt that the administration of oestrogens relieves these symptoms, but they return when the oestrogen therapy is discontinued.

Changes in target organ response

The reduction in ovarian oestrogen production results in involution and regression of target organs (Fig. 21.9).

The most obvious response is the cessation of menstruation. Periods generally exhibit a gradual reduction in both amount and duration, with occasional delays in menstruation. The vaginal walls lose their rugosity and become smooth and atrophic. In severe cases, this may also be associated with chronic infection and atrophic vaginitis. The cervix diminishes in size, and there is a reduction in cervical mucus production. The uterus also shrinks in size, and the endometrium becomes atrophic.

The breasts exhibit parallel changes with involution of breast structure and the disappearance of cyclical breast changes, which may bring considerable relief to some women.

Although it is not in any proper sense an endocrine target organ, the bladder epithelium may also become atrophic with the development of frequency, dysuria and urge incontinence in the absence of any overt urinary tract infection. It is important to recognize these symptoms because they can be relieved by oestrogen replacement therapy.

Epidermal appendages

The skin tends to become thinned and wrinkled after the menopause as a result of oestrogen deprivation; these changes can be reversed by the use of local oestrogen creams or by hormone replacement therapy. There is loss of scalp hair and of pubic and axillary hair. There is an androgen-based increase in the growth of coarse terminal hair so that a slight moustache may develop, and loss of scalp hair sometimes results in partial or complete baldness, but this is uncommon.

Bone changes

Osteoporosis is an important health hazard in the menopausal woman. The loss of trabecular bone is the major disorder. Bone loss occurs at a rate of about 2.5% per year for the first 4 years after the

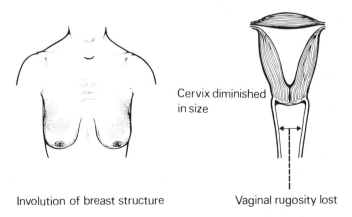

Cervix diminished in size

Involution of breast structure

Vaginal rugosity lost

Fig. 21.9 Characteristic changes in the breasts and genitalia following the menopause.

menopause so that fractures become a major source of morbidity in the menopausal female. Thus, by the age of 65 years, vertebral fractures occur in 25% of all women.

Bone loss is most severe in women who have an artificial menopause. Hip fractures increase in incidence from 0.3/1000 at an age of 45 years to 20/1000 at age 85 years, and there is also a 10-fold increase in Colles' fractures.

Osteoporosis is associated with increased bone resorption with normal bone formation. There is no doubt that there is a net loss of calcium. These changes are associated with oestrogen deficiency and there is little doubt that prolonged and early hormone replacement therapy can prevent the development of osteoporosis. The means by which these effects are achieved remains uncertain. Fractures late in life carry serious implications in relation to life expectation because of the immobilization of the elderly woman.

Cardiovascular complications

There is evidence of an increase in coronary heart disease following the menopause which is not simply an age-related phenomenon. However, hormone replacement therapy with oestrogens does reduce the incidence of coronary heart disease. Serum cholesterol levels rise at the time of the menopause. There is an increase in all lipoprotein fractions, with a decrease in the ratio of the high- to low-density fractions. This is reversed by the administration of hormone replacement therapy. There is no specific association between the menopause and hypertension.

Psychological and emotional symptoms

Many women experience serve emotional disorders at the time of the menopause with depression and anxiety states. The emotional disturbances of the menopause are often associated with feelings of inadequacy and uncertainty about the woman's role with the departure of children from the home. However, there is no doubt that in many women these symptoms are related to oestrogen deficiency and that hormone replacement therapy can return such women to a normal state. The severity of the symptoms should not be underestimated. The depression may be acute and can sometimes result in a successful suicidal attempt. There are many other symptoms ascribed to the menopause, including anorexia, excessive fatigue, nausea and vomiting and bowel disorders.

Treatment of the menopause

Many women pass through the menopause without any symptoms, and there is considerable variation in serum oestradiol levels between individuals after the menopause. Symptoms can often be treated by reassurance and explanation and occasionally by the use of tranquillisers, anti-depressants and sedatives. Flushes sometimes respond to belladonna alkaloids, but respond best to oestrogen therapy.

Hormone replacement therapy

Oestrogen therapy may be given on its own or as a combined or sequential therapy with a progestogen (Fig. 21.10). The type of therapy recommended will depend on whether the uterus has been removed and whether the therapy planned is to be short or long term.

Oral therapy – Ethinyloestradiol or conjugated equine oestrogen (Premarin) is given continuously with concomitant administration of a progestogen in women with an intact uterus to prevent the development of endometrial hyperplasia or malignancy. Progestogens are commonly given for 10–12 days every 4 weeks, to produce a monthly withdrawal bleed, but there is no loss of protective effect when this is reduced to 12-weekly intervals. Those women who have previously stopped their periods and wish to avoid further bleeds can be offered combination therapy which includes continuous progestogen administration with an oestrogen or a compound such as Tibolone.

Parenteral therapy – Oestrogen can also be administered by injection or by subcutaneous implants. This is best achieved with oestradiol benzoate, 100 mg, in a pellet which is inserted in the subcutaneous tissue of the anterior abdominal wall. This is often combined with testosterone, which has the advantage of a mild anabolic effect and of enhancing libido. The pellets usually last for anything up to 6 months and are particularly useful in women who have experienced a surgical menopause. Tachyphylaxis with progressively shorter intervals between implants and the return of symptoms even in the presence of normal or high oestradiol levels can be a problem.

If the implants are given to a woman with an intact uterus, then it is important to give a progestogen, such as norethisterone acetate 5 mg, for the first 7 days of each month. This will provoke withdrawal bleeding as long as active oestrogen absorption occurs.

Topical therapy – Oestradiol can be given percutaneously by self-adhesive patches or gel. Patches

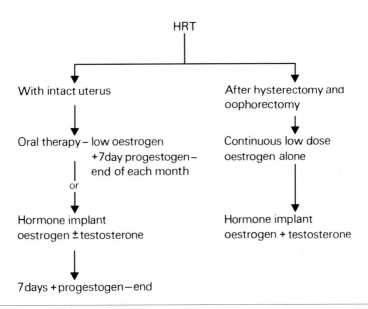

Fig. 21.10 Treatment protocol for the management of menopausal symptoms with the use of hormone replacement therapy (HRT).

are applied to any area of clear, dry skin other than the face or breast, and changed twice a week. The gel is rubbed into the skin once a day. A progestogen can be given either orally or transdermally. This route has the advantage of bypassing liver metabolism, and gives more stable serum hormone levels than with implants. The major complication is one of skin irritation.

Complications – The potential complications of hormone replacement therapy include an increased incidence of carcinoma of the endometrium and possibly of the breast. Some women develop hypertension on oestrogen therapy and, therefore, periodic checks on blood pressure are important. Caution should be taken when there is a history of gall bladder disease.

The development of irregular uterine bleeding is an indication for diagnostic curettage.

Contraindications – Hormone replacement therapy is contraindicated in the presence of endometrial and breast carcinoma, acute thrombotic disease, fibrocystic disease of the breast, uterine fibroids, familial hyperlipidaemia, diabetes and gall bladder disease. However, with the exception of malignant disease of the breast and endometrium, none of the other conditions provide an absolute contraindication, and relief of symptoms may sometimes be more important than other considerations.

In conclusion, hormone replacement therapy relieves menopausal symptoms and reduces osteoporosis and heart disease. Despite a slight increase in breast cancer, there is a net reduction in mortality in women on hormone replacement therapy.

Menopause

- Onset 49–50 years
- FSH rises, oestradiol falls
- Menstrual irregularity with short follicular phase
- Associated with vasomotor instability, atrophic changes in genital tract and skin, osteoporosis, cardiovascular complications
- Hormone replacement therapy (HRT) requires additional progestogens if woman still has uterus
- HRT contraindicated by breast/endometrial carcinoma

BIBLIOGRAPHY

Lachelin G C L 1991 Introduction to clinical reproductive endocrinology. Butterworth/Heinemann, London

Shearman R P 1985 Clinical reproductive endocrinology. Churchill Livingstone, Edinburgh

22 Disorders of the menstrual cycle

AMENORRHOEA

Primary amenorrhoea has been previously described in Chapter 20.

Secondary amenorrhoea is defined as the cessation of menses for 3 or more months.

Aetiology

There are numerous causes of amenorrhoea although the commonest are physiological. Amenorrhoea may result from any disorder of the endocrine or central nervous system or abnormalities of the target organ.

Physiological causes – These include pregnancy, the puerperium, lactation and the menopause.

Pyschogenic factors – Emotional stress is a common cause of amenorrhoea. It often occurs where the environment is changed, as for example when a woman changes her occupation or leaves her home environment for institutional life. This problem usually resolves itself, but may persist for some years.

Pseudocyesis

Pseudocyesis, or false pregnancy, occurs in women who have a strong desire to have a child, but are unsuccessful in conceiving. Cessation of the periods is accompanied by abdominal distension, breast enlargement and occasional galactorrhoea. When confronted with evidence that she is not pregnant, menstruation usually returns and the abdominal distension subsides. Further supportive measures, reassurance and investigation and treatment of the underlying subfertility are also required.

Anorexia nervosa

There is a critical relationship between body weight and menstruation. Thus, if body weight falls be-

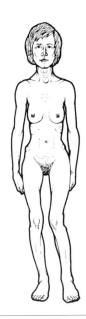

Fig. 22.1 Anorexia nervosa is associated with profound weight loss and amenorrhoea.

tween the 10th and 15th centile, there is a high probability that amenorrhoea will develop. This may result from vigorous dieting, but it is often a manifestation of anorexia nervosa (Fig. 22.1). This condition is characterized by an extreme neurotic aversion to food. There is usually an underlying emotional problem with conflicts over sexuality, obsession with weight loss associated with a persistent refusal to eat adequately, and self-induced vomiting or purgation.

The patient often complains of pain intolerance, and develops a widespread growth of fine body hair. Gonadotrophin and oestrogen levels are low but, unlike panhypopituitarism, other hormone levels are normal. This is a serious condition which results in death in 10–15% of the subjects involved. Early recognition is important because it is essential to supplement dietary replacement with long-term psychiatric therapy.

225

Hypothalamic and pituitary disorders

Hypogonadotrophic amenorrhoea

The commonest condition encountered in this group is one of hypothalamic amenorrhoea. The patient develops amenorrhoea, but has normal prolactin levels and a normal pituitary fossa. This form of amenorrhoea often occurs in women who are underweight and who have a previous history of menstrual irregularity. Gonadotrophin, prolactin and oestradiol levels are all low.

Galactorrhoea–amenorrhoea syndromes

These are associated with hyperprolactinaemia and the presence of pituitary microadenomas. All patients with secondary amenorrhoea should have a prolactin estimation and, if the levels are abnormally raised, radiography of the pituitary fossa is essential. If the film shows evidence of distortion of the sella turcica with 'double flooring' of the pituitary fossa, then further tomographic views must be taken (Fig. 22.2). This condition is also known as the **Chiari–Frommel syndrome**.

Pituitary disorders

Apart from the presence of pituitary adenomas, pituitary amenorrhoea may occur where there is destruction from postpartum damage as in Sheehan's syndrome, or where there is surgically-inflicted damage.

Secondary hypothalamic dysfunction

This condition can be iatrogenic, and is sometimes induced by the administration of sex steroids as in the pill or by the use of psychotropic drugs such as the phenothiazines. These compounds are associated with hyperprolactinaemia. Thyroid and adrenocortical diseases or severe chronic systemic disease may also cause amenorrhoea.

Ovarian insufficiency

Surgical removal of the ovaries or destruction by radiation or infection results in secondary amenorrhoea. Ovarian neoplasms, particularly those associated with excessive production of oestrogen or testosterone, may cause amenorrhoea but constitute only a very small percentage of known causes. Auto-immune disease of the ovaries is a rare condition which sometimes presents as a premature menopause. Polycystic ovarian syndrome (Stein–Leventhal syndrome) usually causes oligomenorrhoea rather than true secondary amenorrhoea.

Failure of uterine response

Damage to the target organ may result in secondary amenorrhoea (Fig. 22.3). This includes surgical removal of the uterus or damage to the endometrium as with Asherman's syndrome. In this condition, overvigorous curettage, particularly when performed in the presence of endometritis, results in the formation of intra-uterine adhesions or synechiae. Destruction of the endometrium may also result from tuberculous infection. Cervical stenosis may cause retention of endometrial products within the uterine cavity – a condition known as **cryptomenorrhoea**.

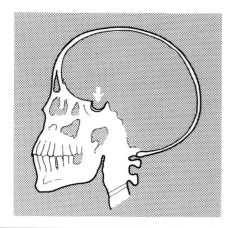

Fig. 22.2 Lateral skull radiograph in the presence of 'double' flooring' of the pituitary fossa (arrow).

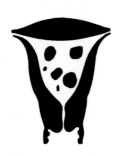 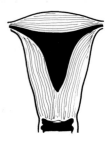

Asherman's syndrome   Cervical stenosis

Fig. 22.3 Abnormalities of the cervix and uterine cavity resulting in secondary amenorrhoea.

Investigations

A great deal of important information can be obtained from a careful history and examination. In the majority of cases nothing abnormal is found on clinical examination. In the absence of clinical evidence of thyroid or adrenal diseases it is unusual to find biochemical evidence. The differential diagnosis is established by the measurement of serum oestradiol, follicle-stimulating hormone and luteinizing hormone, prolactin and progesterone levels.

The administration of medroxyprogesterone acetate 10 mg daily for 5 days will produce withdrawal bleeding only in a functional uterus with an intact endometrium and a patent outflow tract.

Secondary amenorrhoea may result from stenosis of the cervix secondary to previous surgical trauma.

Management

The treatment depends on the cause. Outside of the physiological group, the vast majority of cases are hypothalamic in origin. Most of these will eventually resolve spontaneously. However, the uterus is often small and oestradiol levels are low. This also applies in the 'post-pill' group and, in some cases, it is useful to administer cyclical oestrogen therapy.

Where the amenorrhoea is associated with a desire to conceive, it is appropriate to treat it by the administration of exogenous gonadotrophins, but if amenorrhoea is the only problem then it is inappropriate to stimulate ovulation.

Cryptomenorrhoea

Secondary amenorrhoea may be due to retention of menstrual products because of cervical stenosis, as a result of surgical trauma or infection. This may occur in the presence of malignant disease of the cervix.

Amenorrhoea

- No period for 3 or more months
- Most common cause physiological
- Can also be iatrogenic or associated with chronic illness or body weight < 10th centile
- Drug history, history of previous curettage/cervical surgery

---

DYSMENORRHOEA

Dysmenorrhoea or painful menstruation is the commonest of all gynaecological symptoms.

Primary dysmenorrhoea occurs in the absence of any significant pelvic pathology. It usually develops within the first 2 years of the menarche and is often familial, with a strong likelihood that the attitude of the mother may influence the response of the daughter. Nevertheless, it would be a mistake to underestimate the severity of dysmenorrhoea in some women. The pain is often intense and cramping and can be crippling and severely incapacitating so that it causes a major disruption of social activities. It is usually associated with the onset of menstrual blood loss but may begin on the day preceding menstruation. The pain only occurs in ovulatory cycles, is lower abdominal in nature but sometime radiates down the anterior aspect of the thighs (Fig. 22.4). The pain often disappears or improves after the birth of the first child. Dysmenorrhoea is often associated with vomiting and diarrhoea. Pelvic examination reveals no abnormality of the pelvic organs.

Secondary or **acquired dysmenorrhoea** is caused by organic pelvic pathology and it usually has its onset many years after the menarche.

Any woman who develops secondary dysmenorrhoea should be considered to have organic pathology in the pelvis until proved otherwise.

Pelvic examination is particularly important in this situation and, if the findings are negative,

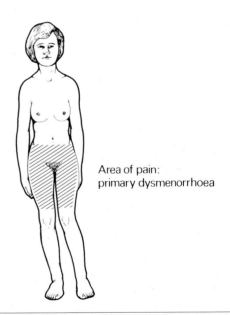

Area of pain: primary dysmenorrhoea

Fig. 22.4 Distribution of pain experienced in dysmenorrhoea; there may also be symptoms of lumbar and sacral backache.

laparoscopy is indicated. Common associated pathologies include endometriosis, adenomyosis, pelvic infections and intra-uterine lesions such as submucous fibroid polyps.

Investigations

A careful history is of great importance in this condition. Pelvic examination may not be helpful in primary dysmenorrhoea but it is advisable to perform either a vaginal or rectal examination to exclude any obvious pelvic pathology. However, in secondary dysmenorrhoea a pelvic examination is essential and, if pelvic pathology is not palpable, laparoscopy is advisable. This is only performed in cases with primary dsymenorrhoea if the condition is particularly resistant to therapy.

Management

Primary dysmenorrhoea

Discussion and reassurance are an essential part of management. Primary dysmenorrhoea tends to present some months after the menarche and is associated with ovulatory cycles, early cycles frequently being anovulatory. The intensity of pain may be aggravated by apprehension and fear, and reassurance that the pain does not indicate any serious disorder may lessen the symptoms. It is also common for the pain to either disappear or substantially lessen after the birth of the first child.

Drug therapy

Dysmenorrhoea can be effectively treated by drugs that inhibit prostaglandin synthesis and hence uterine contractility. These drugs include aspirin, mefenamic acid, naproxen or ibuprofen. As dysmenorrhoea is often associated with vomiting, headache and dizziness, it may be advisable to start therapy either on the day before the period is expected, or as soon as the menstrual flow commences. Mefenamic acid is given in a dose of 250 mg 6-hourly. This drug also reduces menstrual flow in some women with menorrhagia.

If these drugs are inadequate, suppression of ovulation with the contraceptive pill is highly effective in reducing the severity of dysmenorrhoea. Where it is ineffective, then careful consideration should be given to the possibility of underlying pathology.

If all conservative medical therapy fails, then relief may sometimes be achieved by mechanical

dilatation of the cervix or by the surgical removal of the pain fibres to the uterus in an operation known as presacral neurectomy, but these methods of treatment should be approached with considerable caution.

In cases of secondary dysmenorrhoea, the treatment is dependent on the nature of the underlying pathology. If the pathology is not amenable to medical therapy, the symptoms may only be relieved by hysterectomy.

Dysmenorrhoea

- Primary: usually normal pelvic examination and improves spontaneously
- Secondary: endometriosis, infection and intra-uterine lesions
- Management: treat any underlying cause, prostaglandin inhibitors, suppression of ovulation.

DYSFUNCTIONAL UTERINE BLEEDING

This term describes the occurrence of abnormal uterine bleeding for which an organic cause cannot be found. The diagnosis can be made only by excluding any pathology both by examination and by diagnostic curettage. It may, however, be impossible to exclude some types of benign organic disease.

Adenomyosis is associated with invasion of the myometrium by endometrial glands and may cause menorrhagia and dysmenorrhoea, but is not

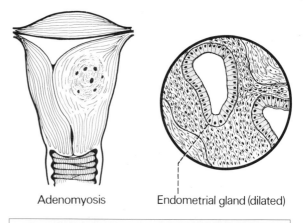

Adenomyosis   Endometrial gland (dilated)

Fig. 22.5 Adenomyosis may cause dysmenorrhoea and menorrhagia and is an important consideration in the differential diagnosis of dysfunctional uterine bleeding (left); histological features (right).

associated with any histological abnormality of the endometrium (Fig. 22.5).

The pathophysiology of dysfunctional uterine bleeding is poorly understood, and therefore classification is generally unsatisfactory. Abnormalities of uterine bleeding most commonly occur at the extremes of menstrual life and particularly in the premenopausal years. These conditions are classified as ovular or anovular.

Ovular dysfunctional uterine haemorrhage
(Fig. 22.6)

The pattern of the menstrual cycle and menstrual loss may be altered by defects of the corpus luteum or by shortening of the follicular phase of development.

Functional epimenorrhoea and epimenorrhagia

Factors which affect the pituitary–ovarian axis will alter the periodicity of the menstrual cycle. The follicular phase is shortened but the luteal phase

tends to remain constant. Changes in the periodicity of the menstrual cycle and, in particular, shortening of the cycle commonly occur:

1. After pregnancy
2. Following the menarche
3. Preceding the menopause.

Functional menorrhagia

Abnormalities of menstrual loss may occur on a regular cyclical basis. The number of days of bleeding may remain constant and the loss become heavy or the number of days of bleeding may become prolonged, although the loss may be slight for many of these days. Two common abnormal forms of ovular dysfunctional bleeding occur:

1. Defective corpus luteum formation – irregular spotting and blood loss occurs for some days preceding the onset of menstruation. The endometrium shows only patchy progestational changes.
2. Defective degeneration of the corpus luteum – slow degeneration of the corpus luteum results in

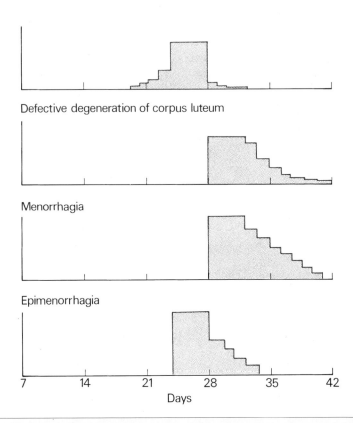

Fig. 22.6 Disturbance of menstrual flow in dysfunctional uterine bleeding.

slight bleeding which persists for several days after completion of the normal period. The endometrium in such patients shows patchy progestational changes in the early proliferative phase.

Estimation of menstrual blood loss is inevitably subjective, and up to 50% of patients presenting with heavy periods will have a blood loss of less than 50 ml/month.

Anovular dysfunctional uterine haemorrhage

Metropathia haemorrhagica

This condition most commonly occurs around the time of the menopause but may also occur in the adolescent female. The history classically involves a period of amenorrhoea followed by prolonged, heavy and irregular bleeding of such severity that it may occasionally be life threatening. The persistence of an unruptured follicular cyst in one ovary results in extended and excessive oestrogen production causing cystic or adenomatous endometrial hyperplasia. The endometrium becomes greatly thickened and when it can no longer be sustained by the continuing high levels of oestrogen it eventually breaks down in a patchy fashion. The haemorrhage commonly follows a period of 6–8 weeks amenorrhoea. Myometrial hyperplasia also occurs so that the uterus is often bulky, the endometrium being up to one centimetre thick and having the characteristic 'Swiss cheese' appearance (Fig. 22.7).

Differential diagnosis

The diagnosis of dysfunctional uterine haemorrhage is made partly on the actual history and findings and partly by excluding other factors. It is, therefore, important to:

1. Obtain an accurate medical and menstrual history.
2. Perform a careful general examination to look for signs of endocrine disorders such as the polycystic ovarian syndrome, hyperthyroidism or myxoedema and Cushing's disease.
3. Perform a pelvic examination to exclude any obvious local pathology.
4. Obtain a cervical smear. In practical terms this is unlikely to be productive, as most malignant lesions of the cervix that cause irregular bleeding are readily apparent on clinical examination. Nevertheless it is an essential part of the pelvic examination in a woman with irregular bleeding in the latter part of her menstrual life.

The cause of abnormal uterine haemorrhage is at least, in part, related to the age of the patient (Fig. 22.8). Around the time of puberty it most commonly results from dysfunctional uterine haemorrhage. During the reproductive years, the commonest causes of abnormal vaginal bleeding are disorders of pregnancy. Near the menopause the incidence of uterine malignancy rises sharply and abnormal bleeding most commonly results from malignancy, benign pelvic tumours and dysfunctional uterine haemorrhage.

Any of these conditions may occur in any age group, but the balance of probabilities may signi-

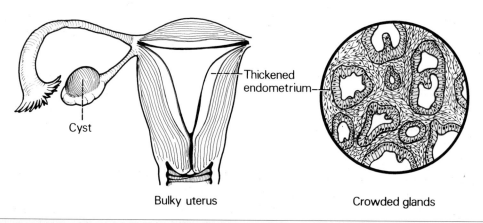

Cyst

Thickened endometrium

Bulky uterus

Crowded glands

Fig. 22.7 Metropathia haemorrhagica – caused by persistent production of high levels of oestrogen (left); histological features (right).

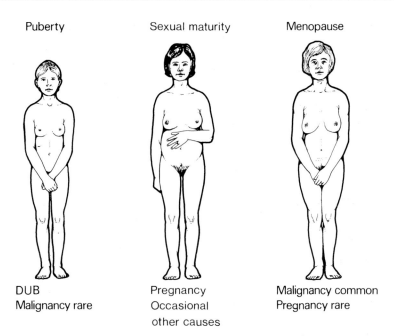

Puberty   Sexual maturity   Menopause

DUB
Malignancy rare

Pregnancy
Occasional
other causes

Malignancy common
Pregnancy rare

Fig. 22.8 Irregular vaginal blood loss poses a different diagnostic and management problem at different ages (DUB, dysfunctional uterine bleeding).

ficantly affect the scope of clinical investigation. In the older age group, examination under anesthesia and diagnostic curettage is essential. The presence of pelvic tumours does not exclude the possibility of uterine malignancy and diagnostic curettage may still be necessary. Uterine pathology such as endometrial polyps and submucous fibroids may be missed at curettage. The diagnosis in such cases may be established by hysteroscopy. General investigations should include a full blood count and clotting screen and thyroid function tests if indicated by the history or examination.

Treatment

The management of dysfunctional uterine haemorrhage depends in part on the age of the female.

Dysfunctional uterine haemorrhage around the menarche

Abnormal uterine haemorrhage around the time of the menarche is nearly always hormonally based as malignant disease at this age is extremely rare. It is therefore reasonable to introduce medical management without initial curettage. Initial assessment should include clinical examination and haemoglobin estimation with a complete blood

picture. It is important to exclude blood dyscrasia and pregnancy. Abnormal bleeding can sometimes be controlled by the combined contraceptive pill with a high dose combination of oestrogen and progestogen. Occasionally, it may be necessary to give a loading dose of oestrogen using a compound such as Premarin (conjugated equine oestrogen) followed by cyclical combined therapy for a period of 3 months. The problem will usually resolve itself after medical treatment but occasionally a therapeutic curettage might be necessary, as well as blood transfusion or iron therapy. Compounds such as Danol may also be given for 3 months on a continuous basis; this compound will completely suppress menstruation.

The use of prostaglandin synthetase inhibitors such as mefenamic acid, ibuprofen and naprosyn, antifibrinolytic agents such as tranexamic acid and capillary-stabilizing drugs such as ethamsylate may reduce menstrual loss by 20–50%.

Perimenopausal dysfunctional uterine haemorrhage

In the older age group, it is essential to perform diagnostic curettage or uterine aspiration to exclude the possibility of uterine malignancy. Once the diagnosis has been established, curettage may itself effect a cure, particularly following a single episode, and is sufficient to resolve the problem in 60% of cases. If the bleeding has been prolonged and irregular, it is sensible to suppress menstruation for 3 months with Danol or to regulate menstrual bleeding and suppress ovulation by using a combined contraceptive pill for three cycles. The prognosis for conservative management is not good if:

1. The uterus is bulky
2. The haemoglobin level is less than 10 g% at presentation
3. Irregular bleeding has persisted for more than 1 year.

Under these circumstances, it may be necessary to proceed to hysterectomy.

Surgical treatment

Endometrial resection or ablation – The endometrium can be removed or destroyed using an operating hysteroscope. The most widely used techniques are laser ablation and endoscopic resection with a diathermy wire loop (Fig. 22.9). The endometrium is prepared by treatment with Danazol or gonadotrophin-releasing hormone analogues for 4–8 weeks prior to surgery. The uterine cavity is distended with an irrigation fluid such as glycine or normal saline. The procedure takes a similar amount of operation time as an hysterectomy, but the sub-

sequent in patient stay and recovery time following discharge are considerably less. There is a risk of intra-operative uterine perforation and, possibly, damage to other organs requiring laparotomy and repair. The other potential complication is of fluid overload from excessive absorption of the irrigation fluid resulting in cerebral or pulmonary oedema. Approximately 40% of patients will become amenorrhoeic, with a further 30–40% achieving a significant reduction in their symptoms. A minority of patients will eventually need further surgery and hysterectomy.

Hysterectomy – This remains the definitive treatment, and is more likely to be appropriate for those women with pelvic pathology such as adenomyosis and fibroids than medical treatment or endoscopic surgery. It is associated with a mortality of 1/10 000. Significant complications occur in 25–40% of patients, and are more common in patients undergoing abdominal hysterectomy.

Complications of hysterectomy

- Haemorrhage
- Damage to other organs (bladder, ureters, bowel)
- Infection (wound, chest)
- Thrombo-embolism
- Fistulas
- Vaginal vault prolapse

The majority of operations are carried out through a transverse lower abdominal or midline incision. **Total abdominal hysterectomy** (TAH). The round ligaments, Fallopian tubes and ovarian vessels are cut and and ligated on each side either medial or distal to the ovaries, depending on whether these are to be conserved (see below). The utero-vesical peritoneum is opened and the bladder reflected off the lower part of the uterus and cervix, so as to displace the ureters away from the uterine vessels, which are then cut and ligated. Finally, the cervical ligaments are cut and the vagina opened around the cervix, allowing removal of the uterus. If there has been no history of cervical disease the cervix can be conserved by removing the uterine corpus above the internal os after the uterine vessels have been ligated, **sub-total hysterectomy**. This may be indicated if other pelvic disease makes dissection of the cervix difficult, in order to reduce the risk of ureteric damage, or because of patient preference.

In **vaginal hysterectomy** the vaginal skin is opened around the cervix and the bladder and

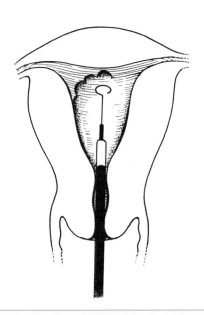

Fig. 22.9 Transcervical resection of the endometrium.

reflected up into the pelvis. The peritoneum over the uterovesical and rectovaginal space is opened, and the cervical ligaments cut and ligated. The uterine and ovarian vessels are ligated, the uterus removed and the peritoneum and vaginal skin closed. Removal of the ovaries is possible but less commonly carried out by this route. The absence of an abdominal wound substantially reduces postoperative morbidity, making this the method of choice for hysterectomy. It is contraindicated where malignancy is suspected. Other relative contraindications include a uterine size of over 14 weeks, endometriosis and lack of uterine descent.

In **laparoscopically assisted vaginal hyster-ectomy** (LAVH) the ovarian and uterine pedicles are cut under laparoscopic control though the abdomen, and the remainder of the operation completed vaginally. This may enable oophorectomy or a vaginal operation to be carried out where a full abdominal procedure might otherwise have been required.

Conservation of the ovaries, if normal, is usually recommended for women under the age of 45 years undergoing hysterectomy for menorrhagia to avoid the onset of a surgically induced early menopause. For women near the menopause this advantage has to be offset against the risk of later ovarian malignancy, and the option of oophorectomy should be discussed.

Dysfunctional uterine bleeding

- Abnormal uterine bleeding with no apparent organic cause
- Pattern of bleeding and age of patient key features in history
- Essential to exclude pregnancy in young patients and malignancy in old
- Treatment by high dose progestogens or Danol®, curettage/hysterectomy/endometrial resection

---

PREMENSTRUAL TENSION

Premenstrual tension or the premenstrual syndrome is a common episodic condition that afflicts many women and can sometimes be incapacitating in its severity. Most women experience some changes in mood during the menstrual cycle and minor symptoms of breast tenderness and weight gain. If these symptoms become severe in the premenstrual week, the condition is defined as the premenstrual syndrome (Fig. 22.10).

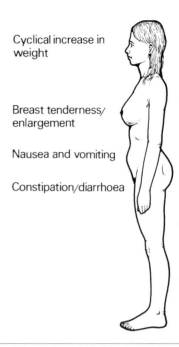

Cyclical increase in weight

Breast tenderness/ enlargement

Nausea and vomiting

Constipation/diarrhoea

Fig. 22.10 Premenstrual syndrome presents with a variety of physical and psychological symptoms that tend to be worse in the week before menstruation.

Symptoms and signs

The condition is commonly precipitated by stress and tension, either at home or at work, and particularly afflicts women during the third decade of life. The common symptoms include:

1. Behavioural changes – there are symptoms of depression and tension often associated with unreasonable outbursts of temper. Suicide occurs more often in the premenstrual week, and minor crimes are also more frequent in the second half of the cycle.
2. Symptoms of bloatedness – many women experience these symptoms. Their clothing feels uncomfortably tight, and this symptom does not subside until the onset of menstruation. Although there is a cyclical increase in weight in both symptomatic and asymptomatic women in the premenstrual week, weight gain is not usually excessive in those with premenstrual tension. The exception is the small group of women who suffer from cyclical oedema, where generalized oedema and oliguria occur in the second half of the cycle.
3. Breast symptoms – breast tenderness, enlargement of the breast and heaviness and pain are features of the syndrome in most women.

4. Gastrointestinal symptoms – nausea and vomiting and constipation or diarrhoea occur occasionally but are not major symptoms.

Pathogenesis

The mechanism of premenstrual tension remains unclear. The difficulty in studying this condition is one of definition as the symptoms are so protean. Various hypotheses have been explored, particularly in relation to the balance between oestrogen and progesterone, to the excessive production of prolactin, aldosterone or antidiuretic hormone, or to hypoglycaemia. None of these hypotheses have been substantiated.

Management

The first important aspect of management is to discuss the symptoms fully and to explore the social background particularly in relation to domestic and work tensions.

Some women lose their symptoms when they take the contraceptive pill, but this is not invariably the case. Progesterone therapy administered as intramuscular injections or suppositories produces relief of symptoms. Bromocriptine is effective only in the relief of breast symptoms.

Diuretics have been widely employed, and most of them produce some relief in symptoms of bloatedness. Of these compounds, the most effective is probably spironolactone given from day 12 to 26 of a 28 day cycle.

Complete suppression of the menstrual cycle will reduce the symptoms but is rarely acceptable as a method of treatment.

The simplest form of treatment is to give pyridoxine 100 mg daily. This produces a reduction in prolactin synthesis, and is a safe and effective form of therapy.

Reassurance and support must be an important and continuing requirement in the treatment of premenstrual tension, and it may be necessary to try a variety of therapies before a satisfactory response can be obtained.

The assessment of any form of therapy is particularly difficult because of a 70–80% placebo response. It is inadvisable to accept the validity of any form of drug therapy that has not been subjected to a placebo-controlled, double-blind trial, as virtually any form of therapy will produce an improvement in symptoms in some women.

Premenstrual tension

- Key features are cyclical changes occurring in the week prior to, and ceasing within 48 hours of, the onset of menstruation
- Most common symptoms are mood changes, breast tenderness, bloating and gastrointestinal changes
- Management involves establishing the diagnosis, counselling, pyridoxine and suppression of ovulation in some cases

---

BIBLIOGRAPHY

Jacobs H S 1985 Clinics in obstetrics and gynaecology. W B Saunders, Eastbourne

O'Brien P M S 1987 Premenstrual syndrome. Blackwell, Oxford

Shearman R P 1985 Clinical reproductive endocrinology. Churchill Livingstone, Edinburgh

Sutton C J G 1995 Advanced laparoscopic surgery. Clinical Obstetrics and Gynaecology 9(4)

Wood E C 1994 Gynaecological operative laparoscopy: current status and future development. Clinical Obstetrics and Gynaecology 8(4)

23 Disorders of sexual function

Disorders of sexual function may be divided into those that have a strictly organic basis and those that are predominantly functional. In most disorders, there are areas of overlap.

DISORDERS WITH AN ORGANIC BASIS

Two conditions have a predominantly organic basis: apareunia and dyspareunia.

Apareunia

This term defines the 'absence' of intercourse or the inability to have intercourse at all.
The common causes are:

1. Congenital absence of the vagina
2. Imperforate hymen
3. Impotence.

The treatment depends on the cause. Surgical treatment by vaginoplasty or by incision of the imperforate hymen is effective. The treatment of impotence will be discussed later in this chapter.

Dyspareunia

Dyspareunia is defined as painful intercourse. It is predominantly but not exclusively a female problem. The aetiology is divided on the basis of whether the condition is superficial or deep and it is therefore particularly important to obtain a concise history.

Superficial dyspareunia (Fig. 23.1)

Pain felt on penetration is generally associated with a local lesion of the vulva or vagina from one of the following causes:

1. Infections – local infections of the vulva and vagina. These commonly include monilial and trichomonas vulvo-vaginitis. Infections involving Bartholin's glands also cause dyspareunia.

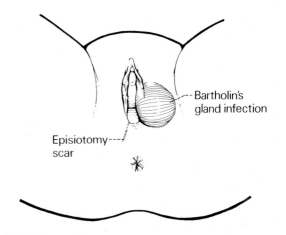

Fig. 23.1 Common causes of superficial dyspareunia.

2. Narrowing of the introitus – this may be congenital with a narrow hymenal ring or vaginal stenosis. It may sometimes be associated with a vaginal septum. The commonest cause of narrowing of the introitus is the over-vigorous suturing of an episiotomy wound or vulval laceration or following vaginal repair of a prolapse.
3. Menopausal changes – atrophic vaginitis or the narrowing of the introitus and the vagina from the effects of oestrogen deprivation may cause dyspareunia. Atrophic vulval conditions such as kraurosis vulvae can also cause pain.
4. Functional changes – lack of lubrication associated with inadequate sexual stimulation and emotional problems will result in dyspareunia. Vaginismus is a condition caused by spasm of the pelvic floor muscles and adductor muscles of the thigh, which results in pain on attempted penetration. This condition will be discussed later in this chapter.

Deep dyspareunia

Pain on deep penetration is often associated with pelvic pathology. Any woman who develops deep dyspareunia after enjoying a normal sexual life should be considered to have an organic cause for her pain until proved otherwise. The common causes of deep dyspareunia include (Figs 23.2 and 23.3):

1. Acute or chronic pelvic inflammatory disease – including cervicitis, pyosalpinx and salpingoophoritis. The uterus may become fixed. Ectopic pregnancy must also be considered in the differential diagnosis in this group.
2. Retroverted uterus and prolapsed ovaries – if the ovaries prolapse into the pouch of Douglas, and become fixed in that position, intercourse is painful on deep penetration.
3. Endometriosis – both the active lesions and the chronic scarring of endometriosis may cause pain.
4. Neoplastic disease of the cervix and vagina – at least part of the pain in this situation is related to secondary infection.

5. Postoperative scarring – this may result in narrowing of the vaginal vault and loss of mobility of the uterus. The stenosis commonly occurs following vaginal repair and, less often, following repair of a high vaginal tear. Vaginal scarring may also be caused by chemical agents such as rock salt which, in some countries, is put into the vagina in order to produce contracture.
6. Foreign bodies – occasionally, a foreign body in the vagina or uterus may cause pain in either the male or female partner. For example, the remnants of a broken needle or partial extrusion of an intrauterine device may cause severe pain in the male partner.

Treatment

Accurate diagnosis is dependent on careful history taking and a thorough pelvic examination. The

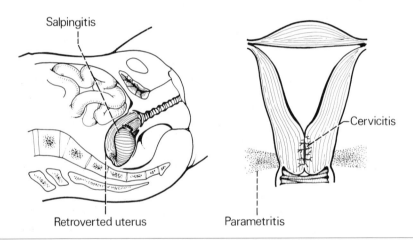

Fig. 23.2   Deep-seated dyspareunia can be caused by a variety of pelvic diseases and uterine displacement.

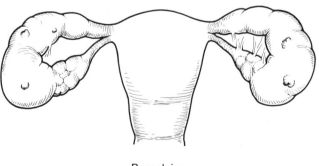

Fig. 23.3   Chronic or acute pelvic inflammatory disease such as pyosalpinx commonly causes dyspareunia.

treatment will therefore be dependent on the cause.

Medical treatment includes the use of antibiotics and antifungal agents for pelvic infection and long-term Danol or progestagen therapy for endometriosis. Surgical treatment includes correction of any stenosis, ventrosuspension of the retroverted uterus, excision of painful scars where appropriate, and reassurance and sexual counselling in functional disorders.

DISORDERS WITH NO ORGANIC BASIS

The most frequently occurring disorders include:

1. Premarital anxiety
2. Frigidity
3. Non-consummation
3. Impotence, including premature ejaculation.

Recognition

Sexual unhappiness finds expression in many different ways. Sometimes it is accompanied by awareness of the underlying disturbance, but often, as in other emotional difficulties, the link between cause and manifestation is obscure even to the sufferer. Sexual problems may therefore appear in the guise of mental or physical illness or disturbances of behaviour and relationships and thus form a part of the working experience not only of doctors but of anyone in the 'caring' professions.

Sexual difficulties underlie many cases of vague ill health in women which defy diagnosis until repeated attempts at communication have been made. Complaints are often ill-defined but affect the life of the patient and her family. Lack of energy, backache and irritability are common problems but, understandably enough, are often treated merely by reassurance and placebos.

The patient's emphasis on a particular aspect of her difficulties is likely to determine the doctor's choice of referral. Since symptoms of anxiety and depression are often present, psychiatric advice is frequently indicated. Sexual problems may be a presenting symptom or a part of a broader symptomatology in mental illness but very commonly there is sexual malfunction in an otherwise sound personality.

Some patients will go to family planning clinics. This approach is likely to be chosen by those women who focus their problems upon contraception and by those who need the reassurance which is implicit in the very existence of these clinics, namely that

sexual intercourse is permissible and respectable when its purpose is love and pleasure rather than procreation.

A gynaecologist will see many such cases. Some will verbalize their problems openly and directly: others will come because they have translated their emotional difficulties into physical terms. Their inability to have the 'right' feelings has found expression as something wrong with the body. In emotional and physical terms the patient is saying 'all is not well with me as a woman'.

Each one of the basic gynaecological symptoms may be wholly or partially determined by organic pathology or by psychogenic distress. When dealing with the fear of abnormality it is as important to look for the cause of the fear as for evidence of abnormality. Dread of cancer or anxiety about a non-existent vaginal discharge may be concealing the patient's real fears.

Dyspareunia means pain associated with intercourse and there may be a physical reason for it. However, particularly in early married life, it is often an expression of sexual uneasiness. Some patients are concerned about the size of the vagina, which seems too large or small. Except for the very rare cases of structural abnormality, the size of the vagina demonstrably depends not upon its anatomy but upon its physiology. It is determined by muscle tone or spasm, which in turn depends upon emotional factors. It is very unusual to find a hymen or a state of vaginismus which will not respond to gentle physical and psychological exploration. Resort to surgery is likely to confirm the patient's fears of abnormality and often leaves the presenting problem unchanged.

There are some unhappy women for whom all feminine functions are burdensome from menarche to menopause. They have painful periods, symptomful pregnancies, difficult labours and a suffering change of life. It would be almost out of character were they to have a joyful sexual life.

Frigidity

Definition

In medical literature the term 'frigidity' is used to describe a variety of conditions which range from a total lack of sexual feeling and response to the infrequent event of orgasm. It seems most realistic to include here all those cases in which a woman expresses overtly, or by implication, dissatisfaction with the quality of her sexual experience. The orientation is thus based on the patient's own expectations and hopes and on her disappointment at their lack of fulfilment.

The problem of frigidity may perhaps be most readily understood in terms of the demands which active participation and pleasure in sexual intercourse make upon any woman. In fact, in feeling she has to be open and approachable, and therefore in a position in which she is undefended, vulnerable and dependent. Orgasm demands that she abandons the self-control imposed by the conventions of everyday life and allows herself to be overcome by feelings which may reach an intensity unknown in any other human activity. On the physical level, she is required to accept her genital organs as good and wholesome and as the source of pleasure and happiness. She is required to put her trust in her man and to regard him as both strong and safe and to find his body wholly acceptable. She has to accept the possibility of pregnancy or the propriety and adequacy of birth control.

This concept provides a map indicating the probable areas of tension. In each of these areas there is likely to be a conflict between the patient's needs and desires on the one hand and her defences on the other.

Secondary frigidity

It is not uncommon for a woman to declare that all was once well with her sexual life, but that later there was a gradual or sometimes sudden decline in her interest and responsiveness. Patient and doctor may well be at a loss to understand or to reverse this change. They are likely to remain so while keeping their attention focused on the presenting symptoms, although of course a careful history may be taken and appropriate examination made. Commonly it is found that other events have taken place in the life of the patient, approximately during the time under scrutiny, which have a particular meaning to this woman. One may call these 'echo situations'. It is as though she had been sensitized in childhood to certain happenings, without obvious effect on her sexual health, but that a further dose of similar trauma had tipped the balance towards loss of sexual pleasure. For example, a major quarrel with a husband may bring to the surface stormy episodes of childhood or a father's leaving home; the death or illness of a parent may re-awaken confused and conflicting feelings relating to that parent during the formative years.

Non-consummation

All that has been said about frigidity applies with equal force to those patients who not only do not enjoy intercourse but are not able to allow it to take place. Cases of impotence in the male are not considered here, but it is noteworthy that many a man who was described as a very poor lover proves himself surprisingly virile when his wife's problems have been overcome. An element must be mentioned which is sometimes encountered in cases of frigidity but which is much more in evidence in non-consummation. This is the element of fantasy.

In contrast to the penis, which is visible, touchable and in everyday use throughout life, the vagina is mysterious and unexplored. The hymen is regarded as almost a sacred barrier guarding not simply a physical structure but also the semimystical concept of virginity.

Reality is not readily available to confront the fantasies which flourish in the soil of sexual immaturity. The mind's eye has a picture which is undefined by structure but determined by feelings and fears scarcely affected by intellectual knowledge. The hymen may be thought of as a rigid wall which will have to be 'broken in' with much pain and bleeding. The vagina appears as tiny and fragile or as an enormous cavity communicating with everything else in the abdomen. Others have feared penetration into the urethra, the anus or the cervical os. Dread of penetration has become intelligible.

Psychopathology

Mature sexuality has a complex derivation, rooted and broadly determined in infancy but affected by events and relationships throughout childhood and adolescence. The relationship which a child forms with its mother in the first months of life provides the foundation for future emotional health and thereby of sexual health also.

The adult gender role appears to be greatly influenced by a child's capacity to find in the parent of the same sex an adequate model for its own development and to retain at the same time a sound relationship with the other parent. A boy, therefore, has to turn from his initial total involvement with his mother to finding a pattern of masculinity in his father, but nevertheless, to maintain a safe and satisfying relationship with his mother. It may be that the commoner occurrence in men of problems of sexual misdirection is partially explained by the difficulties which arise in this complex emotional change. In women, on the other hand, the common problems are those of failure of full development, rather than deviation from the accepted norm.

A study of cases of frigidity and similar sexual problems suggests that the roots of these problems are to be found in several aspects of child development.

The mother–infant relationship

This relationship contains on a pregenital level many elements which may later enrich a sexual relationship. It can provide the first and most deeply felt experience of warmth and tenderness and of physical closeness to another person. The child gives pleasure to its mother by being and not by doing. Its weakness and its needs are accepted without patronage. The body and that which it produces is handled lovingly and without distaste. Many fields of psychological research have provided ample evidence to confirm the damaging effect of interference with this relationship on the personality as a whole.

Later parent–child relationships

In several respects, childhood difficulties are mirrored in future sexual problems. Many patients demonstrate their inability to tolerate dependence upon others and scoff at any sign of weakness. They set themselves high standards of sensible behaviour and rigid self-control. They are unable to accept a childish component of adult personality and attempt to put firm restrictions on all uncontrolled feeling which seems silly or noisy or messy. Often there emerges the picture of a miniature adult, an only child, or the eldest of a family, struggling hard to comply with real or imagined parental demands, tackling the sadness of unsatisfied childish needs by a denial of these needs.

Parental attitudes towards the body and its function also continue to exert their influence from childhood to adolescence, and sometimes into adult life. If these are prudish and prohibitive, it is likely that the child will learn to regard the body, and particularly the genital area, as unpleasant or even dirty. Some women find the vulva and even the breasts ugly and un-touchable. Stern disapproval of masturbation will tend to endow any form of sexual excitement with guilt.

The mother–daughter relationship

Few patients have spoken of their mothers with easy, assured affection. Many have unhesitatingly blamed them for their sexual difficulties, while others have used excessive devotion to veil an intolerable antagonism. Criticisms have been varied and conflicting. Mothers have been accused of making sex seem a 'wife's duty' or frankly disgusting, of being too sexy or not sexy enough, of being too dominating or too submissive, of failing to tell the daughter the facts or of always talking about sex.

Like Homer's mariners who had to find their way between Scylla and Charybdis, mothers have to steer a difficult course in helping their daughters to grow towards mature womanhood by being themselves moral but not prohibitive, encouraging but not seductive, available and supporting but not intrusive. A daughter demands from her mother her blessing for her own sexuality and permission to find pleasure untainted by guilt, rivalry or envy.

The father–daughter relationship

A daughter seeks from her father support and affection which is a tribute to her femininity, but does not obtrude his own sexuality; she needs to see the relationship between her parents as sufficiently secure to withstand any unconscious desire of her own to have her father to herself. She will be greatly helped in establishing her own social and sexual feminine role if she can find in him an example of strength and dependability with whom she knows her mother to be safe and which will form the basis of her own attitude to men.

Difficulties in relationships with men

If there develops during childhood a deeply felt envy of boys, this may lead to a resentful conviction that a man always has the best of things in life and therefore engenders an unwillingness to give pleasure, even though this attitude is likely to defeat her own hopes for fulfilment. Uneasiness in the feminine role is sometimes spoken of as a feeling of being 'used'.

There may be an unconscious attempt to deal with envy by the adoption of a bossy or contemptuous manner or in gentler personalities by treating men like boys or babies. The ways in which such attitudes may hinder the development of healthy sexuality can readily be imagined.

Although in some cases it seems that emotional difficulties are related to defects of personality of one or both parents, the child's contribution to family relationships must not be ignored. However irreproachable parental behaviour and personality may appear to be, it does not necessarily follow that the child will be able to accept them without prejudice or distortion.

Treatment

Congenital absence of sexual drive is unknown and therefore treatment requires to be directed towards understanding and overcoming the obstacles which prevent its free expression. It is hoped to achieve this end by the establishment of a doctor–patient relationship which has within it the potential for bringing about emotional change for the patient.

The way in which the patient enters into the relationship, her attitudes and behaviour enable the doctor to gain insight into her case. A woman's appearance and manner often provide evidence of her difficulty in accepting the feminine role. An attempt is made to understand and to help her to understand the meaning of exaggeration or denial. These patients frequently express themselves in richly symbolic language and this is freely interpreted. Some are withdrawn and hostile and need help to face their underlying conflicts. It is hoped that an atmosphere will be established in which the patient is able to express fears and feelings which had hitherto seemed quite intolerable. Although the treatment relationship which makes this possible is clearly of great importance it is usually built up with surprising rapidity. This may be because the patient enters it on the most intimate level of her personality. Against this background, vaginal examination becomes a significant experience for the patient. When indicated, she is encouraged to examine herself. Often for the first time she becomes aware of her own physical femininity and is able to confront fantasy with a reality which is not only intellectually appreciated, as it might have been through books or lectures, but which is linked by the nature of the treatment to her own feelings.

Prognosis

As a result of treatment, many patients are able to reach complete sexual fulfilment. Others find an increase of warmth and tolerance and a relief of tension, which indicate that the treatment has been worthwhile. Some remain unchanged; among these are those who are unwilling to enter into this type of treatment and do not return after one or two visits. The prognosis is best for cases of nonconsummation, secondary frigidity and frigidity in the young but, commonly, good results are achieved in older women.

Impotence

Under this heading must be considered:

1. Failure to achieve erection
2. Premature ejaculation
3. Inability to ejaculate
4. Lack of sexual interest.

All or any of these may be present from adolescence or have their onset at any time of life after a period of healthy sexuality.

By far the most common causes of all forms of impotence are psychological. Occasionally, a physical origin is found, probably endocrine, metabolic or neurological. It seems reasonable to suppose that where there is a capacity for masturbation, involving full erection and ejaculation, difficulties in intercourse have a psychological basis.

Depression, reactive or endogenous, is an important aetiological or concomitant condition. It appears to be a particularly common cause of loss of sexual interest in cases where this was previously lively.

The woman's contribution to the problem also requires consideration – one may not be dealing with an inability to swim but with an understandable reluctance to jump into cold water!

The effect of ageing is important and interesting. Many men who are troubled by failing sexual energy, or even by an occasional unsuccessful attempt, fear that this is due to a premature ageing process. Since many such men show no other evidence of ageing, it seems more realistic to search for signs of depression or for the kind of situation mentioned above under the heading of secondary frigidity.

Impotence can be understood, as has been suggested in the case of sexual difficulties in women, in terms of the demands which are made upon a man and his response, conscious and unconscious, to those demands. It is required that he should be able to establish a relationship with a woman in which he is willing to give himself to her, feeling confident that he will neither suffer nor inflict pain or damage, that he will be welcomed but not devoured. He requires to be sure of his own power but, at the same time, sure of his capacity to control that power.

His confidence will be based on his past experience of relationships with women and his feelings about himself as a man. A need to settle old scores or a fear that past difficulties will be repeated is likely to present obstacles. The emotional background will have a physical counterpart and he will need to see the penis as strong but not destructive and the vagina as safe.

Treatment is by psychotherapy, somewhat along the lines mentioned earlier. The prognosis is not as good as it is for women.

Dyspareunia

- Painful intercourse
- Pain felt on penetration usually associated with local lesion of vulva/vagina
- Deep dyspareunia commonly due to pelvic inflammatory disease or endometriosis
- Organic disease needs to be excluded in new deep dyspareunia
- Non-organic causes more commonly present as superficial pain

24 Genital tract infections

The female genital tract provides direct access to the peritoneal cavity. Infection may extend to any level of the tract and, once it reaches the Fallopian tubes, is usually bilateral.

The genital tract has a rich anastomosis of blood and lymphatic vessels which serve to resist infection, particularly during pregnancy.

There are other natural barriers to infection which include:

1. The physical apposition of the pudental cleft and the vaginal walls.
2. Vaginal acidity – the low pH of the vagina in the sexually mature female provides a hostile environment for most bacteria. This resistance is weakened in the prepubertal and post-menopausal female.
3. Cervical mucus, which acts as a barrier in preventing the ascent of infection.
4. The regular monthly shedding of the endometrium.

VULVOVAGINITIS

The commonest infections of the genital tract are those that affect the vulva and vagina.

Symptoms

Swelling and reddening of the vulval skin is accompanied by pruritus and occasionally proctitis and dyspareunia. When the infection is predominantly one of vaginitis, the symptoms include vaginal discharge, pruritus, dyspareunia and often dysuria.

Signs

These will depend on the cause. The appearance of the vulval skin is reddened, sometimes with ulceration and excoriation. In the sexually mature female, the vaginal walls may become ulcerated with plaques of white monilial discharge adherent to the skin or, in protozoal infections, the discharge may by copious with a greenish-white frothy appearance.

Common organisms

Protozoal infection include *Trichomonas vaginalis* – a single cell, flagellated organism which may infect the cervix, urethra and vagina. In the male the organism is carried in the urethra or prostate and infection is sexually transmitted.

Candida albicans is a yeast pathogen and occurs naturally on the skin and in the bowel. The white curd-like collections are attached to the vaginal epithelium and bleeding often occurs when removed. These infections are particularly common during pregnancy, in women taking the contraceptive pill or in diabetic women. In each instance, vaginal acidity is increased above normal and bacterial growth in the vagina is inhibited in such a way as to allow free growth of yeast pathogens which thrive well in a low-pH environment.

Diagnosis

The organisms are often seen on the Papanicolaou smear even in the absence of symptoms.

A fresh wet preparation in saline of vaginal discharge will show motile trichomonads. The characteristic flagellate motion is easily recognized and the organism can be cultured.

Candida hyphae and spores can also be seen in a wet preparation (Fig. 24.1) and can be cultured.

Vulvovaginitis

- Commonest infection of genital tract
- Presents as pruritus, dyspareunia or discharge
- Common causes are *Trichomonas* and *Candida*
- Predisposing factors include pregnancy, diabetes, contraceptive pill
- Can be diagnosed by examination of fresh wet preparation of vaginal discharge

---

Herpes genitalis

This condition has become a major cause of concern in recent years.

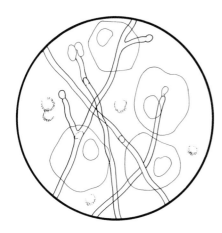

Candida hyphae

Fig. 24.1 *Candida* hyphae and spores in a wet preparation.

The condition is caused by herpes simplex virus type 2, and is a sexually transmitted disease. The local symptoms include vaginal discharge, vulval pain, dysuria and vaginal bleeding.

The lesions include skin vesicles, multiple shallow skin ulcers and inguinal lymphadenopathy (Fig. 24.2). The infection is also associated with cervical dysplasia.

The incubation period for herpes infection is 2–14 days. Recurrences may be triggered by stress, menstruation or intercourse, but are normally of shorter duration and less severe than the primary episode.

Herpes genitalis
- Caused by herpes simplex type 2 virus
- Presents with pain, bleeding and vesicles or shallow ulcers on the vagina/vulva
- Associated with cervical dysplasia
- Tends to be recurrent but with decreasing severity
- Can be transmitted to the neonate during vaginal delivery if active

---

Infections of Bartholin's glands

Bartholin's glands are sited between the posterior part of the labia minora and the vaginal walls, and these two glands secrete mucus as a lubricant during coitus. Infection of the duct and gland results in closure of the duct and formation of a Bartholin's cyst or abscess. The condition is often recurrent and causes pain and swelling of the vulva. Bartholinitis is readily recognized by the site and nature of the swelling.

Bacterial vaginosis

This is due to a number of anaerobic organisms including *Gardnerella*. The patient presents with a frothy green discharge. It may be asymptomatic but is associated with an increased risk of pelvic inflammatory disease, urinary tract and puerperal infections. Diagnosis can be made by detecting an increase in vaginal pH or by a fishy odour produced when 10% potassium hydroxide is added to the discharge.

Vaginal discharge in the child may also be associated with the presence of a foreign body, and this possibility should always be excluded. Gonococcal vulvo-vaginitis is often associated with extensive pelvic infection but may also be asymptomatic or indicated merely by vaginal discharge and dysuria.

The diagnosis can be made by demonstrating the presence of Gram-negative intracellular diplococci and by anaerobic culture of discharge from the cervix and urethra. The herpes virus can be recognized from scrapings and skin biopsy and culture of vesicles in appropriate culture media. Serum antibodies are raised in well-established lesions.

Syphilis

The initial lesion appears 10–90 days after contact with the spirochaete *Treponema pallidum*.

The primary lesion or chancre is an indurated, firm papule which may become ulcerated and has a raised firm edge (Fig. 24.3). This lesion most commonly occurs on the vulva but may also occur in the vagina or cervix. The primary lesion may be accompanied by inguinal lymphadenopathy. The chancre heals spontaneously within 2-6 weeks.

Some 6 weeks after the disappearance of the chancre, the manifestations of secondary syphilis appear. A rash develops which is maculopapular and is often associated with alopecia. Papules occur, particularly in the anogenital area and in the mouth, and give the typical appearance known as **condylomata lata**.

Swabs taken from either the primary or secondary lesions are examined microscopically under darkground illumination, and the spirochaetes can be seen (Fig. 24.3). The serological tests have been described in a previous chapter.

The disease then progresses from the secondary phase to a tertiary phase. It may mimic almost any disease process and affect every system in the body, but the common long-term lesions are cardiovascular and neurological.

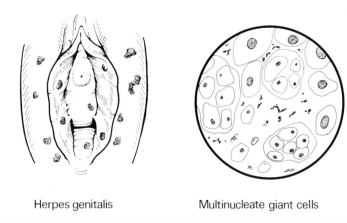

Herpes genitalis   Multinucleate giant cells

Fig. 24.2   Herpetic lesions of the vulva (left) are associated with the presence of multinucleate giant cells in direct smears from the vesicles (right).

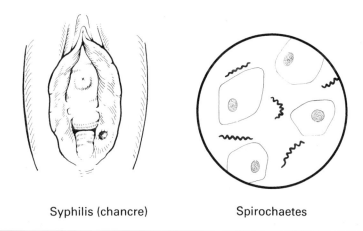

Syphilis (chancre)   Spirochaetes

Fig. 24.3   The typical lesion of primary syphilis is the chancre (left); diagnosis is established by dark-ground illumination of the spirochaetes (right).

Syphilis

- Spirochaete *Treponema pallidum*
- Primary infection occurs 10–90 days after contact
- Secondary symptoms 6 weeks after primary lesion
- Can be diagnosed serologically or by detection of the organism in vesicle fluid
- Responds to penicillin

Granuloma inguinale and lymphogranuloma venereum

Both of these conditions present with infected skin eruptions on the vulva. They are sexually transmitted diseases which are rare in Western Europe but are most commonly seen in tropical countries. Granuloma inguinale is caused by *Calymmatobacterium granulomatis*, and is diagnosed by the recognition of Donovan bodies, bacteria encapsulated in mononuclear leucocytes. Lymphogranuloma venereum is caused by a chlamydial infection and results in a vesiculo-pustular eruption associated with a painful inguinal lymphadenitis and, in the longer term, with vulval lymphoedema which may be gross. It may also cause rectal and vaginal stenosis. The diagnosis is a positive Frei test, which involved the injection of a small volume of antigen intradermally and reading the response of the skin reaction. The histological diagnosis depends on the exhibition of a granulomatous tubercle with central fibrinoid necrosis surrounded by plasma cells.

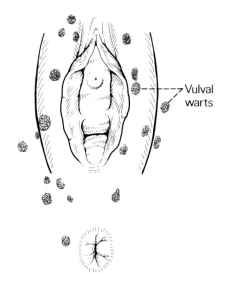

Vulval warts

Fig. 24.4 Warts may be widespread on the vulval and perianal skin.

Vulval warts (condylomata acuminata)

Vulval warts are caused by a papilloma virus. The condition is commonly, although by no means invariably, transmitted by sexual contact.

The warts have an appearance that is similar to those seen on the skin in other sites, and in the moist environment of the vulval skin are often prolific – particularly during pregnancy (Fig. 24.4). There is frequently associated pruritus and vaginal discharge. The lesions may spread to the peri-anal region, and in some cases become confluent and subject to secondary infections.

Treatment of vulval and vaginal infections

When the diagnosis has been established by examination and the bacteriological tests, the appropriate treatment can be instituted.

Vulval and vaginal monilial infections are treated by topical application of nystatin, natamycin clotrimazole, miconazole nitrate, econazole nitrate or candicidin. All these compounds are inserted intravaginally as tablets, pessaries, creams or foams and should be administered over a 14 day period. Recurrent infections can be treated by oral administration of ketoconazole and fluconazole. The patient's partner should be treated at the same time, and any predisposing factors such as poor hygiene or diabetes corrected.

Trichomonas infections and bacterial vaginosis are treated with metronidazole 200 mg taken three times a day for 7 days, and must be taken by both sexual partners if recurrence of the infection is to be avoided. It may be administered as a single dose of 2 g, but high-dose therapy should be avoided in pregnancy. Nimorazole is also an imidazole derivative, and is given as a single 2 g dose or as 1 g every 12 hours for three doses.

Chlamydial infections are treated by oral tetracycline or erythromycin in pregnancy.

Non-specific vaginal infections are common, and are treated with vaginal creams including hydrargaphen, povidone–iodine, diiodohydroxyquinoline or sulphonamide creams.

Gonorrhoea and syphilis are treated in the first instance with penicillin and, if this fails, for example in the case of penicillin-resistant strains of the gonococcus, doxycyline hydrochloride or acrosoxacin can be used.

Infections of the vagina associated with menopausal atrophic changes are treated by the appropriate hormone replacement therapy using an oral or vaginal oestrogen preparation or lactic acid pessaries where oestrogens are contraindicated. The same therapy may be used with the local application of oestrogen creams in juvenile vulvovaginitis.

Infections of Bartholin's gland are treated with the antibiotic appropriate to the organism. If abscess formation has occurred, the abscess should be 'marsupialized' by excising an elipse of skin and sewing the skin edges to wall off the abscess cavity (Fig. 24.5). This reduces the likelihood of recurrence of the abscess.

Vulval warts are treated with either physical or chemical diathermy using podophyllin applied directly to the surface of the warts. Any concurrent vaginal discharge should also receive the appropriate therapy.

Herpetic infections are notoriously resistant to treatment and highly prone to recurrence. The best available treatment is acyclovir administered in tablet form 200 mg five times daily for 5 days or locally as a 5% cream.

INFECTIONS OF THE CERVIX

Infections that affect the vagina also produce acute and chronic cervicitis.

Acute cervicitis

This usually occurs in association with generalized infection of the genital tract, and is diagnosed and

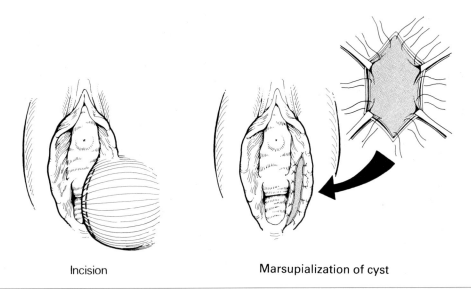

Incision

Marsupialization of cyst

Fig. 24.5 Marsupialization of a Bartholin's cyst or abscess, the incision is made over the medial aspect of the cyst (left) and the lining sutured to the skin (right).

treated according to the microbiology, as described in the management of vulvovaginitis.

Symptoms and signs

Acute cervicitis is associated with purulent vaginal discharge, sacral backache, lower abdominal pain, dyspareunia and dysuria. The proximity of the cervix to the bladder often results in coexistent trigonitis and urethritis, particularly in the case of gonococcal infections. The cervix appears reddened and may be ulcerated as with herpetic infections, and there is a mucopurulent discharge as the endocervix is invariably involved. The diagnosis is established by examination and taking cervical swabs for culture.

Treatment depends on the infecting organism.

Chronic cervicitis

This is an extremely common condition, and is present in about 50–60% of all parous women. In many cases, the symptoms are minimal. There may be a slight mucopurulent discharge which is not sufficient to trouble the woman and may simply present as an incidental finding that does not justify active treatment.

In the more severe forms of the condition, there is profuse vaginal discharge, chronic sacral backache, dyspareunia and occasionally postcoital bleeding. The cervix is often lacerated and there is mucopurulent discharge from the cervical canal. Infection in the ducts of the endocervical glands results in obstruction of these ducts and the development of small retention cysts visible on the ectocervix. These cysts may simply contain mucus, but in more severe infections contain mucopus. They are usually 2–3 mm in diameter but may be as large as 1 cm, and are known as **Nabothian follicles** (Fig. 24.6). Bacteriological culture of the discharge is usually sterile. The condition may cause subfertility because of hostility of the cervical mucus to sperm invasion.

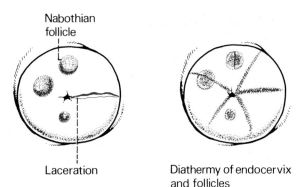

Nabothian follicle

Laceration

Diathermy of endocervix and follicles

Fig. 24.6 Chronic cervicitis with infected Nabothian follicles (left); treatment is by radical cautery and needle diathermy of the follicles (right).

Treatment

Medical treatment is rarely effective in chronic cervicitis because it is difficult to identify an organism and antibiotics do not penetrate the chronic micro-abscesses of the cervical glands. If the cervical swab is negative, then the next most effective management is diathermy of the endocervix in order to cauterize the Nabothian follicles so that the discharge is released.

This procedure is performed under general anaesthesia, as superficial chemical or physical cautery is unsatisfactory.

Following diathermy, an antibacterial cream should be placed in the vagina and the woman advised that the discharge may increase in amount for 2–3 weeks but will then diminish. She should also be advised to avoid intercourse for 3 weeks as coitus may cause secondary haemorrhage.

The two major complications of the procedure are secondary haemorrhage and postcautery stenosis. Stenosis is uncommon in the healthy parous woman but secondary haemorrhage may sometimes occur. Treatment involves packing the vaginal vault with a gauze pack soaked in an antiseptic cream such as proflavine and implementing blood transfusion where necessary. Antibiotic cover should also be given as there will invariably be infection present.

It is occasionally necessary to suture the cervix but this is often difficult because of the oedematous state of the tissue under these circumstances.

Infections of the cervix

- Acute (associated with generalized infection) or chronic
- Discharge, dyspareunia, low abdominal pain or backache, urinary symptoms and postcoital bleeding
- Can cause subfertility
- Difficult to isolate an organism when chronic
- Treatment includes appropriate antibiotics and cautery

Human papilloma virus (HPV)

Certain types of HPV are found in association with neoplastic changes in the cervix.

Types 6 and 11 are associated with low-grade cervical intra-epithelial neoplasia (CIN) and condyloma, whereas serotypes 16, 18 and 23 are associated with all grades of CIN and carcinoma of the cervix. These viruses are identified by their DNA sequences.

Factors which point towards an aetiological role for the virus in carcinoma of the cervix include:

1. Continued expression of the DNA in transferring epithelium
2. Gene products which transform epithelial cells
3. The particular types of HPV associated with carcinoma of the cervix will transform cells in vitro.
4. Women with the type 16 HPV have a 10-fold increased risk of developing CIN.

The immune response to this virus group appears to be relatively ineffective, and anti-HPV titres do not reflect the ability to resist further infection.

HPV DNA is present in 80–90% of cervical tumours, but it must be remembered that 30–40% of normal subjects will also be found to have HPV DNA present in cervical epithelium.

ACUTE INFECTIONS OF THE UPPER GENITAL TRACT

Acute infection of the endometrium, myometrium, Fallopian tubes and ovaries are usually the result of ascending infections from the lower genital tract causing pelvic inflammatory disease (Fig. 24.7).

However, infection may be secondary to appendicitis or other bowel infections, which sometimes give rise to a pelvic abscess. Perforation of the appendix with pelvic sepsis remains a common cause of tubal obstruction and subfertility. Pelvic sepsis commonly occurs during the puerperium and after an abortion. Retained placental tissue and blood provide an excellent culture medium for organisms from the bowel including *Escherichia coli*, *Clostridium welchii* or *C. perfringens*, *Staphylococcus aureus* and *Streptococcus faecalis*.

The principal organism to cause acute salpingitis by sexual transmission is *Neisseria gonorrhoea*. The organism spreads across the surface of the cervix and endometrium and causes tubal infection within 1–3 days of contact. Acute infection may also be caused by *Chlamydia*, which is now the most common cause of sexually transmitted pelvic inflammatory disease.

Pelvic inflammatory disease affects approximately 1% per year of women between 15 and 35 years of age in the developed world. The disease is most common between the ages of 15 and 24 years, and particular risk factors include multiple sexual partners and the use of intra-uterine contraceptive devices.

Symptoms and signs

The symptoms of acute salpingitis include (Fig. 24.8):

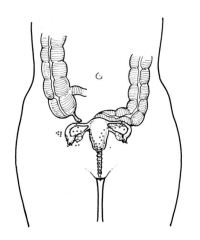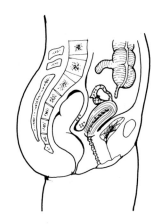

SITES OF INFECTION OF UPPER GENITAL TRACT

Fig. 24.7 Pelvic infections may occur by ascending from the lower genital tract or descending from the bowel or appendix.

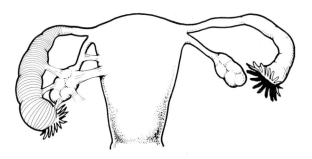

Fig. 24.8 Acute salpingitis with reddened, oedematous Fallopian tubes and pus discharging from the fimbrial ends of the tubes.

1. Acute bilateral lower abdominal pain. Salpingitis is almost invariably bilateral. Where the symptoms are unilateral, an alternative diagnosis should be considered.
2. Purulent vaginal discharge.
3. A pyrexia of 38°C or more, sometimes associated with rigors.
4. Vomiting and diarrhoea.

The signs include:

1. Signs of systemic illness with pyrexia and tachycardia.
2. Signs of peritonitis with guarding or rebound tenderness.
3. On pelvic examination, acute pain on cervical excitation and thickening in the vaginal fornices which may be associated with the presence of cystic tubal swellings due to pyosalpinges or pus-filled tubes. Fullness in the pouch of Douglas suggests the presence of a pelvic abscess.

Differential diagnosis

It is often difficult to establish the diagnosis of acute pelvic infection with any degree of certainty. The differential diagnosis includes:

1. *Tubal ectopic pregnancy* – initially pain is unilateral in most cases. There are often syncopal episodes and signs of diaphragmatic irritation with shoulder tip pain. The white cell count is normal or slightly raised but the haemoglobin level is low, whereas in acute salpingitis the white cell count is raised and the haemoglobin concentration is normal.
2. *Acute appendicitis* – the most important difference in the history lies in the unilateral nature of the condition. Pelvic examination does not usually reveal as much pain and tenderness but it must be remembered that the two conditions sometimes coexist, particularly where the infected appendix lies adjacent to the right Fallopian tube.
3. *Acute urinary tract infections* – may produce similar symptoms but rarely produce signs of peritonism and are commonly associated with urinary symptoms.
4. *Torsion or rupture of an ovarian cyst.*

Investigation

When the diagnosis of acute salpingitis is suspected, the woman should be admitted to hospital. After completion of the history and general examination swabs should be taken from the cervical canal and the urethra and sent to the laboratory for culture and antibiotic sensitivity. An additional endocervical swab should be taken into special media for detection of *Chlamydia* by enzyme-linked immunoassay (ELISA). A midstream specimen of urine should also be sent for culture.

Examination of the blood for differential white cell count, haemoglobin estimation and erythrocyte sedimentation rate may help to establish the diagnosis. Blood culture is indicated if there is a severe pyrexia. The diagnosis of mild to moderate degrees of PID on the basis of history and examination findings is unreliable and where the diagnosis is in doubt, laparoscopy is indicated.

Management

When the patient is unwell and exhibits peritonitis, high-grade fever, vomiting or a pelvic inflammatory mass, she should be admitted to hospital and managed as follows:

1. Fluid replacement by intravenous therapy. Vomiting and pain often result in dehydration.
2. Antibiotic therapy – it is sensible to treat the infection according to the organism and its sensitivity. However, the result of the cultures may not be available for 24 hours and, therefore, treatment should be started with an antibiotic such as cefuroxime and metronidazole given intravenously with oral doxycycline until the acute phase of the infection begins to resolve. Treatment with oral metronidazole and doxycycline should then be continued for 7 and 14 days, respectively.
3. Pain relief with opiate therapy.
4. If the uterus contains an intra-uterine device, it should be removed as soon as antibiotic therapy has been commenced.
5. Bed rest – immobilization is essential until the pain subsides.

Patients who are systemically well can be treated as an out-patient, with a single dose of ciprofloxacin and a 10 day course of doxycycline and reviewed after 48 hours. In all cases it is important to treat the partner and arrange appropriate contact tracings.

Indications for surgical intervention

In most cases, conservative management results in complete remission. However, one episode of acute infection results in tubal obstruction in about 30% of cases, and a further episode gives a 60% obstruction rate.

Laparotomy is indicated where the condition does not resolve with conservative management and where there is a pelvic mass.

In most cases, the mass will be due to a pyosalpinx or tubo-ovarian abscess. This can either be drained or a salpingectomy performed. If a pelvic abscess develops, it can be drained through the posterior fornix of the vagina by performing a posterior colpotomy.

CHRONIC PELVIC INFECTION

Acute pelvic infections may progress to a chronic state with dilatation and obstruction of the tubes forming bilateral hydrosalpinges with multiple pelvic adhesions.

Symptoms

Symptoms are varied but include:

1. Chronic pelvic pain and sacral backache
2. Chronic purulent vaginal discharge
3. Epimenorrhagia and dysmenorrhoea
4. Deep-seated dyspareunia.

Chronic salpingitis is also associated with infection in the connective tissue of the pelvis known as **parametritis**.

Signs

On examination, there is a purulent discharge from the cervix. The uterus is often fixed in retroversion, and there is thickening in the fornices and pain on bimanual examination.

Management

Conservative management of this condition is rarely effective and the problem is only eventually resolved by clearance of the pelvic organs.

CHRONIC TUBERCULOSIS OF THE GENITAL TRACT

Tuberculous salpingitis occurs in 5–10% of women with pulmonary tuberculosis and follows the spread of the tubercule bacillus from the primary lesion in the chest. A chronic granulomatous infection of the tubes will result in tubal obstruction and sterility.

The organism also causes chronic endometritis and the diagnosis can be established by culture and histological examination of the curettings.

Laparoscopic inspection of the tubes can also be employed to effect a diagnosis.

Management

Antibiotic therapy using drugs such as isoniazid, aminosalicylic acid, streptomycin, ethambutol and rifampicin will usually cure the condition but will not often restore fertility.

Upper genital tract infection

- Usually from ascending lower genital tract infection
- Can follow abortion or normal delivery
- Commonly due to *Neisseria gonorrhoea* or *Chlamydia* when sexually transmitted
- Presents as pain, fever, discharge and irregular periods
- Bilateral pain on cervical excitation and raised white cell count
- Differential diagnosis includes ectopic pregnancy, urinary tract infection and appendicitis
- Management includes fluid replacement, antibiotics, analgesia and rest
- Surgery is indicated to confirm diagnosis if in doubt, for drainage of pelvic mass and to clear pelvis in unresponsive chronic disease
- Major cause of infertility worldwide resulting in tubal obstruction in 60% of cases after 2 or more attacks

---

HUMAN IMMUNODEFICIENCY VIRUS (HIV) 1 AND 2

These RNA retroviruses are characterized by their tropism for the human CD4 (helper) T-lymphocyte. The proportion of cells infected is initially low, and there is a prolonged latent phase between infection and clinical signs. Transmission occurs by sex, infected blood products, shared needles, breast feeding and transplacentally. Risk groups include intravenous drug abusers and their partners, the partners of bisexual men, haemophiliacs, prostitutes and immigrants from high-risk areas. Although more common in men in the developed world, anonymous testing shows 0.3% of pregnant women in London to be infected, and it is now the most common cause of death in black females aged 24–35 years in the USA.

The main clinical states can be identified as:

1. A 'flu-like' illness 3–6 months after infection associated with seroconversion
2. Asymptomatic impaired immunity
3. Persistent generalized lymphadenopathy
4. Acquired immunodeficiency syndrome (AIDS)-related complex with pathognomonic infections or tumours.

Common opportunistic infections include *Candida*, herpes simplex, HPV, *Mycobacterium*, *Cryptosporidium*, *Pneumocystis carinii* and cytomegalovirus. Non-infective manifestations include weight loss, diarrhoea, fever, dementia, Karposi's sarcoma and an increased risk of cervical cancer.

The diagnosis is made by detecting antibodies to the virus, although these may take up to 3 months to appear.

HIV infection

- Retrovirus infection of T-helper cells and central nervous system
- Transmitted by sex, blood transfusion or to offspring
- Diagnosis by serology, differential lymphocyte count or opportunistic infection
- Can be asymptomatic, cause generalized malaise and lymphadenopathy or AIDS
- Incidence in heterosexuals increasing

BIBLIOGRAPHY

Johnstone F D 1992 Clinical Obstetrics and Gynaecology. Baillière Tindall, London
Spagne V A, Prior R B 1985 Sexually transmitted diseases. Marcel Dekker, New York

25 Endometriosis and adenomyosis

These two terms describe the presence of endometrium in sites other than the uterine cavity. In endometriosis, the ectopic endometrium occurs in various sites outside the uterine cavity or myometrium. In adenomyosis, the endometrium exhibits aberrant growth by invading the myometrium. The glands remain in communication with the uterine cavity. Adenomyosis is sometimes known as endometriosis interna, and endometriosis as endometriosis externa. Although the two conditions may coexist, they are characterized by different clinical features and do not have a common pathogenesis.

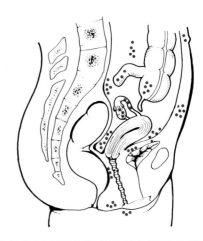

Fig. 25.1 Common sites of endometriotic deposits.

ENDOMETRIOSIS

Pathology

Aberrant endometrial deposits occur in many different sites (Fig 25.1). Endometriosis commonly occurs in the ovaries, utero-sacral ligaments and the recto-vaginal septum. It may also occur in the pelvic peritoneum covering the uterus, tubes, rectum, sigmoid colon and bladder. Remote ectopic deposits of endometrium may be found in the umbilicus, laparotomy scars, hernial scars, the appendix, vagina, vulva, cervix, lymph nodes and, on rare occasions, the pleural cavity.

Ovarian endometriosis occurs in the form of small superficial deposits on the surface of the ovary or as larger cysts known as **endometriomas**, which may grow up to 10 cm in size. These cysts have a thick whitish capsular layer and contain altered blood which has a chocolate-like appearance. For this reason, they are known as **chocolate cysts**. Endometriomas are often densely adherent both to the ovarian tissue and to other surrounding structures.

These cysts are likely to rupture and, in 8% of cases, patients with endometriosis present with symptoms of acute peritoneal irritation (Fig. 25.2).

The microscopic features of the lesions may be of endometrium that cannot be distinguished from the normal tissue lining the uterine cavity, but there is

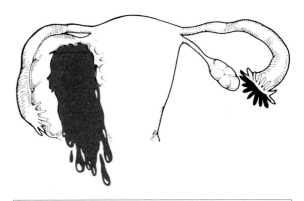

Fig. 25.2 Rupture of an endometriotic cyst causes acute peritonism.

wide variation and, in many long-standing cases, desquamation and repeated menstrual bleeding may result in the loss of all characteristic features of endometrium. Underneath the lining of the cyst, there is often a broad zone containing phagocytic cells with haemosiderin. There is also a broad zone of hyalinized fibrous tissue. One of the characteristics of endometriotic lesions is the intense fibrotic reaction

253

that surrounds them, and this may also contain muscle fibres. The intensity of this reaction often leads to great difficulty in dissection at the time of any operative procedure. The pathogenesis of endometriosis remains obscure. Sampson (1921) originally suggested that the condition was associated with retrograde spill of endometrial cells during menstruation and that some of these cells would implant under appropriate conditions in the peritoneal cavity and on the ovaries. In some cases, the spill would appear to occur from cells lining the Fallopian tubes, giving rise to a condition more appropriately known as **endosalpingiosis**.

This hypothesis does not account for endometriotic deposits outside the peritoneal cavity. An alternative theory suggests that endometrial lesions may arise from metaplastic changes in epithelium surfaces throughout the body.

Symptoms and signs

The disease most commonly presents in the third decade of life and in women of low parity. A substantial number of women are asymptomatic and present only with a history of subfertility. The mechanism of the association between subfertility and endometriosis is unknown, and cannot be explained in most instances by distention or obstruction of the tubes. An alternative explanation is that endometriosis is commonly associated with the LUF syndrome (luteinized unruptured follicles). The commonest symptom is crescendic dysmenorrhoea. Pelvic pain and swelling commence in the week preceding menstruation and dysmenorrhoea persists until the completion of the period. If an endometrioma ruptures, then generalized abdominal pain and peritonism may occur.

If the uterus becomes fixed or there is any adnexal mass adherent in the pouch of Douglas, then deep-seated dyspareunia results. Menstrual disorders are not a common feature of endometriosis, but if the ovaries are extensively involved the cycle may shorten and under these circumstances menorrhagia may also occur.

The symptoms produced by lesions outside the peritoneal cavity depend on the site of the lesion. Involvement of bowel may result in melaena or, if the lesion has caused scarring and fibrosis, in bowel obstruction. Lesions of the bladder may cause haematuria. Cutaneous lesions at the umbilicus, in skin wounds and at the vulva will bleed externally on a cyclical basis. Occasionally lesions in the pleural cavity cause recurrent pneumothorax.

Diagnosis

In a small number of cases, the lesion is visible on the surface, but in most patients nothing abnormal is visible or palpable on pelvic examination. In well-established disease, the uterus is often fixed in retroversion. There is thickening in the utero-sacral ligaments and, if the ovaries are involved, there may be fixed cystic swellings palpable in the pelvis.

The diagnosis can be established only be direct inspection by laparoscopy or at the time of laparotomy. Cysts can be identified by ultrasound or by magnetic resonance imaging. Endometriosis is associated with an elevated serum CA125 level.

Management

Medical therapy

Endometriosis is a difficult condition to treat, and therapy is determined by the presenting symptoms and the nature of the endometriotic lesion. It is often necessary to combine both medical and surgical treatment if the best results are to be obtained.

Endometriotic deposits respond in the same way as normal endometrium. Thus, pregnancy usually induces marked regression of the lesions. However, as the condition is commonly associated with infertility, this is rarely a practical solution to the problem. Medical therapy depends on the concept of inducing a pseudopregnancy, and is most effective in the treatment of small lesions. These effects can be achieved by administration of:

1. Combined oestrogen and progestogen therapy consisting of a high dose of progestogen and a low dose of oestrogen. To prevent 'breakthrough' bleeding, it is necessary to give increasing dosages over a period of 6–9 months.
2. Progestogens–dydrogesterone 10 mg three times daily is usually sufficient to inhibit menstruation and to produce regression of small lesions. A similar effect can be achieved with oral medroxy-progesterone acetate 10 mg three times a day over a 9 month interval.

An alternative approach to therapy is to induce a pseudomenopause, which is probably the most effective method of medical therapy available at the present time.

Danazol is a weak impeded androgen which causes marked gonadotrophin inhibition with minimal overt sex hormone stimulation. This produces suppression of all endogenous stimuli to the endometrium and allows regression to occur in endometriotic deposits.

Given in adequate dosage, the drug induces complete suppression of menstruation, but cessation of therapy results in the resumption of menstruation within 6 weeks. The required dosage is between 200 and 600 mg daily for 6–9 months. The drug may produce side effects which are not tolerable and may necessitate cessation of therapy. These include weight gain, oedema, fatigue, depression, increased hair growth, acne and reduced breast size. In the infertile group, success rates of 30–40% have been reported. In terms of menstrual symptoms, there is a much greater rate of relief but the symptoms often return after cessation of therapy.

Gestrinone, which is a synthetic trienic 19-norsteroid, may be used as an alternative therapy. The drug acts by inhibiting ovarian steroidogenesis, and is taken twice weekly. It has similar side effects to Danazol but in a lower proportion of patients. Gonadotrophin-releasing hormone analogues (GnRHa) are synthetic peptides that bind competitively to pituitary GnRH receptors, causing a down-regulation in the release of follicle-stimulating hormone and luteinizing hormone. These compounds can be administered as monthly depot injections or implants (Leuprorelin, Goserelin) or as a twice-daily nasal spray (Nafarelin, Buserelin). Menopausal side effects such as flushes, vaginal dryness and breast atrophy are common, but androgenic side effects are minimal. Long-term use is limited to 6 months because of a reversible loss of bone density. Recurrence of symptoms occurs in 40–70% of cases compared with figures in different trials of 22–50% with Danazol.

Surgical treatment

Diathermy of small lesions, either at laparotomy or through the laparoscope, is the treatment of choice. Ablation of surface lesions with a carbon dioxide laser is now considered to be the method of choice because of minimal subsequent problems with adhesions.

Skin lesions can be cured by excision.

Where large endometriomatous deposits occur, as with ovarian endometriomas, medical therapy is rarely effective, and it is necessary to resect these lesions. Every attempt should be made to conserve ovarian tissue in these circumstances. If the uterus is fixed in retroversion- and there is dyspareunia, ventrosuspension of the uterus should be performed by shortening the round ligaments and pulling the uterus anteriorly out of the pouch of Douglas. In a limited number of situations where conservation of reproductive potential is important, pain relief can be achieved by presacral neurectomy. This procedure involves surgical transection of the presacral plexus with excision of tissue between the right ureter and superior haemorrhoidal vessels.

If all these procedures fail or there is no desire for conservation of reproductive function, then pelvic clearance is indicated with total hysterectomy and bilateral salpingo-oophorectomy. In the author's experience, hormone replacement therapy under these circumstances does not cause recurrence of the endometriotic lesions.

ADENOMYOSIS

Adenomyosis is a condition characterized by the invasion of endometrial glands and stroma into the myometrium. It is difficult to diagnose until the uterus is subjected to histological examination and, for this reason, the diagnosis is often overlooked.

Symptoms and signs

This condition, unlike endometriosis, occurs in parous women and usually arises in the fourth decade. It is associated with menorrhagia and dysmenorrhoea of increasing severity. On clinical examination, the uterus is symmetrically enlarged and tender. The condition is rare after the menopause.

Pathology

The macroscopic appearances of the uterus are those of diffuse enlargement. Adenomyosis and myomas often co-exist, although the uterus is rarely enlarged to the size seen in the presence of myomas. The posterior wall of the uterus is usually thicker than the anterior wall. The cut surface of the uterus presents a characteristic whorl-like trabeculated appearance, but occasionally circumscribed nodules with dark haemorrhagic spots can be seen in the myometrium.

The microscopic diagnosis is based on the finding of islands of endometrial tissue buried deep within the myometrium. The aberrant endometrium does not respond to progesterone and the appearances are always those of proliferative endometrium. It is very rare for malignant change to occur in these lesions.

The only certain way of diagnosing adenomyosis preoperatively is by the use of magnetic resonance imaging (MRI). The nature of MRI of endometrial tissue can be seen within the myometrium, and provides a high degree of accuracy in diagnosing adenomyosis (Fig. 25.3).

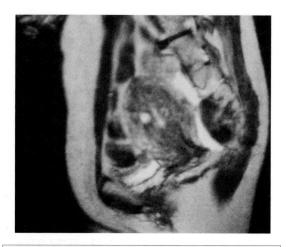

Fig. 25.3 Sagittal view using MRI of a uterus enlarged by adenomyosis.

Treatment

The only satisfactory treatment of this condition is hysterectomy. The ovaries should be conserved, depending on the age of the patient. Conservative therapy with hormone preparations is rarely effective, although symptomatic relief of dysmenorrhoea with prostaglandin synthetase inhibitors is sometimes achieved.

Irradiation of the ovaries is occasionally employed to stop ovarian function, but this therapy should be reserved for women with medical problems that make surgical treatment unusually hazardous. Thus, a radiation menopause may be used in women who are excessively obese or who have a history of severe cardiac disease or thromboembolic disorders.

Endometriosis and adenomyosis

- 'Ectopic' endometrium
- Commonest sites are ovaries, uterosacral ligaments and pelvic peritoneum
- May arise from metaplastic change or implantation
- Presents as subfertility and/or crescendic dysmenorrhoea
- Management is to induce pseudopregnancy or pseudomenopause or surgical excision
- Adenomyosis is invasion of the myometrium by endometrial tissue
- Presents as menorrhagia and dysmenorrhoea

BIBLIOGRAPHY

Chalmers J A 1975 Endometriosis. Butterworths, London
Jordan J A (ed) 1993 Mini-symposium: endometriosis. Current Obstetrics and Gynaecology 3(3): 121–138
Sampson A 1921 Perforating haemorrhagic (chocolate) cysts of the ovary and especially their relation to pelvic adenomas of the endometrial type. Archives of Surgery 3: 245

26 Lesions of the vulva and vagina

BENIGN LESIONS OF THE VULVA

There have been numerous changes in the classification of vulvar disease, and the previous terminology of 'vulval dystrophies' has been discarded.

The following classification is now recommended:

I Non-neoplastic epithelial disorders of skin and mucosa:
1. Lichen sclerosus (lichen sclerosus et atrophicus)
2. Squamous cell hyperplasia (formerly hyperplastic dystrophy)
3. Other dermatoses.

II Classification of vulvar intra-epithelial neoplasia (VIN):
VIN I   Mild dysplasia (formally mild atypia)
VIN II Moderate dysplasia (formally moderate atypia)
VIN III Severe dysplasia (formally severe atypia).

This classification is based on histological appearances. The typical appearances are still described as leucoplakia and kraurosis vulvae under the general heading of squamous cell hyperplasia, and other dermatoses include psoriasis, lichen planus, lichen simplex chronicus, *Candida* infection and condyloma acuminatum. Mixed epithelial conditions may occur, and it is recommended that both descriptions should be used under these circumstances. However, this range of terminology has now largely been abandoned, and where there is histological evidence of cellular atypia, lesions should simply be classified on the basis of histological appearance.

Where there is histological evidence of cellular atypia, the lesion should be classified as vulvar intra-epithelial neoplasia. The clinical appearances of these conditions are described under a descriptive classification which is useful only in so far as it describes the clinical appearance of these lesions.

Non-neoplastic epithelial disorders

Lichen sclerosus (lichen sclerosus et atrophicus)

The typical lesions of this condition, sometimes known as lichen sclerosus et atrophicus, are white papules which progress to atrophic plaques. The condition affects the perineum and peri-anal skin. The atrophic changes lead to a progressive loss of normal anatomy accompanied by fusion of the labia and adhesion formation with vaginal stenosis (Fig. 26.1).

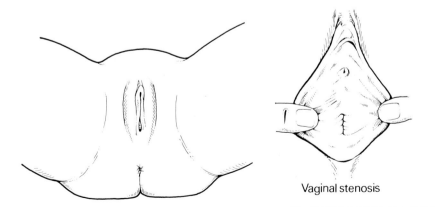

Vaginal stenosis

Fig. 26.1   Atrophic vulval changes (left) result in stenosis of the vaginal introitus (right).

Other dermatoses

Vulval skin can be affected by a wide range of conditions that affect other skin surface and these include allergic dermatitis, psoriasis, intertrigo and lichen planus.

Aetiology

The cause of non-neoplastic epithelial disorders is unknown. These conditions are associated with a high incidence of autoimmune disorders including pernicious anaemia, hypothyroidism and hyperthyroidism.

The epithelial disorders are associated with malignant change in about 5% of cases, the development of which is always preceded by atypical changes.

Treatment

It is important to inspect the vulva with good light and magnification, and biopsy the skin to establish an accurate diagnosis. Common infections, such as by *Trichomonas* and *Candida*, should be excluded, and a full history of onset, previous treatments, other skin complaints and illnesses such as diabetes should be taken. General advice on hygiene and potential irritants, clothing and barrier creams should be given. Treatment is medical with long-term follow-up for early detection of malignant change. The mainstay of treatment is topical steroids using short courses of high-potency creams such as betnovate for exacerbations and low-potency creams such as 0.1% hydrocortisone for maintenance. Testosterone cream is of limited value because of its short shelf life. If all conservative therapy fails, it may be necessary to remove the affected skin by simple vulvectomy or excision biopsy or laser ablation of visible lesions. However, the conditions have a tendency to reoccur.

Benign tumours of the vulva

Benign cysts of the vulva include sebaceous cysts, epithelial inclusion cysts and Wolffian duct cysts, which arise from the labia minora and the peri-urethral region, and Bartholin's cysts which have been described elsewhere. A rare cyst may arise from a peritoneal extension along the round ligament, forming a hydrocele in the labium major. Benign solid tumours include fibromas, lipomas and hidradenomas. Fibromas may reach an enormous size (Fig. 26.2). True squamous papillomas appear as

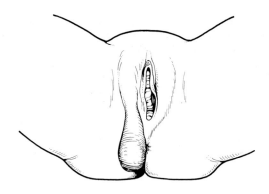

FIBROMA OF VULVA

Fig. 26.2 Vulval fibroids are usually pedunculated and may be very large.

warty growths and rarely become malignant. All of these lesions are treated by simple biopsy excision.

Vulval and vaginal trauma

Injuries to vulva and vagina may result in severe haemorrhage and haematoma formation. Vulval bruising may be particularly severe because of the rich venous plexus in the labia, and commonly results from falling astride. Lacerations of the vagina are often associated with coitus.

Vulval haematomas often subside with conservative management, but will sometimes need drainage. It is important to suture vaginal lacerations and to be certain that the injury does not penetrate into the peritoneal cavity.

Benign vulval lesions

- Cause unknown/auto-immune
- Usually presents as pruritus
- Classified by appearance or histology
- Associated with malignant change in 5% cases
- Need to exclude malignancy, infection, diabetes and other systemic conditions

---

NEOPLASTIC LESIONS OF THE VULVA

Vulval intraepithelial neoplasia (VIN) is a condition which is characterized by disorientation and loss of epithelial architecture extending through the full thickness of the epithelium but not penetrating the basement membrane. There is an association with similar changes to the cervix (CIN) and in the peri-anal region (PAIN). Forty per cent of cases occur in women under the age of 41 years. It was originally known as **Bowen's disease**. A further variant which arises from the apocrine glands is known as **Paget's disease**. The appearance of the lesions is variable, but they are papular and raised and may be white, grey, dull red or various shades of brown and may be localized or widespread. These conditions are rare, with an incidence of 0.53 per 100 000, and commonly occur in women over the age of 60 years. This condition is associated with adenocarcinoma of the apocrine glands in one-third of cases.

Management

The only satisfactory treatment of this condition is local excision. It is important to establish the diagnosis by biopsy and to search for any other sites of intra-epithelial neoplasia, which are commonly found in association with the vulval lesion, particularly the cervix and vagina. Other methods of treatment include cryosurgery and the use of the carbon dioxide laser and, in some cases, the local application of 5-fluorouracil cream.

There is a 15% risk of progression to invasive disease, so that long-term follow-up with excision biopsy of suspicious lesions is essential.

Carcinoma of the vulva

Carcinoma of the vulva accounts for 2–3% of female malignancies. Ninety-two per cent of the lesions are squamous cell carcinomas, 5% are adenocarcinomas, 1% are basal carcinomas and 0.5% are malignant melanomas (Fig. 26.3). The lesions may occur at any age, but are commonest after the age of 65 years.

Predisposing conditions include VIN and lichen sclerosus, and there is an association with chronic vulvitis, diabetes, hypertension and obesity.

Symptoms

The patient with vulval carcinoma experiences pruritis and notices a raised lesion on the vulva which may ulcerate and bleed. Malignant melanomas are usually single, hyperpigmented and ulcerated. The tumour most frequently develops on the labia majora but may also grow on the prepuce of the clitoris, the labia minora, Bartholin's glands and in the vestibule of the vagina. Carcinoma of the vulva most commonly occurs in the sixth and seventh decades.

Natural history

The disease tends to progress from an area of VIN through carcinoma in situ to invasion. Spread occurs both locally and through the lymphatic system (Figs 26.4 and 26.5). The lymph nodes involved are the superficial and deep inguinal nodes and the femoral nodes (Fig. 26.4). Pelvic lymph nodes, except in primary lesions involving the clitoris, have usually only secondary involvement. In particular, the external iliac and obturator nodes are involved. Blood vascular spread is late and rare. The disease usually progresses slowly and the

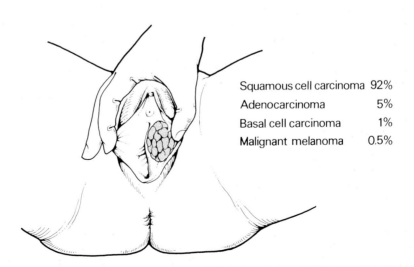

Squamous cell carcinoma 92%
Adenocarcinoma 5%
Basal cell carcinoma 1%
Malignant melanoma 0.5%

Fig. 26.3 Carcinoma of the vulva occurs at any site but is commonly a squamous cell lesion.

259

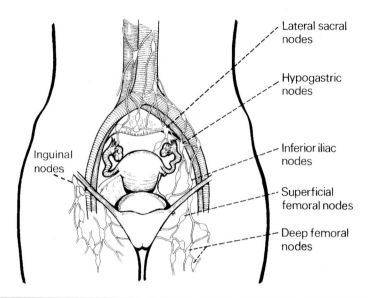

Fig. 26.4 Lymphatic drainage of the vulva.

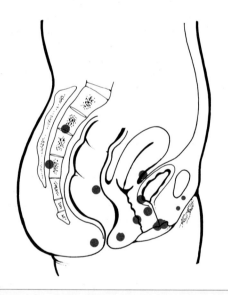

Fig. 26.5 Sites of spread of vulval carcinoma.

terminal stages are accompanied by extensive ulceration, infection, haemorrhage and remote metastatic disease. In some 30% of cases, lymph nodes are involved on both sides.

Classification

The most widely used classification of carcinoma of the vulva is the FIGO classification, and is described as follows:

Stage I Tumour confined to the vulva – 2 cm or less in diameter. Nodes are not involved.

Stage II Tumour confined to the vulva – more than 2 cm in diameter. Nodes are not involved.

Stage III Tumour of any size with:
1. Adjacent spread to the lower urethra and/or the vagina, the perineum and the anus, and/or
2. Unilateral lymph node involvement.

Stage IV Tumour of any size with:
A. Infiltrating the bladder mucosa or the rectal mucosa, or both, including the upper part of the urethral mucosa and/or bilateral lymph node involvement.
B. Fixed to the bone or other distant metastases. Fixed or ulcerated nodes in either one or both groins.

Therapy

Stages I to III should be treated with radical vulvectomy. This procedure involves extensive removal of the vulval and bilateral inguinal nodes and pelvic lymphadenectomy (Fig. 26.6). Radiotherapy has a limited role to play in advanced lesions in elderly patients.

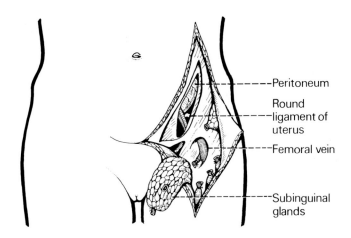

Fig. 26.6 Block dissection of the lymph nodes in surgical treatment of malignant disease of the vulva.

Complications of radical vulvectomy include wound breakdown and lymphoedema (30%), secondary bleeding, thrombo-embolism and psychological morbidity. Response to chemotherapy (bleomycin) is generally poor.

Prognosis

Stages I and II have a good 5 year salvage rate, with 100% survival in stage I, 80% in stage II, and 30–40% in stages III and IV.

Malignant melanoma and adenocarcinoma have a poor prognosis, with a 5 year survival of 5%.

Malignant vulval lesions

- Commonest in 6th decade
- 2–3% of female cancers
- Premalignant changes occur in 0.5/100 000 women
- Majority are squamous (92%) or adenocarcinomas (5%)
- Present with pruritus, bleeding lesions
- Spreads by local invasion and via inguinal and femoral nodes
- Staged according to size, lymph node involvement and spread
- Good prognosis if confined to vulva at presentation

BENIGN TUMOURS OF THE VAGINA

Vaginal cysts

Congenital

Cysts arise in the vagina from embryological remnants; the commonest varieties are those arising from Gartner's duct (Wolffian duct remnants). These are not rare and occur in the antero-lateral wall of the vagina. They are usually asymptomatic and are found on routine examination.

Histologically, the cysts are lined by cuboidal epithelium, but sometimes a flattened layer of stratified squamous epithelium is seen.

Treatment – The cysts are treated by simple surgical excision and rarely give rise to any difficulties.

Vaginal inclusion cysts

Inclusion cysts arise from inclusion of small particles or islands of vaginal epithelium under the surface. The cysts commonly arise in episiotomy scars and contain yellowish thick fluid within the cyst. They are treated by simple surgical excision.

Endometriosis

Endometriotic lesions may appear anywhere in the vagina, but occur most commonly in the posterior fornix. The lesions may appear as dark brown spots or reddened ulcerated lesions. The diagnosis is established by excision biopsy. If the lesions are multiple, then medical therapy should be instituted as for lesions in other sites.

Solid benign tumours

These lesions are rare but may represent any of the tissues that are found in the vagina. Thus, polypoid tumours may include fibromyomas, myomas, fibromas, papillomas and adenomyomas. These tumours are treated by simple surgical excision.

NEOPLASTIC LESIONS OF VAGINAL EPITHELIUM

Vaginal intra-epithelial neoplasia

Vaginal intra-epithelial neoplasia (VAIN) is usually multicentric and tends to be multifocal and associated with similar lesions of the cervix. The condition is asymptomatic and tends to be discovered because of a positive smear test or during colposcopy for abnormal cytology, often after hysterectomy. There is a risk of progression to invasive carcinoma, but the disease remains superficial until then, and can be treated by surgical excision, laser ablation or cryosurgery.

Vaginal adenosis

This is the presence of columnar epithelium in the vaginal epithelium and has been found in adult females whose mothers received treatment with diethylstilboestrol during pregnancy. The condition commonly reverts to normal squamous epithelium, but in about 4% of cases the lesion progresses to carcinoma in situ. It is therefore important to follow these women carefully with serial cytology.

MALIGNANT VAGINAL TUMOURS

Primary malignancies of the vagina are very rare. The lesions include squamous cell carcinomas and sarcomas and, rarely, chorio-epitheliomas.

Vaginal tumours

- Benign tumours are commonly, embryological remnants, inclusion cysts or endometriotic
- Primary malignancy rare, squamous carcinomas arising in upper third
- Common site for spread from cervix and uterus
- Presents as pain, bleeding and fistula formation
- Spreads by local invasion and lymphatics
- Usually treated by radiotherapy
- Increased incidence in young women whose mothers were given diethylstilboestrol in pregnancy
- Premalignant changes associated with CIN

Carcinoma of the vagina

Invasive carcinoma of the vagina may be a squamous carcinoma or, occasionally, an adenocarcinoma. Primary lesions arise in the sixth and seventh decades, but are rare in the UK. In recent years, there has been an increase in adenocarcinomas in young women, which has been associated with the administration of diethylstilboestrol during the pregnancies of their mothers. These tumours are of the clear-cell or mesonephric variety.

Secondary deposits from cervical carcinoma and endometrial carcinoma are relatively common in the upper third of the vagina and can sometimes occur in the lower vagina due to lymphatic spread.

Symptoms

The symptoms include irregular vaginal bleeding and offensive vaginal discharge when the tumour becomes necrotic and infection supervenes. Infection may also cause pain, and local spread into the rectum, bladder or urethra may result in fistula formation.

The tumour may appear as an exophytic lesion or as an ulcerated, indurated mass.

Method of spread

Tumour spread, as previously stated, occurs by direct infiltration or by lymphatic extension. Lesions involving the upper half of the vagina follow a pattern of spread similar to that of carcinoma of the cervix. Tumours of the lower half of the vagina follow a similar pattern of spread to that of carcinoma of the vulva.

Clinical staging

Carcinoma of the vagina is classified as follows:

Stage 0 – intra-epithelial carcinoma
Stage I – limited to the vaginal walls
Stage II – involves the subvaginal tissue, but has not extended to the pelvic wall
Stage III – the tumour has extended to the lateral pelvic wall
Stage IV – the lesion has extended to involve adjacent organs (IVa) or has spread to distant organs (IVb).

Treatment

The diagnosis is established by biopsy of the

tumour, and careful evaluation of tumour extension and staging is made before commencing treatment.

The primary method of treatment is by radiotherapy – both by external beam therapy and by interstitial γ ray sources.

Surgical treatment includes radical vaginectomy, and anterior or posterior exenteration, but this is rarely used as the primary therapy.

Prognosis

Results of treatment depend on the initial staging and on the method of therapy. Stages I and II have a 5 year survival of around 60%, and this figure falls to 30–40% for stages III and IV. Adenocarcinoma of the vagina, which often occurs in young females, also responds well to irradiation.

Sarcoma botryoides

This is a rare tumour of mixed mesodermal origin which occurs in young females of age 2–3 years. The tumour grows rapidly and may appear at the introitus as a grape-like mass. Combined treatment with radiotherapy and surgery seems to offer the best prospect for cure and may allow conservation of the bladder and rectum, although it is not possible to conserve reproductive function.

BIBLIOGRAPHY

Shaw R W, Souter W P, Stanton S L 1992 Gynaecology. Churchill Livingstone, Edinburgh

Lesions of the cervix

EXAMINATION OF THE CERVIX

Routine examination of the cervix involves direct inspection with a good light and exposure with a bivalve or Sims' speculum. The size, shape and consistency of the cervix should be noted and the nature of any discharge recorded. The external cervical os is circular in shape, and in parous women the os is a transverse slit. The nature of the epithelium should be observed, as it will vary according to the hormonal status of the woman. The normal ectocervix

is covered with stratified squamous epithelium and the endocervical canal by columnar epithelium. The junction between these two epithelia is known as the **squamocolumnar junction**, and it may be placed at any point across the cervix. The area adjacent to the squamocolumnar junction is the transformation zone, and it is in this area that most abnormal changes occur.

The term **cervical erosion** or **cervical ectopy** is used where the endocervical epithelium appears to advance on to the ectocervix and gives a bright red velvety appearance (Fig. 27.1). In fact, this reflects

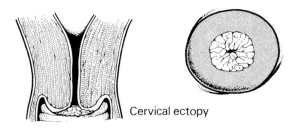

Cervical ectopy

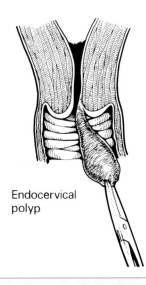

Endocervical polyp

Fig. 27.1 Common benign lesions of the cervix include cervical ectopy or 'erosion' (top) and cervical polyps (below).

no more than the dynamic behaviour of the transformation zone and the squamocolumnar junction. During pregnancy and adolescence, and in some women on oral contraception, the endocervical epithelium advances outwards, whereas at the menopause, shrinkage occurs with diminution of the exposed area of the transformation zone.

In most cases, cervical ectopy is asymptomatic, but it is sometimes associated with leucorrhoea and postcoital bleeding.

The term **cervical ectropion** describes the eversion of the cervix associated with bilateral laceration following parturition. The endocervical mucosa rolls out from the cervical canal and may give rise to symptoms similar to those of cervical ectopy.

MANAGEMENT

These conditions are benign and should be treated only where they produce symptoms. Treatment of cervical ectopy is by radial diathermy or cryosurgery. Squamous epithelium grows along the tracks of diathermy wounds, and epithelial growth covers and replaces the endocervical epithelium. For 2 weeks after treatment, the discharge may worsen with separation of the cauterized epithelium, but within a month the symptoms will either recede or disappear.

The complications of the procedure are:

1. Secondary haemorrhage and infection
2. Cervical stenosis.

Occasionally, it may be necessary to excise the endocervical mucosa and the laceration and thereby refashion the cervix, a procedure known as **trachelorrhaphy**.

BENIGN NEOPLASMS OF THE CERVIX

Cervical polyps

Benign polyps (Fig. 27.1) arise from the endocervix, and are pedunculated with a covering of endocervical epithelium and a central fibrous tissue core. The polyps present as bright red, vascular growths which may be identified on routine examination: the presenting symptoms may include irregular vaginal blood loss or postcoital bleeding.

Less frequently, the polyps arise from the squamous epithelium, when the appearance will resemble the surface of the vaginal epithelium.

Treatment

The only treatment is surgical, with ligation of the pedicle and excision of the polyp.

Cervical fibroids

Cervical leiomyomas are similar to fibroids in other sites of the uterus. They are commonly pedunculated, but may be sessile and grow to a size that will fill the vagina and distort the pelvic organs.

Symptoms are similar to those caused by other cervical polyps and, in addition, the attempted extrusion of fibroid polyps may cause colicky uterine pain, particularly at the time of menstruation.

Treatment is by surgical excision. Many of these lesions have a thick pedicle which must be transfixed and ligated before excision of the polyp.

Malignant change in the form of sarcomatous degeneration is extremely rare and is no more frequent than sarcomatous change arising in the myometrium.

Benign lesions of the cervix

- Extension of the endocervical epithelium on to the ectocervix is a normal physiological variant
- Ectropion is cervical eversion revealing the endocervical mucosa
- Benign polyps commonly arise from the endocervix
- Fibroids may arise from the cervix
- Benign lesions may be asymptomatic or present as vaginal bleeding or discharge

---

MALIGNANT LESIONS OF THE CERVIX

Screening for cervical cancer

Squamous cell carcinoma is a sexually transmitted disease, and all women who have had sexual intercourse are at risk. Screening by cervical cytology follows specific national recommendations in the UK which are as follows:

1. First smear – at the age of 20 years
2. Second and subsequent smears – at 3-yearly intervals up to the age of 65 years
3. After 65 years – regular smears not required.

Technique

It is essential to obtain a good view of the cervix. The speculum should be introduced with a minimum of artificial lubricant. Cells are taken from around the cervix from the whole of the transformation zone by taking a smear with a 360° sweep using an Aylesbury spatula. Although pre-invasive lesions arising from the endocervical epithelium (cervical intraglandular neoplasia, CIGN) can be identified by cervical cytology, the method is primarily for screening for squamous lesions and cannot reliably exclude endocervical disease.

Cytology

Apart from assessing the cells for signs of malignant change, a smear from the upper third of the vagina can also be used for assessment of hormone status.

The specimen is spread immediately on to a clear glass slide in a thin even layer. The slide is fixed with 95% alcohol alone or in combination with 3% glacial acetic acid. Fixation requires 30 minutes in solution, and the preparation is then stained using the Papanicolaou technique. With this method, the nuclei stain blue, the superficial cell cytoplasm pink and the intermediate parabasal cell cytoplasm stains blue/green. The squamous epithelium of the vagina and cervix is composed of four layers as follows (Fig. 27.2):

1. *Basal cells* – these lie on the basement membrane and are not usually exfoliated.
2. *Parabasal cells* – these cells are oval in shape and have a centrally placed nucleus with a cytoplasm that is basophilic.
3. *Intermediate squamous cells* – these cells are polygonal in shape and have a basophilic cytoplasm, except in the presence of infection when it becomes

eosinophilic. The cells lie singly or in clumps with either a flattened or a folded appearance.
4. *Superficial or mature squamous cells* – polygonal cells with a pyknotic nucleus and a cytoplasm that is eosinophilic.

Endocervical cells, which are tall and cylindrical, may also be seen as well as endometrial cells. Hormone status is assessed by counting the number of squamous cells with a pyknotic nucleus in relation to the rest of the squamous cell population, and this is known as the **karyopyknotic index** (KPI). The KPI is high (50–60%) in the proliferative phase of the cycle and low (0–10%) in the secretory phase.

Characteristic appearances of malignant cells

Malignant cells show nuclear enlargement at the expense of cytoplasmic mass (Fig. 27.3). The nuclei may assume a lobulated outline. There is increased intensity of staining of the nucleus and an increase in the number of mitotic figures.

Dyskaryosis

The term 'dyskaryosis' describes those cells that lie between normal squamous and frankly malignant cells and exhibit degrees of nuclear changes consistent with malignancy.

The correlation between cytology and histological changes in the cervix is poor, with up to 50% of women with mild dyskaryosis having cervical intra-epithelial neoplasia (CIN) II or greater (Table 27.1). The overall false-negative rate varies from 2 to 26%. CIN will be detected in 2–3% of the screened population.

The British Society for Clinical Cytology introduced in 1986 the following classification for cervical smears:

1. Unsatisfactory for assessment
2. Negative
3. Nuclear changes bordering on mild dyskaryosis
4. Dyskaryotic cells:
   Mild
   Moderate
   Severe
5. Severe dyskaryosis with features suggesting the possibility of invasion.

Colposcopy

The presence of dyskaryosis or malignant cells on cytology is an indication for examination by colposcopy. A borderline smear will be repeated after

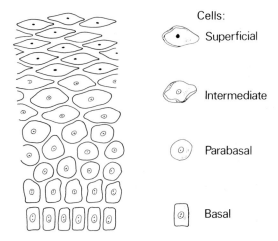

Cells:

Superficial

Intermediate

Parabasal

Basal

Fig. 27.2 Cell layers in the stratified squamous epithelium of the cervix and vagina.

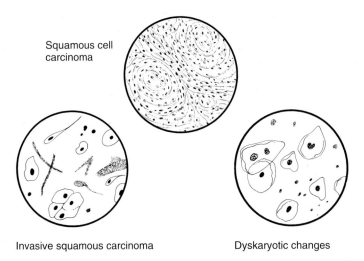

Squamous cell carcinoma

Invasive squamous carcinoma

Dyskaryotic changes

Fig. 27.3 Invasive carcinoma (top) is associated with 'tadpole' and 'fibre' cells in the smear (bottom left); the histology commonly shows layers of non-keratinizing squamous epithelium, although in some lesions keratinization can be seen; dyskaryotic appearances include nuclear changes consistent with malignancy but have normal cytoplasm (bottom right).

Table 27.1 The relationship between cervical cytology and histology

Cytology	CIN II + (%)
Normal	0.1
Borderline	20–30
Mild dyskaryosis	50
Moderate dyskaryosis	50–75
Severe dyskaryosis	80–90 (5% carcinoma)

Cervical screening

- 3-yearly interval from 20 to 65 years of age
- Malignant change suggested by an increased nuclear:cytoplasmic ratio, mitotic figures and intense nuclear staining
- Dyskaryosis represents lesser degrees of abnormality
- Appearance of exfoliated cells varies with hormonal status and infection
- Abnormal cytology requires colposcopy

6 months, and if borderline changes persist colposcopy is also advised. In some centres, colposcopy for mild dyskaryosis is also deferred until after two successive smears 6 months apart are abnormal.

Colposcopy involves the examination of the cervix with a binocular microscope. This enables biopsy of abnormal epithelium and treatment of intra-epithelial neoplasia. The findings on colposcopy are described by the following appearances:

1. **Atypical transformation zone** –
   a. Acetowhite epithelium
   b. Mosaic
   c. Punctation
   d. Leucoplakia
   e. Atypical vessels – suggestive of early invasion.
2. **Malignant epithelium** – An increase in vascular development. The vessels make sharp angulation and have a bizarre pattern. The surface is irregular, raised and nodular, and there is often a large complex lesion.

Pathophysiology

The junction of the squamous epithelium which lines the ectocervix and the columnar glandular epithelium of the endocervix, the **squamo-columnar junction** (SCJ), moves in relation to the anatomical external cervical os. Changes in oestrogen such as occur during puberty, pregnancy or whilst on the pill will move the SCJ outwards, exposing columnar epithelium to the lower pH of the vagina. This reacts by undergoing transformation back to squamous epithelium by a process of **squamous metaplasia**. The area that lies between the current SCJ and that reached as it moves outwards across the ectocervix is known as the **transformation zone**, and it is in this area that most pre-invasive lesions occur.

It follows then that an adequate colposcopic examination requires that all of the SCJ is visualized in order that the entire transformation zone can be inspected.

Neoplastic cells have an increased amount of nuclear material in relation to cytoplasm and less surface glycogen than normal squamous epithelium. They are associated with a degree of hypertrophy of the underlying vasculature. These features are exploited in colposcopic examination. When exposed to 5% acetic acid the nuclear protein will be coagulated, giving the neoplastic cells a characteristic white appearance, but they will not react with Schiller's iodine unlike the normal squamous epithelium, which will stain dark brown. The increased capillary vascularity may be visible through the epithelium as red dots or punctation or a 'crazy paving' mosaic pattern.

Colposcopic appearances

1. Wart virus changes – characterized by acetowhite epithelium but with an irregular, poorly defined border and 'satellite lesions' usually without any vessel changes.
2. Cervical intraepithelial neoplasia – an area of acetowhite epithelium with a well-defined border often associated with punctation or mosaicism.
3. Invasive disease – differs in having a hard, raised, friable area with irregular abnormal looking vessels.

Colposcopy cannot be used reliably in the diagnosis of intraglandular neoplasia or lesions more than 5 mm up the endocervical canal.

Cervical intra-epithelial neoplasia (CIN)

This is a histological diagnosis of changes in the squamous epithelium characterized by varying degrees of loss of differentiation and stratification and nuclear atypia. It may extend up to 5 mm below the surface of the cervix by involvement of crypt epithelium in the transformation zone, but does not extend below the basement membrane. The aetiology is the same as that of invasive disease, but with a peak incidence 10 years earlier. It is classified as CIN I, II or III. Of cases of CIN I, 25% will undergo progression to higher-grade lesions over 2 years, but up to 50% will regress to normal. Approximately a third of CIN III lesions will progress to invasive disease if not adequately treated.

Cervical intraglandular neoplasia (CIGN) is the equivalent lesion in the columnar epithelium of the endocervix, and the pre-invasive stage of cervical adenocarcinoma. It comprises 10–15% of non-invasive cervical neoplasia and co-exists with CIN in two-thirds of cases. Up to 50% of lesions will have no glandular abnormality on cervical cytology and are diagnosed as an incidental finding on treatment for CIN.

Treatment

It is now well established that treatment of CIN can prevent the development of invasive disease and reduce deaths from cervical cancer. This forms the basis of the cervical screening programme. The area of CIN is delineated by colposcopy, and the diagnosis confirmed by colposcopically directed biopsy. The abnormal area can then be ablated using electro-coagulation diathermy or carbon dioxide laser. More commonly, it will be removed as part of an excision of the transformation zone using a diathermy loop (LLETZ) or laser. This can be carried out under colposcopic direction as an out-patient procedure after infiltration of the ectocervix with local anaesthetic.

Glandular lesions, or squamous lesions extending up the cervical canal should be treated by cone biopsy. This procedure involves excision of a cone of cervical tissue which includes any abnormal epithelium on the ectocervix defined by the application of iodine solution and extends to the full length of the cervical canal. This can be carried out using scalpel (under general anaesthetic), loop diathermy or laser. Additional sutures to occlude the cervical branch of the uterine artery may be required for haemostasis (Fig. 27.4).

Complications of cone biopsy

The commonest complication is haemorrhage. This may be primary, i.e. within 12 hours of operation, or secondary, usually between the 5th and 12th post-

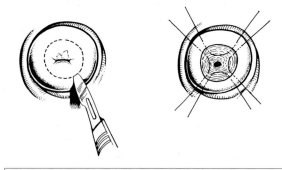

Fig. 27.4 Cone biopsy of the cervix (left); four mattress sutures are usually adequate to control bleeding from the cervical stump (right).

operative day. Haemorrhage may be profuse, but can be controlled by compression with vaginal packing or by resuturing the cervix. Secondary haemorrhage is commonly associated with infection and the management therefore includes blood transfusion and antibiotic therapy.

Later complications include cervical stenosis with dysmenorrhoea and hematometra. Cone biopsy may also cause cervical incompetence and subsequent midtrimester abortion.

Hysterectomy

Hysterectomy is indicated where:

1. Excision is not completed by cone biopsy
2. Persistent abnormal smears follow cone biopsy
3. Other disorders such as fibroids or prolapse are present
4. Hysterectomy is to be used for sterilization.

Follow-up

Approximately 5% of patients with CIN will have residual or recurrent disease. Follow-up is by cytology, usually with 2 smears in the first 12 months after treatment, then annually for a further 4 years before returning to the 3-yearly screening programme.

Cervical cancer

Cervical cancer is the second commonest female cancer worldwide. In many countries this is the most common cause of death from cancer in women. In the UK the annual incidence is 12/100 000 with 3000 new cases and 1200 deaths per year. Cervical cancer has a direct relationship to sexual activity. Associated risk factors are early age of first intercourse, number of partners, smoking and infection with human papillomavirus types 16, 18 and 33.

Age distribution

Incidence increases with age with a peak at 60–64 years. However, the distribution is bimodal with a secondary peak at 35–39 years.

Pathology

There are two types of invasive carcinoma of the cervix. Sixty per cent of lesions are squamous and 40% adenocarcinomas. Histologically the degree of invasion may be:

- Early stromal with isolated pseudopodia only below the basement membrane
- Microinvasive where invasion is less than 3 mm below basement membrane
- Invasive where invasion is more than 3 mm below the basement membrane.

Classification

The following classification is used for carcinoma of the cervix (Fig. 27.5):

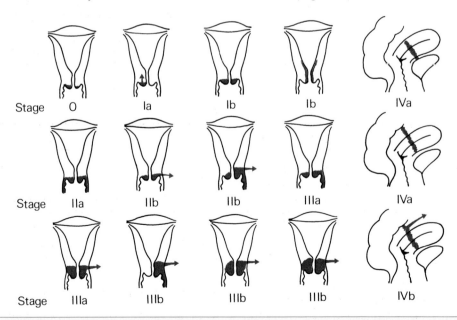

Fig. 27.5 Stages of carcinoma of the cervix. Lateral arrow indicates extension into the parametrium.

Stage I Carcinoma confined to the cervix (extension to the corpus does not advance the stage):

Stage IA – Divided into IA1 early stromal invasion only and IA2 – microinvasion – where the tumour extends less than 3 mm from the base of the epithelium with a horizontal spread of no more than 7 mm.

Stage IB – invasion of more than 3 mm depth or 7 mm area but is still confined to the cervix.

Stage II Carcinoma extends beyond the cervix but does not reach the pelvic side wall or lower third of the vagina:

Stage IIA – no obvious parametrial involvement, upper two-thirds of the vagina involved.

Stage IIB – obvious parametrial involvement, but not reaching the pelvic side wall.

Stage III Carcinoma extends to the pelvic side wall or lower third of the vagina. Includes all cases of hydronephrosis/nonfunctioning kidney unless this is known to be due to another cause:

Stage IIIA – tumour extends to lower third of the vagina.

Stage IIIB – extension to pelvic side wall or hydronephrosis.

Stage IV Carcinoma extending beyond the true pelvis or involving the bladder or rectal mucosa:

Stage IVA – involvement of bladder or rectum.

Stage IVB – spread to distant organs.

The spread of tumour

Cervical carcinoma spreads by direct local invasion and by the lymphatics and blood vessels. Lymphatic spread occurs in approximately 40% of women with stage I and II disease and preferential spread occurs to the external iliac, internal iliac and obturator nodes. Secondary spread may also occur to inguinal, sacral and aortic nodes. Bloodborne metastases occur in the lungs, liver, bone and bowel.

Clinical features

Stage Ia disease is asymptomatic at the time of presentation and is detected at the time of routine examination for cervical cytology. The common presenting symptoms from invasive carcinoma of the cervix include postcoital bleeding, foul-smelling discharge, which is thin and watery and sometimes blood-stained, and irregular vaginal bleeding when the tumour becomes necrotic. Lateral invasion into the parametrium may involve the ureters, leading eventually to ureteric obstruction and renal failure. Invasion of nerves and bone produces excruciating and persistent pain, and involvement of lymphatic channels may result in lymphatic occlusion with intractable oedema of the lower limbs.

The tumour may also spread anteriorly or posteriorly to involve the bladder or rectum, respectively. Involvement of the bladder produces symptoms of frequency, dysuria and haematuria; if the bowel is involved, tenesmus, diarrhoea and rectal bleeding may occur. The neoplasm may initially grow within the endocervix, producing a cylindrical, barrel-shaped enlargement of the cervix with little external manifestation of the tumour.

The exophytic tumour grows over the vaginal portion of the cervix and appears as a cauliflower-like tumour. The tumour eventually sloughs and replaces the normal cervical tissue and extends on to the vaginal walls.

Death occurs from uraemia following bilateral ureteric obstruction or from sepsis and haemorrhage with generalized cachexia and wasting.

Cervical cancer

- More common in lower social class, smokers, early first intercourse and multiple partners
- Associated with herpes and human papilloma virus infection
- May be asymptomatic or present with vaginal bleeding, pain, and bowel or bladder symptoms
- Spreads by local invasion and iliac/obturator nodes
- Treatment is radical hysterectomy for early stage disease, radiotherapy otherwise
- 5 year survival varies from 10 to 90% depending on stage

Investigation

The diagnosis is established histologically by biopsy of the tumour. Careful evaluation and staging should be completed by vaginal and rectal examination and by cystoscopy, proctoscopy, intravenous urography, and lung and skeletal radiography.

Treatment of invasive carcinomas

Treatment is by surgery or radiotherapy or a combination of both methods. *Local excision* carried out by

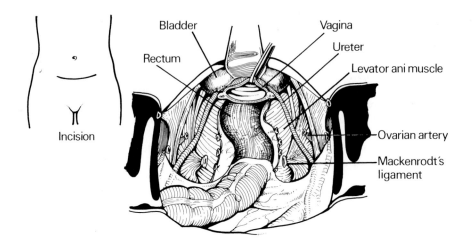

Fig. 27.6 Wertheim's hysterectomy involves block dissection of the pelvic lymph nodes and excision of the uterus, tubes, ovaries and upper third of the vagina.

cone biopsy is an option for patients with stage IA lesions who wish to preserve fertility.

Radical hysterectomy and pelvic lymph node dissection – Radical hysterectomy (Wertheim's hysterectomy) includes removal of the uterus, upper third of the vagina, internal and external iliac and obturator lymph nodes (Fig. 27.6). The ovaries may be conserved. This method of treatment is appropriate for patients with stage I disease. Complications include haemorrhage, infection, pelvic haematomas and damage to the ureters or bladder which may result in fistula formation in 2–5% of cases. However, the incidence of vaginal stenosis is less than that after radiotherapy so coital function is better preserved, making it the treatment of choice in the younger woman.

Radiotherapy – This is to treat other stages of cervical cancer and those patients with bulky stage Ib disease or who are unfit for surgery. Survival stage for stage is similar to that for surgery. Adjuvant radiotherapy is also used for those patients who have been found to have lymph node involvement at the time of surgery.

Radiotherapy is administered by local insertion of a source of radium, caesium or cobalt-60 into the uterine cavity and the vaginal vault and external beam radiation to the pelvic side wall. Complications include the effects of excessive radiation on normal tissues, and may lead to radiation cystitis, proctitis as well as fistula formation and vaginal stenosis.

Results of treatment – The results for 5 year survival in cancer of the cervix vary from centre to centre, but in good radiotherapy centres one can expect figures of:

Stage I	85%
Stage II	60%
Stage III	30%
Stage IV	10%

The comparable survival figure for stage Ib using radical surgery is 90%.

A combination of limited radiation and subsequent radical surgery after 4–6 weeks has produced similar figures, with a 5 year survival in stage I disease of 77% and in stage IIa of 69%.

Recurrent cervical lesions exhibit a poor response to chemotherapy.

Where local recurrence involves the bladder or rectum, but does not extend to other structures, curative excision may occasionally be achieved by radical excision or exenteration including total cystectomy and removal of the rectum.

Vaginal and cervical clear-cell adenocarcinoma

These tumours have been described in relation to DES exposure, and occur on both the vagina and the cervix. They are found in young females born to women who received diethylstilboestrol during pregnancy. The tumours respond to radiation or radical surgery, and there is an overall 5 year survival rate of 70%. The tumour is commonly preceeded by vaginal adenosis. The condition is rare in the UK.

BIBLIOGRAPHY

Coppleson M 1992 Gynecologic oncology, 2nd edn.
    Churchill Livingstone, Edinburgh, vol 1
Jordan J A, Singer A 1976 The cervix. W B Saunders,
    London
Soutter W P 1992 Premalignant disease of the lower genital
    tract. In: Shaw, Soutter, Stanton (eds) Gynaecology.
    Churchill Livingstone, Edinburgh, ch 34

28 Lesions of the uterus and Fallopian tubes

This chapter relates to conditions of the body of the uterus and excludes lesions of the uterine cervix. Some disorders of function have been described in Chapter 22.

CONGENITAL ANOMALIES

The formation of the uterus results from the fusion of the two Müllerian ducts; this fusion gives rise to the upper two-thirds of the vagina, the cervix and the body of the uterus. Congenital anomalies arise from the failure of fusion or absence or partial development of one or both ducts. Thus, the anomalies may range from a minor indentation of the uterine fundus to a full separation of each uterine horn and cervix. These conditions are also commonly associated with vaginal septa.

Symptoms and signs

The majority of uterine anomalies are asymptomatic but are usually diagnosed in relation to complications of pregnancy. However, the presence of a vaginal septum may result in dyspareunia and postcoital bleeding.

The presence of a double uterus may also be established at routine vaginal examination when a double cervix may be seen. The separation of the uterine horns is sometimes palpable on bimanual vaginal examination, but in most cases the uterus feels normal and there is a single cervix. The uterus may be palpable as lying obliquely in the pelvis when only one horn of the uterus is present. The abnormality of the uterine horns and one cervix is known as **uterus bicornis unicollis** (Fig. 28.1).

Partial atresia of one horn of the uterus, or a septate vagina resulting in obstruction to menstrual outflow from one horn of the uterus, may result in a unilateral haematocolpos and haematometra with retrograde spill of menstrual fluid. In this case, the patient may present with symptoms of dysmenorrhoea and will have a palpable mass arising from the pelvis.

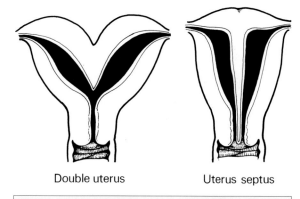

Double uterus   Uterus septus

Fig. 28.1 Common congenital abnormalities of the uterus include uterus bicornis unicollis (double uterus, one cervix) (left) and the subseptate uterus (uterus septus) (right).

The complications of pregnancy include:

1. Recurrent abortions of increasing gestational age – this problem is usually associated with the subseptate uterus and is not common in the unicornuate uterus or in uterus bicornis bicollis
2. Premature labour
3. Malpresentation (Fig. 28.2)
4. Retained placenta (Fig. 28.3).

Diagnosis and management

As many cases are asymptomatic, the diagnosis may arise only as a coincidental finding and requires no treatment or intervention. If there is a history of two or more consecutive abortions, then active surgical intervention is indicated.

Where the diagnosis is suggested by the history, further investigation should include hysterography and hysteroscopy.

Surgical treatment

Surgical reconstruction of a double uterus should be confined to women who have experienced two or

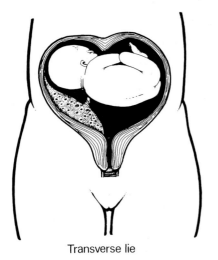

Transverse lie

Fig. 28.2 Malpresentation and a subseptate uterus.

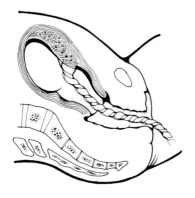

Retained placenta

Fig. 28.3 Retention of the placenta as a feature of congenital abnormalities of the uterus.

more consecutive abortions and where the abnormality is one of uterus bicornis unicollis, or there is an uterine septum.

The operation of plastic reconstruction of the uterus with unification of two uterine horns or excision of the uterine septum is known as **metroplasty** (Fig. 28.4).

An incision is made across the fundus of the uterus between the utero-tubal junctions, but taking care not to involve the intramural portion of the tube. The cavities are then reunited by suturing the surfaces together in the antero-posterior plane. If there is a septum, it is simply divided by diathermy and the cavity is then closed by suturing the transverse incision in the antero-posterior plane.

An alternative surgical management is to divide the septum by diathermy through a hysteroscope inserted through the cervix. Before undertaking a surgical procedure for the treatment of any uterine anomaly, it is essential to perform an intravenous pyelogram, as there is a high incidence of congenital urinary tract abnormalities in these cases, including ureteric reduplication and unilateral renal agenesis.

Abnormalities of uterine position

The uterus normally rests in an anteverted position, but in some 10% of the female population the uterus is retroverted. In some women, this is associated with first-degree descent of the cervix; in other words, it represents an early phase of uterine prolapse. If the uterus is retroverted and mobile, it is of no significance, and represents a variant of normal. However, if the uterus is fixed in retroversion, the condition is often associated with significant pelvic disease such as endometriosis or chronic pelvic inflammatory disease.

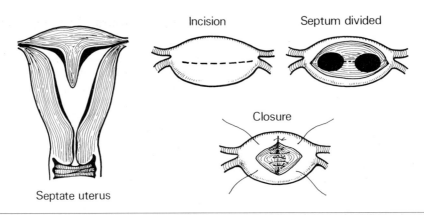

Incision   Septum divided

Closure

Septate uterus

Fig. 28.4 Metroplasty (right) for the reunification of a bicornate uterus or the division of a uterine septum (left).

Management

Where the condition is asymptomatic, no treatment is indicated. If it is associated with deep-seated dyspareunia or sacral backache, then the uterus can be fixed in anteversion by a surgical procedure known as ventro-suspension, which involves shortening the round ligaments by plication. It is advisable to test the relationship between the retroversion and the symptoms by first correcting the retroversion with a Hodge pessary before proceeding to surgical treatment. If correction of the position does not improve the symptoms, then it is unlikely that relief will be obtained from surgical procedures unless there is specific pathology which holds the uterus in fixed retroversion.

Congenital abnormalities of the uterus

- Due to failure of Müllerian ducts to fuse or develop
- Usually asymptomatic unless menstrual flow obstructed
- May cause recurrent abortion, malpresentation or retained placenta
- May be associated with abnormalities of the renal tract

BENIGN TUMOURS OF THE UTERUS

Endometrial polyps

The commonest benign tumours of the endometrium are endometrial polyps (Fig. 28.5). These occur at any age, but are found most frequently in the premenopausal decade.

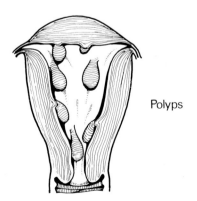

Polyps

Fig. 28.5 Multiple endometrial polyps may be a cause of profuse and irregular bleeding.

Symptoms

Irregular bleeding and menorrhagia result from necrosis of the surface of the polyp and interference with normal endometrial shedding. Occasionally, protrusion of the polyp through the cervix may result in postcoital bleeding. Attempts by the uterus to expel the polyp may cause colicky, dysmenorrhoeic pain.

Signs

The diagnosis must be anticipated on the history, because it is unusual to be able to establish a diagnosis on the basis of the physical signs. If the polyp protrudes through the cervix, it has a bright red appearance, but is difficult to distinguish from an endocervical polyp.

Pathology

Endometrial polyps consist of a fine fibrous tissue core covered by columnar epithelium. They may be covered by functional endometrium that responds to ovarian steroids or by immature endometrium that exhibits no progesterone response even when the surrounding endometrium is in the phase of marked secretory activity. Occasionally, malignant change occurs in endometrial polyps, but there is no increase in such incidence over that seen in normal endometrium.

Treatment

These tumours are usually diagnosed at uterine curettage, and are commonly cured by cervical dilatation and uterine curettage.

Benign tumours of the myometrium

It is estimated that some 20% of women over the age of 30 years have uterine myomas or 'fibroids'. These tumours are derived from smooth muscle tissue and vary enormously in size from microscopic growths to tumours that may weigh as much as 30–40 kg. They may be single or multiple, and may occur in the cervix or in the body of the uterus. The site of the tumour has a considerable effect on the symptoms. Subserosal fibroids may become pedunculated, and submucous fibroids may project into the cavity of the uterus and form a fibroid polyp (Fig. 28.6). Interstitial or intramural growths may result in uniform enlargement of the uterus but can also cause irregular or nodular distention. Large

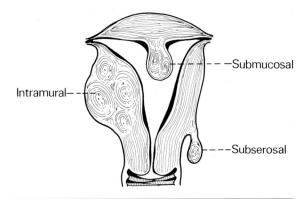

Intramural

Submucosal

Subserosal

Fig. 28.6 Uterine fibroids produce symptoms which are determined by the site of the fibroids.

subserosal tumours frequently become adherent to the omentum and eventually derive an additional blood supply. The tumour may then become separated from the uterus and form a **parasitic** or **wandering fibroid**.

The aetiology of fibroids is not known, but some 25–35% of women with myomas are sterile, and the tumours occur more frequently in black than in white women. Pregnancy causes enlargement, and the menopause is associated with involution.

Histopathology

Myomas consist of whorled masses of unstriped muscle cells. There is always some admixture of connective tissue, but the true nature of myomas is that of a smooth muscle benign tumour.

Pathological changes

Secondary changes may occur in fibroids. These changes include:

1. *Hyaline degeneration* – a common finding in most fibroids. Scattered islands of muscle cells are found intact in broad expanses of hyaline degeneration.
2. *Cystic degeneration* – this is an extension of hyaline degeneration with liquefaction of some areas of the fibroid and cyst formation.
3. *Calcification* – this provides evidence of degeneration and is associated with circulatory impairment. It is therefore commonly seen in fibroids after the menopause; in its most extreme form the fibroid is converted into a stony mass.
4. *Infection and abscess formation* – these are rare complications which are particularly likely to affect

submucous fibroids following septic abortions or occasionally following tumours, particularly if radiotherapy is used.
5. *Necrobiosis* – impairment of blood supply is particularly likely to occur in pedunculated subserous fibroids, but there are special forms of necrosis such as red degeneration, which is seen in pregnancy. The cut surface of the tumour has a dull reddish hue and the appearance is associated with aseptic degeneration and local haemolysis.
6. *Sarcomatous change* – the incidence of malignant change in fibroids has been variably reported to be between 0.13 and 1%.

Symptoms and signs

Fifty per cent of women with fibroids are asymptomatic and may be discovered during routine pelvic examination – either at the time of cervical cytology or in the management of a pregnancy.

Where symptoms do occur, they are often related to the site of the fibroids. The common presenting symptoms are:

1. *Menstrual disorders* – submucous and intramural fibroids commonly cause menorrhagia. They do not influence the length of the menstrual cycle. Submucous fibroids may cause irregular vaginal bleeding particularly if the surface of the fibroid becomes necrotic or ulcerated, or if endometrial carcinoma is also present.
2. *Pain* – colicky uterine pain may occur with pedunculated fibroids as the uterus attempts to expel them. Pain may also occur during pregnancy if red degeneration occurs or if torsion of a subserous fibroid results in necrosis of the tumour. The pain will be persistent until necrosis is complete.
3. *Pressure symptoms* – a large mass of fibroids may become apparent because of palpable enlargement of the abdomen or because of pressure on the bladder or rectum.
4. *Complications of pregnancy* – submucous fibroids interfere with nidation and therefore cause recurrent abortion.
5. *Infertility* – fibroids are found in 3% of women with infertility, and up to 30% of women with uterine fibroids will have difficulty in conceiving. The mechanism may be mediated by both mechanical and hormonal effects.

The diagnosis may be confirmed by ultrasound scans of the pelvis or by radiological diagnosis if the fibroid is calcified.

Management

Small uterine fibroids are a common finding in asymptomatic women, but if they exceed 10 cm in size the tumour should be removed because of the difficulty of excluding the diagnosis of an ovarian tumour. Progestogens and non-steroidal anti-inflammatory drugs have no effect on the size of fibroids, but may be of value in controlling menstrual loss. A reduction of up to 50% in size can be achieved using gonadotrophin-releasing hormone analogues. However, the long-term usage of these drugs is limited by their effect on bone density. They may be of value in reducing the size and vascularity of fibroids prior to myomectomy. Where the preservation of reproductive function is not important, the surgical treatment of choice is by hysterectomy. In younger women or where the preservation of reproductive function is important, the removal of the fibroids by surgical excision or myomectomy is indicated. This procedure involves incision of the pseudocapsule of the fibroid, enucleation of the bulk of the tumour and closure of the cavity by interrupted absorbable sutures. Myomectomy is associated with greater morbidity than hysterectomy because of the occurrence of haematoma formation in the cavity of the excised fibroid and also because of infection. It is also impossible to be certain that all fibroids are removed without causing excessive uterine damage; there is always a possibility that residual seedling fibroids may grow and lead to recurrence of the fibroids.

Endoscopic resection of some submucous or subserous fibroids can be performed using the hysteroscope or laparoscope respectively. This is associated with a lower morbidity and a recurrence rate comparable to the open procedure.

Benign uterine tumours

- Commonest are endometrial polyps and fibroids
- 20% of women over 30 years old have fibroids
- Symptoms depend on size and site and include menstrual disorders, pressure symptoms and complications of pregnancy
- May undergo secondary change including necrosis or malignant change (0.13–1%)
- Management depends on size and need to preserve reproductive function

---

MALIGNANT DISEASE OF THE UTERUS

Endometrial carcinoma

Adenocarcinoma of the endometrium is a common gynaecological tumour with an annual incidence of 13 per 100 000 women in the UK which presents after the menopause in two-thirds of all cases. Cancer of the body of the uterus is the predominant genital tract malignancy in women over the age of 50 years. The peak age of incidence occurs at the age of 61 years, and the disease is rare below the age of 35 years.

There are specific risk factors associated with an increased incidence of corpus carcinoma (Fig. 28.7):

1. *Obesity* – This is a strong risk factor; approximately half of the women who develop endometrial carcinoma are grossly overweight.
2. *Parity* – The incidence of corpus carcinoma is twice as high in nulliparous women.
3. *Late menopause* – The incidence is significantly increased in women who have a menopause after the age of 50 years.

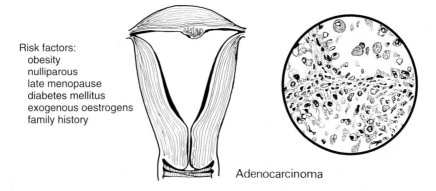

Risk factors:
  obesity
  nulliparous
  late menopause
  diabetes mellitus
  exogenous oestrogens
  family history

Adenocarcinoma

Fig. 28.7 Endometrial adenocarcinoma: there are a number of risk factors associated with it (left); histological features (right).

4. *Diabetes mellitus* – Abnormalities of glucose tolerance are associated with a twofold increase in the incidence of endometrial carcinoma and there is also an increased incidence of hypertensive disease, although this is probably a secondary association.
5. *Exogenous oestrogens* – Unopposed oestrogen action, particularly as used for hormone replacement therapy in the menopause, is associated with an increased incidence of endometrial carcinoma. The addition of a progestogen for 7 days of each month can reduce this risk, and the combined OCP reduces the incidence of the disease.
6. *Family history* – First-degree relatives have an increased risk of endometrial carcinoma, and there may be an increased risk in families with a strong history of breast and gut adenocarcinomas. Rarely, an autosomal dominant pattern of inheritance can be identified similar to that seen in some breast and ovarian cancer families.
7. *Endometrial hyperplasia* – Prolonged stimulation of the endometrium with unopposed oestrogen may lead to hyperplasia of the endometrium with periods of amenorrhoea followed by heavy or irregular bleeding. If this is associated with cellular atypia, there is a 20–30% risk of an eventual progression to endometrial carcinoma.

Symptoms

The commonest symptom is postmenopausal bleeding. However, in the premenopausal woman, endometrial carcinoma is associated with irregular vaginal bleeding and menorrhagia. A serous blood-stained and offensive discharge may also accompany the history of abnormal bleeding.

Pathology

Adenocarcinoma of the endometrium may occur in a diffuse form and cover the whole surface of the endometrium, or it may be circumscribed in the form of a localized polypoid growth. The microscopic appearances include changes in the architecture with the development of closely packed polyhedral cells with dark-staining nuclei and considerable numbers of mitoses. In many tumours, the cells may retain their normal characteristics. The stromal cells almost always show marked reactive inflammatory infiltration with round cells and leucocytes. The virulence of the tumour is related to the degree of histological dedifferentiation. Endometrial cancer grows locally for a long period of time and expands the uterus. The tumour spreads by direct invasion into the myometrium and then transcervically, transtubally and by spillage of carcinomatous material. Lymphatic spread is the primary method of extrauterine extension and involves the external and internal iliac nodes and the aortic nodes. In lesions involving the fundus of the uterus, spread may occur along the lymphatics of the round ligament and metastasize to the superficial or deep inguinal nodes.

The most common histological pattern is endometrioid. Clear cell serous and mixed patterns are found less commonly with serous papillary lesions having a poor prognosis irrespective of stage or differentiation.

Staging

The FIGO classification of endometrial carcinoma takes into account the distribution of the tumour and the depth of penetration of the myometrium and histological grading (Fig. 28.8).

Stage I Carcinoma confined to the corpus:
Stage IA – superficial
Stage IB – penetrating less than half the depth of the myometrium
Stage IC – penetrating into the outer half of the myometrium but not breaching the serosal surface.

Stage Ⅰ   Ⅱ   Ⅲ   Ⅳ

Fig. 28.8 Staging of carcinoma of the body of the uterus.

Stage II The carcinoma involves the cervix but does not extend outside the uterus:
Stage IIA – involving glands only
Stage IIB – involving the cervical stroma.

Stage III The tumour has extended outside the uterus but not the pelvis:
Stage IIIA – positive cytology
Stage IIIB – vaginal metastases
Stage IIIC – abdominal nodes involved.

Stage IV The tumour extends beyond the pelvis:
Stage IVA – spread to bladder and rectum
Stage IVB – spread to distant organs or inguinal nodes.

The tumours are further grouped according to the degree of differentiation:

G1 – Highly differentiated
G2 – Differentiated with solid areas
G3 – Solid or undifferentiated adenocarcinoma.

Diagnosis

The diagnosis of the tumour is established by endometrial biopsy. This should be accompanied by hysteroscopy to identify focal abnormalities that might otherwise be missed by blind curettage. This can be carried out as an out-patient procedure or under general anaesthesia. Where ultrasound assessment of endometrial thickness is less than 3 mm a significant endometrial lesion is unlikely. Invasion of carcinoma into the rectum or bladder can be recognized by cystoscopy and proctoscopy. The most accurate method of determining the depth of invasion of an endometrial carcinoma is by magnetic resonance imaging where the tumour can be clearly seen to breach the non-resonant subendometrial layer.

Treatment

Stage IA and IB G1 tumours with low-risk histology can be treated surgically by total hysterectomy and bilateral salpingo-oophorectomy. For other stage I lesions, hysterectomy should be followed by adjuvant external beam and vault radiotherapy 6–8 weeks later. Stage II lesions with microscopic disease can be treated in the same way, but patients with macroscopic disease should have an extended hysterectomy with aortic and pelvic lymph node sampling and adjuvant radiotherapy. Stage III tumours are treated by debulking the tumour followed by radiotherapy. Stage IV tumours are treated with irradiation and progestational agents such as medroxyprogesterone and megestrol acetate or, in some cases, chemotherapy.

Prognosis

Seventy per cent of recurrences occur within 3 years. Adverse prognostic factors include old age, node involvement, poor differentiation, positive cytology and serous or clear-cell tumours.

Sarcoma of the uterus

These tumours, arising from the stroma of the endometrium, account for 3% of uterine tumours. They usually present between the ages of 45 and 50 years with vaginal discharge and bleeding and are more common in Blacks.

Pathology

Endometrioid stromal sarcoma is found in association with adenomyosis and endometriosis. It can be classified as low or high grade, depending on the number of mitotic figures and similarity to the non-glandular elements of the endometrium. Sarcomas contain elements of both epithelium and stroma. The epithelial elements are usually endometrioid but can be squamous or a mixture. The stromal elements are either heterologous (chondroblastoma, osteosarcoma, fibrosarcoma) or homologous (leiomyosarcoma, presarcoma).

Treatment

This is by hysterectomy with removal of as much macroscopic disease as possible followed by radiotherapy. Prognosis for low-grade stromal sarcomas is similar to that for endometrioid tumours, but poor for others with a 20–30% 5 years survival.

Leiomyosarcoma

These smooth muscle tumours arise in the myometrium of the uterus. They are uncommon (0.7/1000 000) with a peak incidence 10 years later than that for fibroids. From 5 to 10% arise in existing fibroids, and they are classified according to the degree of differentiation. They may present with pain, postmenopausal bleeding or a rapidly growing 'fibroid' but are often asymptomatic and diagnosed following hysterectomy for fibroids. Treatment is by hysterectomy and bilateral salpingo-oophorectomy. Adjuvant radiotherapy and chemotherapy reduces the risk of local recurrence, but does not improve long-term survival.

Case study
Leiomyosarcoma in a young woman

A 26-year-old woman presented for investigation of subfertility and was found to have a 3 cm diameter fibroid arising from the posterior surface of her uterus. This was not considered to be the cause of her difficulties in conceiving, and shortly after laparoscopy she conceived. The pregnancy was uneventful except that she developed episodes of abdominal pain, and the fibroid showed rapid growth and enlarged to fill the pouch of Douglas. Because of the obstruction caused by the fibroid which had enlarged to a diameter of 10 cm, it was necessary to delivery the child by Caesarean section. In the 6 weeks after delivery, the patient continued to complain of pain and, unexpectedly, the fibroid did not regress. Ten weeks after delivery, a myomectomy was performed with a difficult removal of an adherent, necrotic fibroid in the pouch of Douglas. Histology showed numerous mitotic figures with a highly malignant leiomyosarcoma and, despite a further laparotomy, radiotherapy and chemotherapy, the woman died from widespread metastatic disease 8 weeks later. This was a very rare event but demonstrates the rapid blood-borne metastatic disease associated with this type of sarcoma, which has an exceedingly poor prognosis.

Endometrial carcinoma

- Disease of postmenopausal women
- Risk factors include obesity, nulliparity, late menopause, glucose intolerance and unopposed oestrogens
- Commonly presents as postmenopausal bleeding
- Spreads by direct invasion but tends to remain localized within the uterus initially
- Well-differentiated early stage disease can be treated by hysterectomy alone; more advanced lesions require radiotherapy ± progestational agents
- Has 90% 5 year survival if diagnosed early

TUMOURS OF THE FALLOPIAN TUBES

Primary Fallopian tube cancers are extremely rare, accounting for 0.16–1% of all gynaecological malignancies. The mean age at diagnosis is 52 years, with a range of 18–80 years. The symptoms include abnormal vaginal bleeding and a canary-yellow discharge. Tubal cancers are predominantly adenocarcinomas, which are histologically similar to epithelial ovarian tumours and are best treated by radiotherapy. In fact, most of these tumours are first diagnosed at the time of laparotomy and are therefore surgically excised with subsequent treatment with radiotherapy.

SALPINGITIS ISTHMICA NODOSA

This is a special form of chronic salpingitis, and generally represents the residue of chronic interstitial salpingitis.

The condition is characterized by the presence of one or more nodules in the isthmic portion of the tube. These nodules are usually small but may expand to a size of 2 cm.

Treatment of this rare condition is by excision of the Fallopian tubes. Once again, this diagnosis is usually established as a coincidental finding at laparotomy.

BIBLIOGRAPHY

Coppleson M 1992 Gynecologic oncology, 2nd edn. Churchill Livingstone, Edinburgh, vol 2
Wyann R M 1977 Biology of the uterus. Plenum Press, New York

29 Lesions of the ovary

Ovarian enlargement is commonly asymptomatic, and the silent nature of malignant ovarian tumours is the major reason for the advanced stage of presentation. Ovarian tumours may be cystic or solid, functional, benign or malignant. There are common factors in the presentation and complications of ovarian tumours and it is often difficult to establish the nature of a tumour without direct examination.

Symptoms

Tumours of the ovary that are less than 10 cm in diameter rarely produce symptoms. The common presenting symptoms include:

1. Abdominal enlargement: in the presence of malignant change, this may also be associated with ascites (Fig. 29.1).
2. Symptoms from pressure on surrounding structures such as the bladder and rectum.
3. Symptoms relating to complications of the tumour (Fig. 29.1). These include:

a. **Torsion** – acute torsion of the ovarian pedicle results in necrosis of the tumour. There is acute pain and vomiting followed by remission of the pain when the tumour has become necrotic.
b. **Rupture** – the contents of the cyst spill into the peritoneal cavity and result in generalized abdominal pain.
c. **Haemorrhage** – haemorrhage into the tumour is an unusual complication but may result in abdominal pain and shock if the blood loss is severe.
d. **Hormone-secreting tumours** – these may present with disturbances in the menstrual cycle. In androgen-secreting tumours the patient may present with signs of virilization.

Signs

On examination, the abdomen may be visibly enlarged. Percussion over the swelling will demonstrate central dullness and resonance in the flanks. These signs may be obscured by gross ascites. Small

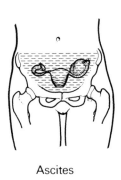

Ascites

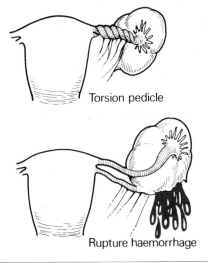

Torsion pedicle

Rupture haemorrhage

Fig. 29.1 Common complications of ovarian tumours which precipitate a request for medical advice.

tumours can be detected on pelvic examination and will be found by palpation in one or both fornices. However, as the tumour enlarges, it assumes a more central position and, in the case of dermoid cysts, will often be anterior to the uterus. Most ovarian tumours are not tender to palpation; if they are painful the presence of infection or torsion should be suspected. Benign ovarian tumours are palpable separately from the uterine body and are usually freely mobile.

FUNCTIONAL CYSTS OF THE OVARY

These cysts occur only during menstrual life and rarely exceed more than 6 cm in diameter.

Follicular cysts

These form the commonest functional cysts in the ovary and may be multiple and bilateral (Fig. 29.2). The cysts rarely exceed 4 cm in diameter, the walls consisting of layers of granulosa cells and the contents of clear fluid, which is rich in sex steroids. These cysts commonly occur during treatment with clomiphene or pergonal. They may produce prolonged unopposed oestrogen effects on the endometrium, resulting in cystic glandular hyperplasia of the endometrium. Multiple follicular cysts commonly arise from ovarian hyperstimulation.

Management

These cysts regress spontaneously, but if they have not involuted after 60 days then the diagnosis should be revised. The size and growth of the cysts can be monitored by ultrasound scans.

The prolonged and heavy menstrual loss caused by unopposed oestrogen action can be offset by the administration of a progestogen for 1 week followed by 'medical curettage', or through surgical intervention by cervical dilatation and uterine curettage.

Lutein cysts

There are two types of luteinized ovarian cysts (Fig. 29.3):

1. *Granulosa lutein cysts* – functional cysts of the corpus luteum may be 4–6 cm in diameter and occur in the second half of the menstrual cycle. Persistent production of progesterone may result in amenorrhoea or delayed onset of menstruation. These cysts often give rise to pain, and they therefore present a problem in terms of differential diagnosis as the history and examination findings mimic tubal ectopic pregnancy. Occasionally, haemorrhage occurs into the cyst, which may rupture and lead to a haemoperitoneum The cysts usually regress spontaneously and require surgical intervention only when they give rise to symptoms of intra-abdominal haemorrhage.

2. *Theca lutein cysts* – these commonly arise in association with high levels of chorionic gonadotrophin and are therefore seen in cases of hydatidiform mole. The cysts may be bilateral and, on occasion, will give rise to haemorrhage if they rupture. Once the cysts have been formed, they can be detected by ultrasound scans. They usually undergo spontaneous involution, but surgical intervention may be necessary if there is significant haemorrhage from the ovaries.

Polycystic ovary syndrome

Polycystic ovary syndrome (PCOS) (Table 29.1) is associated with the **Stein–Leventhal syndrome** in

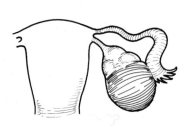
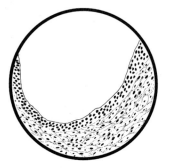

Fig. 29.2 Follicular cysts are common and are generally associated with menstrual irregularity (left); histological features (right).

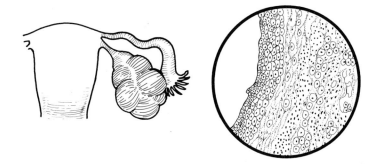

Fig. 29.3 Lutein cysts are a less common variant of functional ovarian cysts; regression is usually spontaneous (left); histological features (right).

which multiple cysts occur in the ovaries and are associated with hirsutism, oligomenorrhoea or amenorrhoea, subfertility and changes in body habitus with obesity (Fig. 29.4). The ovaries are clinically enlarged and are palpable vaginally.

On direct inspection, the ovaries have smooth, white surfaces. There is sometimes luteinization of the theca interna cells and focal stromal luteinization.

Biochemical investigations (Fig. 29.5) indicate abnormally raised luteinizing hormone (LH) levels and absence of the LH surge. Oestrogen and follicle-stimulating hormone (FSH) levels are normal, and as a result there is an increase in the LH:FSH ratio. There may be increased secretion of testosterone and of Δ^4-andronstenedione and dehydroepiandrosterone.

Pathogenesis

Although the cause of PCOS remains obscure, the underlying disorder in androgen biosynthesis may be a central event — exposure of small antral follicles to excessive androgen stimulation. Inappropriate exposure of antral follicles to excessive concentrations of androgens results in inhibition of FSH release and may result in polycystic changes in the ovaries. The primary sources of androgen may be from the ovary or from the adrenals. The excretion of dehydroepiandrosterone – an exclusive adrenal

steroid – is elevated in up to 50% of all women with PCOS. The principal androgens raised in PCOS in the ovary include testosterone and androstenedione, and the production will not be suppressed by adrenal steroids but can be suppressed by gonadotrophin-releasing hormone agonists. It has also been suggested that primary deregulation of the enzyme cytochrome P450c17α, which converts progesterone to 17α-hydroxyprogesterone, may form the basis of the disease. Insulin and insulin-like growth factor significantly increases the production of testosterone and androstenedione from ovarian theca cells. Twenty per cent of women with PCOS develop non-insulin-dependent diabetes by the age of 30 years.

Diagnosis

The diagnosis of PCOS is based on ultrasound scan of the ovaries using a vaginal probe and a hormone profile including measurement of FSH/LH, testosterone and androstenedione.

Treatment

Treatment depends on the underlying problem. If the problem is primarily one of subfertility, then clomiphene citrate or human menopausal gonadotrophin can be used to stimulate ovulation. Prolonged unopposed oestrogen action may result in the development of hyperplastic endometrium, which may undergo malignant change. If this occurs, the tumour will often regress following the administration of a progestational agent such as medroxy-progesterone acetate or megestrol acetate.

Weight reduction needs to be emphasized where there is a problem with obesity, as there is evidence to show that weight reduction alone can improve the menstrual pattern, endocrine profile and fertility. Hirsutism can be treated by the use of depilatory aids and electrolysis, but the presence of hirsutism,

Table 29.1 Features of polycystic ovary syndrome		
Oligomenorrhoea/amenorrhoea	}	Abnormal androgen production
Hirsutism/acne		
Obesity		
Infertility		
Ultrasound – ovaries		Size > 8 cm
		8 ovarian cysts
		< 8 mm diameter
		Echogenic ovarian stroma

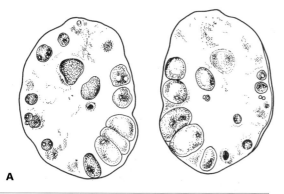

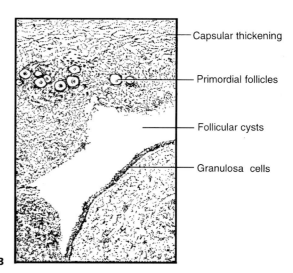

- Capsular thickening
- Primordial follicles
- Follicular cysts
- Granulosa cells

Fig. 29.4 Polycystic ovaries: **A** the capsule of the ovary is thickened and there are numerous small cysts in the ovarian cortex; **B** ovarian section.

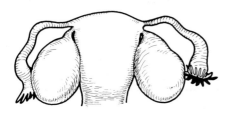

LH ↑
LH surge absent
Δ⁴ - Androstenedione ↑
Dehydroepiandrosterone ↑
Normal oestradiol levels
Normal FSH levels

Fig. 29.5 Biochemical features of the Stein–Leventhal syndrome.

acne and alopecia may also respond to antiandrogens such as cyproterone acetate combined with an oestrogen such as ethinyloestradiol given on a cyclical basis. Surgical management of PCOS includes resection of a wedge of ovarian tissue or drilling of the ovary with laparoscopic needle point diathermy or laser puncture of the ovarian surface.

Functional ovarian cysts

- Usually <6 cm size
- May arise from follicles, corpus luteum or as a result of exogenous gonadotrophins
- Can produce sex steroids and affect menstruation
- Can be monitored by ultrasound
- Usually regress spontaneously
- Require surgical intervention if the source of significant IP bleeding

---

These procedures appear to restore normal ovarian function, although the mechanism remains unclear.

BENIGN NEOPLASTIC LESIONS

These tumours may be cystic or solid and arise from specific cell lines in the ovary. The full World Health Organization classification of ovarian tumours illustrates the complexity of tumours arising from the ovary; only the commoner ones will be discussed in this section.

Epithelial tumours

Serous cystadenomas

These cysts in conjunction with the mucinous cystadenomas form the commonest group of cystic ovarian tumours. The cysts may be unilocular, lined by a layer of cuboidal epithelium, or multilocular with papillary growths extending from both internal and external surfaces of the tumour (Fig. 29.6). It is often difficult to differentiate between benign and malignant appearances. The wall of the tumour sometimes contains calcified granules known as **psammoma bodies**.

The growths may be bilateral and may be large enough to fill the peritoneal cavity.

Treatment – the tumours often replace all normal ovarian tissue; if this is the case, the whole ovary should be removed. If the tumour is small, it may be possible to perform a local resection and to conserve ovarian tissue. If both ovaries are extensively involved or there is reason to believe that the tumours are malignant, it is bet-

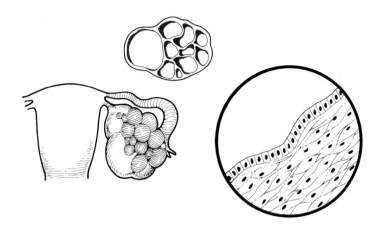

Fig. 29.6 Serous cystadenomas consist of single or multiple cysts lined by cuboidal epithelium and papillary growths extending from both internal and external surfaces of the tumour (left); section through a multiple cyst (top); histological features, showing cuboidal epithelium (right).

ter to perform bilateral oophorectomy and hysterectomy.

Mucinous cystadenomas

These tumours are multilocular and often reach enormous dimensions, with tumours weighing in excess of 100 kg recorded in the literature (Fig. 29.7). The fluid content consists of mucin, and the epithelium lining the cysts presents a characteristic appearance of an epithelium of tall columnar cells with a pseudostratified appearance. This appearance is similar to the epithelium lining the endocervix. The demarcation between epithelial cells and stroma is sharply defined. There is little tendency to form papillae. These tumours are less likely to become malignant than the serous variety.

Management – The only treatment is to remove the tumour surgically. Care should be taken to avoid rupture of the cysts because mucinous epithelium may implant in the peritoneal cavity giving rise to a condition known as **pseudomyxoma peritonei**. Huge amounts of gelatinous material may accumulate in the peritoneal cavity.

Brenner cell tumours

Brenner cell tumours are commonly solid and occur in women after the age of 50 years (Fig. 29.8). They are only rarely malignant. The histological features of these tumours include nests of epithelial cells surrounded by fibromatous connective tissue groundwork.

The cut surface of the tumour is similar to that of an ovarian fibroma apart from a rather yellowish tinge. The tumours are occasionally bilateral and can be safely treated by local excision.

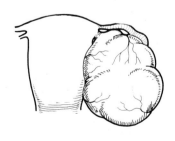
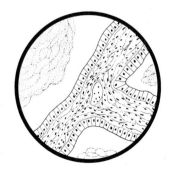

Fig. 29.7 Mucinous cystadenomas are multiocular and often achieve enormous dimensions (left); histological features: the epithelium is columnar and stratified and the contents are mucinous (right).

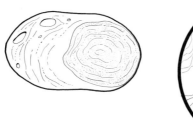
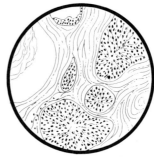

Fig. 29.8 Brenner cell tumours are solid and rarely malignant (left); histological features include nests of epithelial cells surrounded by fibrous connective tissue (right).

Sex cord stromal tumours

Hormone-secreting tumours of the ovary are a small but important group.

Granulosa cell tumours

Arising from ovarian granulosa cells, these tumours produce oestrogens and are the commonest of the hormone-secreting tumours, constituting some 3% of all solid ovarian tumours. Approximately 25% exhibit the characteristics of malignancy. As granulosa cell tumours can present at any age, the symptoms will depend on the age of occurrence. Tumours arising before puberty produce precocious sexual development and, in women of the reproductive age, prolonged oestrogen stimulation results in cystic glandular hyperplasia, and irregular and prolonged vaginal bleeding. Fifty per cent of cases occur after the menopause and present with postmenopausal bleeding. If the tumour is histologically benign, the surgery should be limited to ovariectomy. If there is evidence of malignancy, pelvic clearance is indicated.

Thecomas or **theca cell tumours** arise from the spindle-shaped thecal cells, but are often mixed with granulosa cells and are oestrogen secreting. The presence of a thecoma in one ovary is commonly associated with diffuse thecomatosis in the contra-lateral ovary.

Arrhenoblastomas or androblastomas

These are tumours of Sertoli–Leydig cells. They are rare androgen-secreting tumours that occur most frequently in the decade between 20 and 30 years of age. The clinical manifestations include the onset of amenorrhoea, loss of breast tissue, increasing facial and body hirsutism, deepening of the voice and enlargement of the clitoris. The diagnosis is established by the exclusion of virilizing adrenal tumours and the identification of a tumour in one ovary. The condition is treated by excision of the affected ovary. Approximately 25% of these tumours are malignant.

Germ cell tumours

Tumours of germ cell origin may recapitulate stages resembling the early embryo.

Mature cystic teratoma (dermoid cyst)

Benign cystic teratomas account for 12–15% of true ovarian neoplasms. They are the commonest cystic ovarian neoplasm found in young women, and contain a large number of embryonic elements such as skin, hair, adipose and muscle tissue, bone, teeth

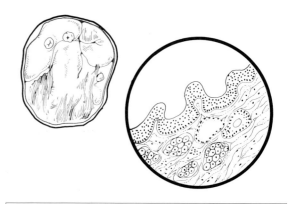

Fig. 29.9 Dermoid cysts are the commonest true ovarian neoplasms in the young female (left); histological features (right).

and cartilage (Fig. 29.9). Some of the components can be recognized on radiography.

These tumours are often chance findings as they are commonly asymptomatic unless they undergo torsion or rupture when the release of sebaceous material causes an acute chemical peritonitis. Dermoid cysts tend to be anterior to the uterus. They are bilateral in 12% of cases, and, although usually benign, become malignant in approximately 2%. Some specialized elements in these tumours become predominant. The growth of thyroid tissue (**struma ovarii**) may induce a state of hyperthyroidism.

Management – these cysts should be excised from the ovary with conservation of ovarian tissue. They are frequently bilateral and it is important to examine both ovaries before proceeding to surgical excision.

Fibromas

These solid tumours of the ovary are rare. They are associated with the presence of ascites or hydrothorax – a condition known as **Meig's syndrome**.

Tumour-like conditions

This group includes **endometriotic cysts**, pregnancy **luteomas** and **germinal cell cysts**. The treatment depends on the nature of the tumour and normally involves simple excision of the cysts.

Endometriotic cysts

Endometriomas contain chocholate-coloured fluid representing the accumulation of altered blood, and have a thick fibrous capsule. The lining may consist of endometrial cells, but in old cysts these may disappear. Management has already been discussed in a previous chapter. The local excision of the endometrium from the ovary should be followed by treatment with a progestogen or Danol for 6 months postoperatively.

Benign ovarian neoplasia

- May be solid, cystic or mixed
- Commonly present as asymptomatic abdominal mass but occasionally by hormone effects or pain
- Mostly serous or mucinous epithelial tumours but germ cell tumours more common in younger patients
- Differential diagnosis include endometriosis, functional cysts and malignant tumours

---

MALIGNANT OVARIAN TUMOURS

Ovarian cancer is the fourth commonest cause of death from malignant disease. It follows breast, large intestine and lung in frequency, and makes up for approximately 5% of all cancer deaths in women. There are approximately 17 per year new cases of ovarian cancer for every 100 000 women in England and Wales (OPCS figures). The 5 year survival figure is approximately 25–30%. The poor survival rate is attributable to late diagnosis and the resistant nature of many of these tumours.

Aetiology

The cause of ovarian cancer is not known, but there are several factors which are associated with the disease. For example, the long-term use of the contraceptive pill reduces the incidence of ovarian cancer. Denmark has the highest age-adjusted death rate for ovarian cancer in the world at 11.12 per 100 000 population, and the lowest rate occurs in Japan at 1.88 per 100 000.

Although the cause of epithelial ovarian cancer remains unknown, there are now several well-defined factors associated with the disease.

Genetic

One per cent of cases of ovarian cancer occur in women whose families show an autosomal dominants pattern of inheritance of ovarian or breast and ovarian cancer. Female members of these families have a 40% lifetime risk of developing the disease. Many of these women have been shown to have defects in the *BRCA1* gene locus on chromosome 17, although the exact nature of the defect varies between different families. Women with only a single affected relative also have a 2–3-fold increased relative risk of getting ovarian cancer.

Parity and fertility

Multiparous women are at 40% less risk than nulliparous women of developing ovarian cancer, whereas women who have had unsuccessful treatment for infertility seem to be at increased risk. The use of the contraceptive pill may produce up to a 60% reduction in the incidence of the disease in long-term pill users.

Symptoms and signs

The symptoms of ovarian cancer are vague and insidious, and as a result 75% of cases present at an advanced stage. There are no signs that this situation is changing, and this seems to be an instance where early diagnosis as a means of improving survival carries little prospect for the future. It is more likely that the future will depend on discovering an effective form of therapy. The common symptoms include:

1. **Abdominal pain** – this varies according to the site of involvement.
2. **Abdominal distension** – enlargement of the abdomen results from the growth of the tumour itself and the presence of associated ascites. The fluid is often blood stained and contains malignant cells shed from the tumour.
3. **Abnormal uterine haemorrhage** – some sex cord tumours produce oestrogens, but hormone production is not confined to these tumours. Cystadenocarcinomas also produce oestrogens and may cause uterine haemorrhage due to the effect of the oestrogen on the endometrium.
4. **Hormonal effects** – some germ cell tumours may contain enough thyroid tissue to cause hyperthyroidism. Sex cord stromal tumours may present with virilization as a result of androgen secretion.

Pathology

Primary ovarian carcinoma

The distribution of histological type of ovarian cancers is as follows:

1. **Epithelial type** – Tumours of this type, such as serous and mucinous cystadenocarcinomas, make up 85% of cases; 15–20% of these cases are of borderline malignancy. All can be papillary solid or exophytic. They are described by their gross morphological features, the proportion of stromal tissue they contain and their degree of differentiation:
   a. *Serous cystadenocarcinoma* – This is the most common histological type of ovarian carcinoma (40%), and is usually unilocular. They may be bilateral. These tumours are more likely to contain solid areas than their benign counterpart.
   b. *Mucinous cystadenocarcinomas* – These multicystic tumours are malignant in 20% of cases. They are characterized by mucin-filled cysts lined by columnar glandular cells, and may be associated with tumours of the appendix and gall bladder. The cysts are commonly multilocular.
   c. *Endometrioid cystadenocarcinomas* – These tumours resemble endometrial adenocarcinomas and are associated with uterine carcinomas in 20% of cases.
   d. *Clear-cell cystadenocarcinoma* – This is the most common ovarian malignancy found in association with ovarian endometriosis. The unilocular thin-walled cysts are lined by epithelium with a typical hobnail appearance and clear cystoplasm.
   e. *Brenner or transitional cell cystadenocarcinoma* – This tumour is often found in association with mucinous tumours, but has a better prognosis than similar tumours arising from the bladder.

Tumours of low malignant or borderline potential account for 10–15% of primary epithelial carcinomas, and occur in any of the histological types already mentioned, but are most commonly associated with mucinous tumours. There are cytological changes of malignancy including cellular atypia with increased mitosis and multilayering but without invasion. They may present as stage III disease, but have a significantly better prognosis than invasive disease with a 5 year survival of greater than 95% for stage I lesions. There is a 10–15% incidence of late recurrence.

2. **Sex cord stromal tumours** – These tumours are relatively rare as they make up only 6% of primary ovarian cancers:
   a. *Granulosa cell tumours* – These solid, unilateral, haemorrhagic tumours are the most common oestrogen secreting lesions, although some epithelial tumours also secrete oestrogens. They are characterized histologically by the presence of Call–Exner bodies.
   b. *Sertoli–Leydig cell tumours* – Approximately 25% of these tumours are malignant, and, as with benign tumours, they may present with signs and symptoms of androgen excess.
3. **Germ cell tumours** –
   a. *Dysgerminomas* – These solid tumours may be small or large enough to fill the abdominal cavity. The cut surface of the tumour has a greyish-pink colour, and the microscopic appearance is characteristic. The tumour consists of large polygonal cells arranged in alveoli or nests separated by septa of fibrous tissue. The 5 year survival rate is only 27%.
   b. *Teratomas* – The malignant or immature form of teratoma is most commonly solid, unilateral and heterogenous with multiple tissue elements. These tumours may produce human chorionic gonadotrophin, α-fetoprotein or thyroxine.

c. *Endodermal sinus or yolk sac tumours* – Although these tumours make up only 10–15% of germ cell tumours, they are the most common germ cell tumour in children. They are solid, encapsulated tumours containing microcysts lined by flat mesothelial cells.

Secondary ovarian carcinomas

The ovaries are a common site for secondary deposits (metastases) from primary sources in the breast, genital tract, gastrointestinal system and haematopoietic system. **Krukenberg's tumours** are metastatic deposits from the gastrointestinal system. They are solid growths that are almost always bilateral and retain the shape of the ovary. The cut surface is variegated in appearance and, although predominantly solid, it often contains areas of cystic degeneration.

The stroma is often richly cellular and may appear to be myomatous. The epithelial elements occur as clusters of well-marked acini with cells exhibiting mucoid change. These cells are often known as **signet cells**. Secondary ovarian tumours may be much larger than the primary lesion, and tumour

deposits in the liver, in particular, suggest primary malignancies in the bowel.

The mechanism by which tumour deposits occur in the ovary is not clear, but there are four possible methods that are likely:

1. Direct implantation of cancer cells on the surface of the ovary after transcoelomic spread from the primary site
2. Lymphatic metastasis
3. Blood-borne spread
4. Extension of tumour by direct spread from contiguous structures.

The same principles apply to the spread of primary ovarian tumours.

Staging of ovarian carcinoma
(Fig. 29.10)

Staging of ovarian carcinoma is important in determining both prognosis and the method of management. Ideally, it should be staged at the time of laparotomy with inspection and biopsy of the peritoneum and diaphragm, cytological examination of any peritoneal fluid and selective sampling of the

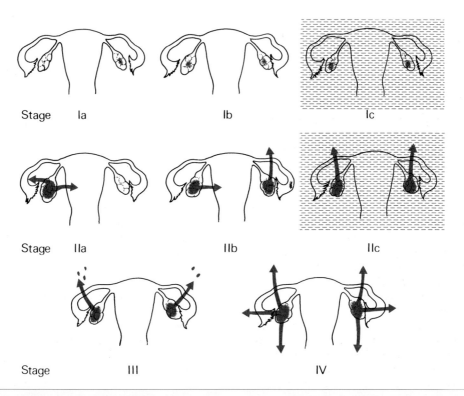

Fig. 29.10 Staging of ovarian carcinoma.

pelvic and paraaortic lymph nodes. Up to 20% of apparently stage I and II lesions will have nodal involvement.

FIGO classification of ovarian carcinoma

Stage I   Growth limited to the ovaries:

Stage IA – growth limited to one ovary, no ascites and no tumour present on the external surface; capsule intact

Stage IB – growth limited to both ovaries, no ascites and no tumour present on the external surface; capsule intact

Stage IC – stage 1A or 1B where there is tumour on the surface of either ovary; or with ruptured capsules or with ascites containing malignant cells or positive peritoneal washings.

Stage II   Growth involving one or both ovaries with pelvic extension:

Stage IIA – extension and/or metastases to the uterus and tubes

Stage IIB – extension to other pelvic tissues

Stage IIC – stage IIA and IIB with tumour on the surface of either ovary or positive peritoneal washings or malignant ascites.

Stage III   Growth involving one or both ovaries with peritoneal implants outside the pelvis or positive retroperitoneal or inguinal lymph nodes:

Stage IIIA – microscopic seeding of abdominal peritoneal surfaces

Stage IIIB – macroscopic disease outside the pelvis less than 2 cm in diameter.

Stage IIIC – abdominal implants greater than 2 cm and/or positive nodes.

Stage IV   Growth involving one or both ovaries with distant metastases including parenchymal (but not superficial) liver metastases and pleural effusions containing malignant cells.

Management

Treatment is based on surgical excision or debulking and chemotherapy.

Stage IA and IB tumours which are well or moderately differentiated can be treated with abdominal hysterectomy, bilateral salpingo-oophorectomy, omentectomy and careful inspection and sampling of peritoneal surfaces and retroperitoneal lymph nodes.

Stage IC, II and poorly differentiated tumours also merit treatment with cytotoxic drugs.

Stage III and IV surgical treatment should aim to remove all macroscopic disease or, failing this, to leave no tumour deposits of greater than 2 cm in diameter. Subsequent prognosis is proportional to the amount of disease remaining after primary surgery, and such optimal debulking should be possible in up to 75% of tumours in experienced hands. Surgery is followed by chemotherapy.

Chemotherapy

This is indicated in all but well or moderately differentiated stage 1A tumours. The platinum-based drugs cisplatin and carboplatin are currently the mainstay of treatment. These are given parenterally at monthly intervals for up to 6 months. The main side effects are marrow suppression, neurotoxicity and renal toxicity (less with carboplatin). The overall response rate is 60–80%, and this is further improved if combined therapy with alkylating agents such as cyclophosphamide is used. Although chemotherapy prolongs median survival and the disease-free interval, it has had little impact on 5 year survival.

Radiotherapy

This can be given as external beam or by intraperitoneal instillation of phosphorus-32 but is less widely used.

Borderline tumours

These can be treated by unilateral oophorectomy in young women wishing to preserve their reproductive capacity, although careful, long-term follow-up is required.

Germ cell tumours

These are more common in young women, and chemotherapy may be curative without hysterectomy.

These patients should, therefore, be referred to specialist gynaecological oncology centres for treatment.

Follow-up and treatment of recurrence

This is carried out by measurement of tumour markers, clinical examination and imaging. Further surgery after chemotherapy (interval debulking) or for recurrence does not appear to improve survival but may be of palliative value. The response to further chemotherapy depends on the interval between original treatment and recurrence. Where this is short, response is poor, although some platinum-resistant tumours will respond to Taxol. In the absence of effective second line treatment, the routine use of second-look staging operations has no value.

Malignant ovarian tumours

- Fourth commonest cause of cancer deaths in women
- Affect 1 in 75 women by the age of 75 years
- Cause unknown.? 'super-ovulation'
- 75% cases present with advanced disease
- Most cases are epithelial in type
- Prognosis depends on stage at diagnosis and extent of residual disease after initial surgery
- 5-year survival 25–30%
- Incidence increases with age
- Shows an autosomal dominant pattern of inheritance in 1% cases

---

Prognosis

The overall 5-year survival is 25–30%, and this figure has remained distressingly constant over recent decades. Five year survival figures depend on the stage and on whether the tumour has or has not been completely removed (Table 29.2).

Table 29.2 Survival, stage and tumour removal (5 year survival, %)

Stage	Incomplete tumour excision	Complete tumour excision
I	–	62
II	15	50
III	8	30
IV	5	–

Table 29.3 Survival rates for stage I tumours

Stage	5 year survival (%)
Stage IA low potential malignancy	95
Stage IA carcinomas	69
Stage IB low potential malignancy	92
Stage IB carcinomas	43
Stage IC carcinomas	40

Case study
Malignant ovarian tumour

A 39-year-old woman with two children attended a gynaecological clinic accompanied by her general practitioner. She had no gynaecological symptoms but requested abdominal hysterectomy and removal of her ovaries on the basis of her family history. She was one of seven sisters, and she produced copies of the death certificates of three of her sisters, all of whom died from ovarian cancer. The request was agreed, and pelvic clearance was performed. The histology of her ovaries was normal. This procedure was performed in the mid-1970s, and whilst this woman was in hospital recovering from her surgery, news came through to the ward that a fourth sister had been admitted to hospital with advanced ovarian cancer, from which she subsequently died. The two remaining sisters were located and offered pelvic clearance. One had a small Brenner cell tumour and subsequently died from bowel carcinoma. The remaining sister, along with the original sister, have both survived.

The impact of eruption of the tumour through the capsule is seen in the difference in survival in the various grades of stage I lesions (Table 29.3).

The only real prospect for survival in ovarian carcinoma is early diagnosis and complete surgical excision.

BIBLIOGRAPHY

Coppleson M 1992 Gynecologic oncology, 2nd edn. Churchill Livingstone, Edinburgh, vol 1

Rajkhowa M, Clayton N 1995 Polycystic ovary syndrome. Mini-symposium: molecular genetics in obstetrics and gynaecology. Current Obstetrics and Gynaecology 5(4): 191–200

30 Disorders of supports of the uterus and vagina

The position of the vagina and uterus depends on various fascial supports and ligaments derived from specific thickening of areas of the fascial support (Fig. 30.1).

The anterior vaginal wall is supported by the pubocervical fascia, which extends from the posterior surface of the pubic symphysis to the cervix and upper vagina. The posterior vaginal wall is supported by the fibrous tissue of the rectovaginal septum and the tonus of the pelvic floor and, in particular, the integrity of the levator ani.

The uterus is supported indirectly by the supports of the vaginal walls, but directly by the cardinal or transverse cervical ligaments, which extend from the lateral pelvic wall to the upper part of the vagina and the lower part of the cervix. The uterosacral ligaments, which comprise the thickening of the pelvic floor fascia, extend from the sacrum to the lower parts of the cervix and the upper third of the vagina. The round and broad ligaments also provide weak support to the vagina and uterus. Indirect support of the vagina and uterus is provided by the integrity of the pelvic floor and the levator ani.

DEFINITIONS OF PROLAPSE

Cystocoele and urethrocoele

Prolapse of the anterior vaginal wall may affect the urethra, **urethrocoele**, and the bladder, **cystocoele** (Fig. 30.2). On examination, the urethra and bladder can be seen to descend and bulge into the anterior vaginal wall and, in severe cases, will be visible at the introitus of the vagina.

A **rectocoele** is formed by a recto-vaginal hernia, which can be seen as a visible bulge of the rectum through the posterior vaginal wall. It is often associated with deficiency and laxity of the pelvic floor.

An **enterocoele** is formed by a prolapse of the recto-uterine pouch, i.e. the pouch of Douglas, through the upper part of the vaginal vault (Fig. 30.2). The condition may occur in isolation but usually in association with uterine prolapse. An enterocoele may also occur following hysterectomy when there is inadequate support of the vaginal vault.

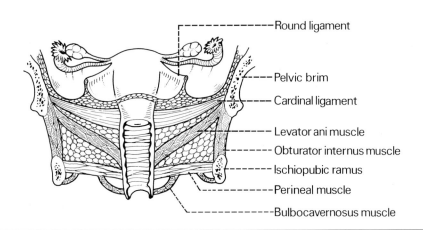

Fig. 30.1 Supports of the uterus, cervix and vagina.

Round ligament
Pelvic brim
Cardinal ligament
Levator ani muscle
Obturator internus muscle
Ischiopubic ramus
Perineal muscle
Bulbocavernosus muscle

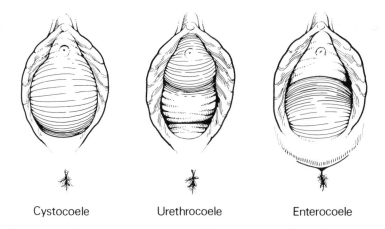

Cystocoele   Urethrocoele   Enterocoele

Fig. 30.2   The clinical appearance of cystocoele, urethrocoele and enterocoele.

Uterine prolapse

Descent of the uterus may occur in isolation from vaginal wall prolapse but more commonly occurs in conjunction with it. First-degree prolapse of the uterus often occurs in association with retroversion of the uterus and descent of the cervix into the lower third of the vagina (Fig. 30.3).

If the cervix descends to protrude through the vaginal introitus, the prolapse is defined as second degree.

The term **procidentia** is applied to third-degree prolapse where the cervix and the body of the uterus and the vagina protrude through the introitus. The word actually means prolapse or **falling** but is generally reserved for the description of **total** or third-degree prolapse.

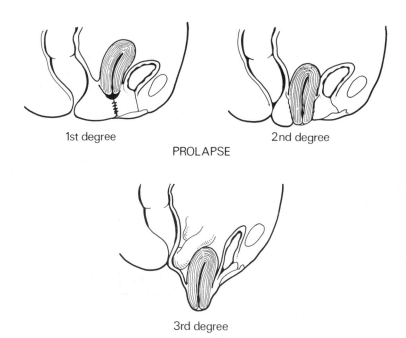

1st degree   2nd degree

PROLAPSE

3rd degree

Fig. 30.3   Classification of uterine prolapse.

SYMPTOMS AND SIGNS

Mild degrees of prolapse are common in parous women and may be asymptomatic. However, symptoms generally depend on the severity and site of the prolapse.

There are some symptoms which are common to all forms of prolapse and these include:

1. A sense of fullness in the vagina associated with dragging discomfort
2. Visible protrusion of the cervix and vaginal walls
3. Sacral backache.

Symptoms are often multiple and related to the nature of prolapse.

Urethrocoele and cystocoele

Specific symptoms relating to the urinary tract depend on the effect the prolapse has on the bladder neck. The loss of the posterior urethrovesical angle is often associated with stress incontinence, i.e. the involuntary loss of urine following raised intra-abdominal pressure. If the angle between the bladder and urethra becomes exaggerated, then there may be incomplete emptying of the bladder and this will be associated with double micturition, the desire to repeat micturition immediately after apparent completion of voiding, or recurrent urinary tract infection as a result of incomplete emptying of the bladder. The sensation of incomplete emptying or difficulty in initiating micturition can be relieved by replacing the cystocoele digitally or by the use of a vaginal pessary or tampon.

Signs

The diagnosis is established by examination with a Sims' speculum so that the vaginal wall can be seen. When the patient is asked to strain, the bulge in the anterior vaginal wall can be seen and often appears at the introitus. It is important to culture a specimen of urine to exclude the presence of infection. The differential diagnosis is limited to cysts or tumours of the anterior vaginal wall, and diverticulum of the urethra or bladder.

Rectocoele

The prolapse of the rectum through the posterior vaginal wall is commonly associated with a deficient pelvic floor, disruption of the perineal body and separation of the levator ani. It is predominantly a problem that results from overdistension of the introitus and pelvic floor during parturition.

Symptoms

The symptoms that relate in particular to rectocoele are difficulties with evacuation of faeces and the awareness of a reducible mass bulging into the vagina and through the introitus.

Signs

Examination of the vulva usually shows a deficient perineum, a lax introitus, and the rectum bulging into the posterior vaginal wall.

Enterocoele

Herniation of the pouch of Douglas usually occurs through the vaginal vault, either through the posterior fornix or through the vaginal vault if the uterus has been removed. It is often difficult to distinguish between a high rectocoele and an enterocoele as the symptoms of vaginal pressure are identical. Occasionally, but rarely, the enterocoele occurs anterior to the vaginal vault and may mimic a cystocoele.

A large enterocoele may contain bowel and may be associated with incarceration and obstruction of the bowel.

Uterine prolapse

Descent of the uterus is initially associated with prolongation of the cervix and descent of the body of the uterus. The symptoms are those of pressure in the vagina and, ultimately, complete protrusion of the uterus through the introitus. At this stage, the prolapsed uterus may produce discomfort on sitting, and decubitus ulceration may result in haemorrhage. Cervical prolongation often leads to confusion in staging the degree of prolapse as it may appear to be in a more advanced stage than actually exists.

Urinary tract infection is common because of compression of the ureters and consequent hydronephrosis due to incomplete emptying of the bladder.

PATHOGENESIS OF UTERO-VAGINAL PROLAPSE

Prolapse may be congenital or acquired:

1. *Congenital* – Uterine prolapse in young or nulliparous women is due to weakness of the

supports of the uterus and vaginal vault. There is a minimal degree of vaginal wall prolapse.

2. *Acquired* – The commonest form of prolapse is acquired under the influence of multiple factors. This type of prolapse is both uterine and vaginal, but it must also be remembered that vaginal wall prolapse can also occur without any uterine descent. Predisposing factors include:

   a. *High parity* – Uterovaginal prolapse is a condition of parous women. The pelvic floor provides direct and indirect support for the vaginal walls and when this support is disrupted by laceration or overdistension it predisposes to vaginal wall prolapse.

   b. *Raised intra-abdominal pressure* – Tumours or ascites may result in raised intra-abdominal pressure, but a more common cause is a chronic cough.

   c. *Hormonal changes* – The symptoms of prolapse often worsen rapidly at the time of the menopause. Cessation of oestrogen production leads to thinning of the vaginal walls and the supports of the uterus. although the prolapse is generally present before the menopause, it is at this time that the symptoms become noticeable and the degree of descent visibly worsens.

MANAGEMENT

The management of prolapse is medical or surgical.

Prevention

Good surgical technique in supporting the vaginal vault at the time of hysterectomy reduces the incidence of later vault prolapse. Avoiding a prolonged second stage of labour, encouraging pelvic floor exercises after delivery and the use of hormone replacement therapy after the menopause may all help to reduce the risk of prolapse in later life.

Medical treatment

Many women have minor degrees of utero-vaginal prolapse which are asymptomatic. If the recognition of the prolapse is a coincidental finding, then the woman should be advised against any surgical treatment.

Minor degrees of prolapse are common after childbirth and should be treated by pelvic floor exercises or by the use of a pessary. Operative intervention is contraindicated for at least 6 months after delivery, as the tissues remain vascular and may undergo further spontaneous improvement.

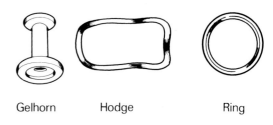

Gelhorn   Hodge   Ring

Fig. 30.4 Various type of vaginal pessaries used in the conservative management of utero-vaginal prolapse.

Symptoms associated with cystocoele after the menopause are often improved by hormone replacement therapy.

Where short-term support is required or the general health of the woman makes operative treatment dangerous, then both vaginal wall and uterine prolapse can be treated by using vaginal pessaries or splinters. It is, however, necessary to have some pelvic floor support if a pessary is to be retained.

The most widely used pessaries are (Fig 30.4).

1. *Ring pessary* – This pessary consists of a malleable plastic ring which may vary in diameter from 60 to 80 mm. The pessary is inserted in the posterior fornix and behind the pubic symphysis. Distension of the vaginal walls tends to support the vaginal wall prolapse.

2. *Hodge pessary* – This is a rigid, elongated curved ovoid which is inserted in a similar way to the ring pessary and is principally useful in uterine retroversion.

3. *Gelhorn pessary* – This pessary is shaped like a collar stud and is used in the treatment of severe degrees of prolapse.

The main problem with long-term use of pessaries is ulceration of the vaginal vault.

Surgical treatment

Surgical treatment of a cystocoele is by anterior colporrhaphy (Fig. 30.5). The operation consists of a surgical excision of the excess vaginal wall and buttressing of the pubocervical fascia. In the presence of stress incontinence due to loss of the posterior urethrovesical angle, this angle is reconstructed by placing buttressing sutures under the bladder neck. These are described as **Kelly's sutures**.

Rectocoele is repaired by posterior colpoperineorrhaphy with reconstruction of the pelvic floor,

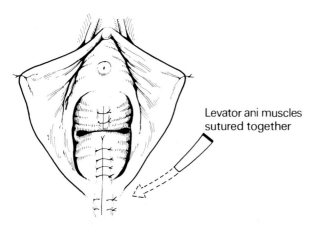

Levator ani muscles
sutured together

Fig. 30.5 Anterior and posterior colporrhaphy.

reapposition of the levator muscles and excision of the redundant vaginal skin.

Where there is an enterocoele, the hernial sac is opened and transfixed at its neck with excision of the redundant tissue.

The treatment of choice for uterine prolapse is vaginal hysterectomy with or without repair of the vaginal walls. If preservation of reproductive function is required, then the uterus can be conserved by simply excising the cervix and suturing the cardinal ligaments in front of the cervical stump. This procedure is known as a **Manchester** or **Fothergill repair**. The vaginal skin is then sutured into the cervical stump.

Vault prolapse occurring after hysterectomy can be treated by suspending the vaginal vault from the anterior longitudinal ligament of the sacrum using a synthetic mesh. This procedure is known as sacrocolpoplexy.

Complications

The immediate complications of vaginal hysterectomy or repair include haemorrhage, haematoma formation, infection and urinary retention. The long-term complications are those of dyspareunia and vaginal stenosis. Inadequate supportive tissue may result in recurrence of the prolapse of the vaginal vault.

Prolapse

- May involve anterior or posterior vaginal wall with varying degrees of uterine descent
- Predisposing factors include high parity, chronically raised intra-abdominal pressure and hormonal changes
- Symptoms depend on degree of prolapse and whether bowel or bladder neck involved
- May present as renal failure
- May undergo spontaneous improvement up to 6 months postpartum
- Treatment of choice is surgical repair ± hysterectomy
- No treatment required for asymptomatic minor degrees of prolapse

---

BIBLIOGRAPHY

Howkins J, Hudson C N 1983 Shaw's textbook of operative gynaecology. Churchill Livingstone, Edinburgh

31 Disorders of the urinary tract

STRUCTURE AND PHYSIOLOGY OF THE LOWER URINARY TRACT

The urinary bladder is a hollow muscular organ with an outer adventitial layer, a smooth muscle layer known as the detrusor muscle and an inner layer of transitional epithelium.

The innervation of the bladder contains both sympathetic and parasympathetic components (Fig. 31.1). The sympathetic fibres arise from the lower two thoracic and upper two lumbar segments of the spinal cord, and the parasympathetic fibres from the second, third and fourth sacral segments. The urethra consists of a muscle coat lined by epithelium continuous with the bladder epithelium. The muscle coat consists of a mixture of smooth muscle with an outer sleeve of striated muscle. The bladder neck does not contain a smooth muscle sphincter. The majority of muscle fibres in the bladder neck enter obliquely or longitudinally into the wall of the urethra.

During micturition, the pressure in the bladder rises to exceed the pressure within the urethral lumen and there is a fall in urethral resistance. The tonus of muscle fibres around the bladder neck is reduced by central inhibition of the motor neurones in the sacral plexus.

The ureter is 25 cm long. It runs along the transverse processes of the lumbar spine, anterior to the psoas muscle, is crossed by the ovarian vessels and enters the pelvis anterior to the bifurcation of the common iliacs. From there it runs anterior to the internal iliac vessels to the ischial spines where it turns medially to the cervix. It turns again anteriorly 1.5 cm lateral to the vaginal fornix, crossing below the uterine vessels to enter the posterior surface of the bladder.

COMMON DISORDERS OF BLADDER FUNCTION

The common symptoms of bladder dysfunction include:

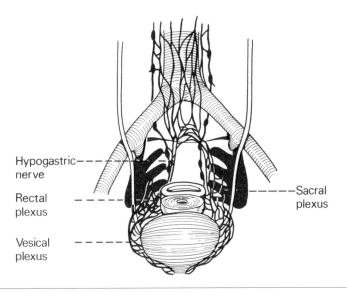

Hypogastric nerve

Rectal plexus

Vesical plexus

Sacral plexus

Fig. 31.1 Sympathetic and parasympathetic innervation of the bladder.

1. Urinary incontinence
2. Frequency of micturition
3. Dysuria
4. Urinary retention.

Incontinence of urine

The involuntary loss of urine may be associated with bladder or urethral dysfunction or fistula formation. The types of incontinence include:

1. **True incontinence** – continuous loss of urine through the vagina; it is commonly associated with fistula formation but may occasionally be a manifestation of urinary retention with overflow.
2. **Stress incontinence** – the involuntary loss of urine that occurs during a brief period of raised intra-abdominal pressure related to pelvic floor weakness, and in 30% of cases with detrusor instability. Examination reveals the involuntary loss of urine during coughing with descent of the anterior vaginal wall and reduction of the posterior urethro-vesical angle. Digital elevation of the anterior vaginal wall leads to correction of the condition. Loss of support to the anterior vaginal wall is frequently associated with reduced pelvic floor support.
3. **Urge incontinence** – the problem of sudden detrusor contraction with uncontrolled loss of urine. The condition may be due to idiopathic detrusor instability or associated with urinary infection, obstructive uropathy, diabetes or neurological disease. It is particularly important to exclude urinary tract infection.
4. **Mixed urge and stress incontinence** – a substantial number of women with urge incontinence also have true stress incontinence and if the latter is corrected, the detrusor instability will disappear.

The bladder fills at 1–6 ml/min. The intravesical pressure remains low because of compliance of the bladder wall as it stretches and reflex inhibition of the detrusor muscle. At the same time the internal urethral meatus is closed by tonic contraction of the rhabdosphincter and the tone of the urethral mucosa. During rises in intra-abdominal pressure such as coughing or sneezing, continence is maintained by transmission of the pressure rise to the proximal urethra (which lies normally within the intra-abdominal space) and an increase in the levator tone.

Urinary frequency

Urinary frequency is an unsuppressible desire to void more than seven times a day or more than once a night. If affects 20% of women aged between 30 and 64 years, and can be caused by pregnancy, diabetes, pelvic masses, renal failure, diuretics, excess fluid intake or habit, although the most common cause is urinary tract infection.

The commonest cause of frequency of micturition is urinary tract infection. However, enhanced bladder contractility may occur without the presence of infection. Reduced bladder capacity may also result in frequency of micturition. The symptom may also develop because of anxiety concerning involuntary loss of urine.

Dysuria

This symptom results from infection. Local urethral infection or trauma causes burning or scalding during micturition, but bladder infection is more likely to cause pain suprapubically after micturition has been completed. It is always advisable to perform a vaginal examination on any woman who complains of scalding on micturition because urethritis is associated with vaginitis and vaginal infection.

Urinary retention and outflow obstruction

Acute urinary retention is not the common problem seen in the ageing male. It is, however, seen:

1. After vaginal delivery and episiotomy
2. Following operative delivery
3. After vaginal repair procedures – particularly those operations that involve posterior colpoperineorrhaphy
4. In the menopause – spontaneous obstructive uropathy is more likely to occur in menopausal women
5. In pregnancy – a retroverted uterus may become impacted in the pelvis towards the end of the first trimester
6. When inflammatory lesions of the vulva are present
7. As a result of untreated over-distension of the bladder (such as following delivery), neuropathy or malignancy.

DIFFERENTIAL DIAGNOSIS

The diagnosis is initially indicated by the history. Continuous loss of urine indicates a fistula, but not all fistulas leak urine continuously. The fistulous communication usually occurs between the bladder and vagina, **vesico-vaginal fistula**, and the ureter and vagina, **uretero-vaginal fistula**. Fistula formation results from:

1. Surgical trauma
2. Obstetric trauma associated with obstructed labour
3. Malignant disease
4. Radiotherapy.

There are other types of fistulas with communications between bowel and urinary tract and between bowel and vagina, but these are less common.

Recto-vaginal fistulas have a similar pathogenesis with the additional factor of perineal breakdown after a third degree tear.

Urinary fistulas are localized by:

1. Cystoscopy
2. Intravenous urogram
3. Instillation of methylene blue via a catheter into the bladder; the appearance of dye in the vagina indicates a vesico-vaginal fistula.

The differential diagnosis between stress and urge incontinence is more difficult and is often unsatisfactory. Adequate pre-operative assessment is important if the correct operation is to be employed or if surgery is to be avoided.

The cystometrogram

Pressure is measured intravesically and intrarectally because intrarectal pressure represents intra-abdominal pressure and is subtracted from the intravesical pressure to give a measure of detrusor pressure. The volume of fluid in the bladder at which the first desire to void occurs is usually about 150 ml. A strong desire to void occurs at 400 ml in the normal bladder. Values at a lower volume reflect an abnormally sensitive bladder associated with chronic infection. There should be no detrusor contraction during filling, and any contraction that occurs under these circumstances indicates **detrusor instability**. An underactive detrusor shows no contractions on filling and indicates an abnormality of neurological control. The average bladder has a capacity of 250–550 ml, but capacity is a poor index of bladder function. Thus, cystometry is a useful method for assessing detrusor muscle function or detrusor instability which may result in urge incontinence.

Pressure/flow studies (Fig. 31.2) enable a measurement to be made of the rate of flow in relation to intravesical pressure and hence indicate if there is any bladder neck obstruction. Normal flow may occur in the presence of a bladder neck obstruction if there is a powerful detrusor muscle.

Detrusor overactivity is indicated by high resting urethral pressure, good voluntary increase in urethral pressure, good ability to stop midstream, the presence of good detrusor muscle power, frequent strong bladder contractions and small volumes of urine on frequency/volume charts.

In the presence of urethral incompetence, there is low resting urethral pressure, no voluntary increase in urethral pressure, inability to stop midstream, decreased pressure transmission to the abdominal urethra and large volumes in the frequency/volume

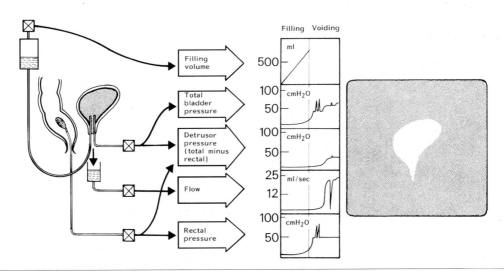

Fig. 31.2 Bladder flow studies in the investigation of lower urinary tract symptoms.

measurements. There is not always a clear-cut demarcation between the two conditions as there may be a mixture of both stress and urge incontinence. Nevertheless, it is important to differentiate between the predominant influence of bladder neck weakness and stress incontinence, and detrusor instability and urge incontinence.

Fistulas

- May present as continuous urinary or faecal incontinence
- Commonly related to surgery but may occur after radiotherapy, childbirth or in association with malignancy
- May heal with conservative treatment if small

MANAGEMENT

Urinary tract fistulas

In Western European countries, most urinary tract fistulas result from surgical trauma. The commonest fistulas are vesico-vaginal (Fig. 31.3 left) or uretero-vaginal, and result from surgical trauma at the time of hysterectomy or sometimes following Caesarean section (Fig. 31.3).

A vesico-vaginal fistula will usually become apparent in the first postoperative week. If the fistula is small, closure may be achieved spontaneously.

The patient should be treated by catheterization and continuous drainage. If closure has not occurred after 2–3 months, the fistula is unlikely to close

spontaneously, and surgical closure is recommended. The timing of further surgery is still a subject of controversy. Until recently, a delay of 6 months had been recommended, but there is increasing evidence that good results can be obtained with early surgical intervention. However, the fistulous site should be free of infection.

Surgical closure may be achieved vaginally by meticulous separation of the edges of the fistula and closure in layers of the bladder and vagina (Fig. 31.3 right). Postoperative care includes continuous catheter drainage for 1 week and antibiotic cover. An abdominal approach to the fistula can also be used and has some advantages in allowing the interposition of omentum in cases where there is a large fistula.

Uretero-vaginal fistulas are usually treated by reimplantation of the damaged ureter into the bladder.

Stress incontinence

- Presents as involuntary loss of urine on raised intra-abdominal pressure
- Commonly associated with prolapse of bladder neck outside the abdominal cavity
- Associated with detrusor instability in up to 30% of cases
- Is indicated by a low resting urethral pressure, decreased pressure transmission to abdominal urethra and inability to stop midstream during cystometry
- Treatment is surgical by elevation of the bladder neck

Stress incontinence

Once the true nature of stress incontinence has been established, then surgical correction should be

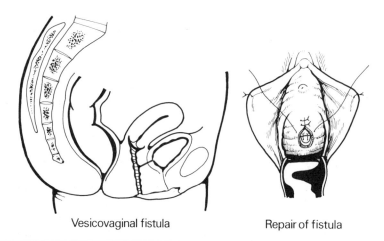

Vesicovaginal fistula   Repair of fistula

Fig. 31.3 True incontinence is associated with a fistulous opening between bladder and vagina: the vesico-vaginal fistula (left); it can be closed by either the vaginal or the abdominal route (right).

attempted. A large number of operative procedures have been described and advocated. In the presence of anterior vaginal wall prolapse, **anterior repair** with the placement of buttressing sutures at the bladder neck has the virtue of simplicity. It will certainly relieve the prolapse, but the results are variable as far as the stress incontinence is concerned, with relief in about 40–50% of cases.

Where there is minimal prolapse, then the following procedures are used:

1. *Marshall–Marchetti–Krantz procedure* – the bladder neck and trigone are elevated by suturing the para-urethral and paravesical tissues to the periosteum on the back of the pubic symphysis. This creates a valve-like effect at the bladder neck.
2. *Burch colposuspension* – the bladder neck is elevated by suturing the upper lateral vaginal walls to the ilio-inguinal ligaments.
3. *Sling procedures* – fascial strips from the anterior abdominal wall or inert synthetic materials attached to the anterior abdominal wall are placed in a sling under the bladder neck and cause urethral closure when the sling is stretched (Fig. 31.4).
4. *Stamey procedure* – a Mersilene strip is introduced per vaginum using a large specialized needle and is fixed to the anterior abdominal wall. The procedure has the advantage of simplicity with minimal incision size and a rapid recovery with a short convalescence time.

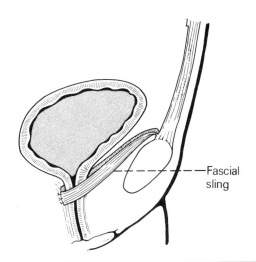

Fig. 31.4 Stress incontinence may be treated by a procedure such as the Aldridge sling that supports the vaginal neck .

5. *Laparoscopic colposuspension* – bladder neck elevation by suturing the upper lateral vaginal walls to the iliopectineal ligaments under laparoscopic control.

All of these procedures have a higher success rate in curing stess incontinence but have a significant surgical complication rate and often cause detrusor instability as well as other urinary symptoms due to incomplete bladder emptying.

The unstable bladder

The features of the unstable bladder arc those of frequency of micturition and nocturia, urgency and urge incontinence.

When confronted with this history, it is important to obtain some indication of the frequency as related to fluid intake and output. A chart should therefore be kept by the patient to clarify this aspect.

The assessment of predisposing factors includes urine culture, urinary flow rates and urodynamic studies.

Treatment will obviously be directed at the cause so that the presence of urinary tract infection necessitates the administration of the appropriate antibiotic therapy. Postmenopausal women with atrophic vaginal epithelium and symptoms of urgency and frequency often respond to replacement therapy with low dose oestrogens.

Detrusor instability of unknown aetiology

If the problem arises at a cerebral level, then psychotherapeutic measures are indicated. Bladder drill involves a regime of gradually increasing the voiding interval on a recorded pattern. This is effective in the short term but the relapse rate is high.

The placebo response rate in detrusor instability is more than 40% and spontaneous remissions occur.

Drug treatment

The alternative approach is to use anticholinergic drugs which act at the level of the bladder wall. The most effective drugs are oxybutynin, propantheline and imipramine. The addition of tranquilizers and hypnotics may also help. Oxybutynin is prescribed in a dose of 5 mg three times daily and has a direct local anaesthetic effect on the bladder. As an anticholinergic drug, it also has side effects such as mouth dryness and blurring of vision.

Detrusor instability

- Presents as frequency, urgency, nocturia and incontinence
- Usually idiopathic but needs to be distinguished from obstructive uropathy, diabetes, neurological disorders and infection
- May occur in combination with true stress incontinence and improve when this is treated
- High resting urethral pressure and frequent strong bladder contractions at low volumes on cystometry
- Management includes bladder drill, anticholinergics and treatment of infection

---

Surgical treatments are not commonly used, but include bladder overdistension, bladder transection and transvesical injection of 6% aqueous phenol into the trigone.

Bladder outlet obstruction

Primary bladder neck obstruction in the female probably results from the failure of the vesical neck to open during voiding, and can be treated either with α-adrenergic blocking agents or by urethral dilatation. Secondary outlet obstruction is usually associated with previous surgery for incontinence and may respond to urethral dilatation but the results are not particularly good.

The neuropathic bladder

Loss of bladder function may be associated with a variety of conditions that affect the central nervous system. These conditions may also be associated with alteration in bowel function, sexual dysfunction and loss of function of the lower limbs.

Presentation

The neuropathic bladder is a reflection of dysergy between the activity of the detrusor muscle and the bladder sphincter. This results in a variety of disorders ranging from the 'automatic bladder', retention with overflow at high or low pressure and total stress incontinence. It may also be associated with renal failure.

Aetiology

The causation may be suprapontine such as a cerebrovascular accident, Parkinson's disease or a cerebral tumour. Infrapontine causes include cord injuries or compression, multiple sclerosis and spina bifida. Peripheral autonomic neuropathies that affect bladder function may be idiopathic or diabetic and, occasionally, secondary to surgical injury.

Diagnosis

The diagnosis is established by a systematic search for the cause involving cystometry, urinary flow rate studies, neurological screening, brain scan, pyelography and renal isotope scans.

Management

The management clearly depends on establishing the cause, but symptomatically it also involves non-surgical management using absorptive pads and clean intermittent self-catheterization. Anticholinergic drugs also have a place for some patients. Surgical treatment include the use of artificial sphincters and sacral nerve stimulators.

Conclusions

The important feature in the management of urinary tract disorders in the female is to ensure that the underlying nature of the symptoms is defined before embarking on any surgical treatment.

Simple medical measures such as bladder drill, pelvic floor exercises and anticholinergic drug therapy may give adequate relief of symptoms when administered in the appropriate situation. Surgical treatment is predominantly of value in the correction of fistulas and in the support of the bladder neck where stress incontinence is present.

BIBLIOGRAPHY

Khullar V, Cardozo L 1995 Drugs and the bladder. Current Obstetrics and Gynaecology 5(2): 110–116
Monga A K, Stanton S 1994 The Burch colposuspension. Current Obstetrics and Gynaecology 4(4): 210–214
Raz S 1985 Gynaecological urology. Clinics in Obstetrics and Gynaecology 12(2)

32 Psychological aspects of obstetrics and gynaecology

M. R. Oates

This chapter describes the psychological and psychiatric sequelae of the most common conditions and procedures found in gynaecology – miscarriage, therapeutic termination of pregnancy, hysterectomy and sterilization. It also addresses the psychological issues involved in the new assisted reproduction technologies.

PSYCHIATRIC MORBIDITY IN GYNAECOLOGICAL PATIENTS

Termination of pregnancy, sterilization and hysterectomy have in the past acquired a reputation for causing psychiatric morbidity and psychological distress. However, the available modern evidence from prospective studies using standardized psychiatric assessments would suggest that this reputation is largely unfounded and that these procedures are not causally related to either an increased rate of psychiatric morbidity nor, indeed, to long term psychological distress. This is in marked contrast to childbirth which has consistently been found to be related to an excess of serious psychiatric morbidity.

Nonetheless, the available evidence suggests that psychiatric morbidity in gynaecological patients before surgery is higher than in the general population and than in other areas of medicine. Short-lived states of psychological distress, essentially healthy, are also commonplace in the few weeks following the event.

Neurotic psychiatric disorder (excluding alcoholism) is more common in women than in men in a general practice setting. Amongst women, in a general practice population, there is an excess of psychiatric morbidity, and in those complaining of premenstrual tension, menstrual problems such as menorrhagia and dysmenorrhoea and those suffering from perimenopausal symptoms, hot flushes and sweating. There is also an increased likelihood of referral to a gynaecologist if menstrual and psychiatric problems co-exist. It is possible that the association of psychiatric morbidity with menstrual complaints and also with childbirth may largely contribute to the excess of psychiatric morbidity amongst women, particularly in a general practice population. It is, therefore, not surprising that psychiatric morbidity in gynaecological out-patient clinics is also high – higher than that of women in the general population and higher than that in patients attending general medical and surgical clinics.

With the exception of gynaecological emergencies such as ectopic pregnancies, ruptured ovarian cysts or gynaecological neoplasms, the majority of gynaecological conditions present because of the subjective experience of quantitative variation in normal physiology. For example, premenstrual and perimenopausal phenomena and menstrual problems, or because of problems with fertility. In the past it was thought by some clinicians that these symptoms themselves were of psychogenic origin. A more recent explanation, however, is that at all stages in the chain leading from presentation to gynaecological surgery, the gynaecological disorders themselves are distressing and lead to secondary emotional problems.

DISORDERS RELATED TO EARLY PREGNANCY

Miscarriage

The loss of a pregnancy in the first trimester is a very common event affecting up to 20% of all confirmed pregnancies. In Western Europe most women confirm their pregnancies considerably earlier than in previous generations. A spontaneous miscarriage is often regarded medically as not serious, and is rarely investigated when it occurs for the first time. Follow-up is often left in primary care, and few women receive gynaecological attention or an explanation of their loss. Although there is no evidence to associate miscarriage with an overall increased risk of psychiatric morbidity, almost half of all women are considerably distressed at 6 weeks following miscarriage, and often feel angry, alone and guilty. Women who have had a previous miscarriage and no live child, women who have had a previous termination of pregnancy and those with a previous psychiatric history are most at risk of becoming depressed in the months that follow miscarriage. Women who have had many miscarriages are particularly vulnerable, and should probably receive gynaecological support and counselling.

Women who lose pregnancies in the second and third trimesters face the same risks of postpartum 'mood disorder' as a delivered population, and their grief reactions are usually more severe. They will, therefore, be considerably distressed, with the features of a typical grief reaction for up to 6 months following the loss of their pregnancy. Their psychological recovery may be assisted by granting their pregnancy the dignity afforded to a full-term infant with a burial, naming, etc. However, rigid 'grieving procedures' should be avoided even for full-term stillborn infants. Women and their partners should be allowed the flexibility to manage their baby's death in the way that they find most suitable.

Therapeutic termination of pregnancy

In Great Britain, approximately the same number of confirmed pregnancies are therapeutically terminated as spontaneously aborted. Over 80% of these are the majority of first-trimester therapeutic terminations of pregnancy, of which 80% are allowed under the so-called 'psycho-social' clauses of the Abortion Act 1967 (see Ch. 20). Most of these early terminations of pregnancy will be conducted by surgical or vacuum extraction under general anaesthetic. There will always be personal anecdotes of long-term distress and regret, and the majority of women who find themselves with an unwanted pregnancy are very distressed. Despite this, evidence shows that the majority of women do not experience medium- to long-term psychological sequelae, nor is there any evidence of an increase in the rate of psychiatric morbidity. The available evidence is that the rate of psychiatric morbidity following termination of pregnancy decreases.

Risk factors for adverse sequelae of first trimester abortion

Being married and having children prior to a termination can lead to problems of guilt and regret. Women in such circumstances need careful counselling before proceeding with the termination. Ambivalence, coercion, previous terminations of pregnancy, past psychiatric history and termination associated with sterilization are risk factors for psychiatric morbidity.

Later terminations of pregnancy

The number of women having terminations of pregnancy after 12 weeks for psycho-social reasons is falling. Second-trimester terminations now account for less than 8% of all therapeutic terminations of pregnancy. The minority of these women are having therapeutic abortions for psycho-social reasons, the majority for fetal abnormality. Unlike first-trimester abortions, later terminations of pregnancy are associated both with marked psychological distress and an increased rate of psychiatric disorder. Thirty-nine per cent of women having an abortion for fetal abnormality are depressed at 3–9 months, although the rates fall to normal at 1 year. For women undergoing this procedure for psycho-social reasons, the cause for the increased rate of distress and morbidity is likely to be found in the delay in presenting for termination. The very young, the mentally handicapped and the chronically mentally ill may be found in this group, as well as those who have experienced marked ambivalence about their pregnancies. The situation for women having a termination of pregnancy because of fetal abnormality is different. These are usually older women who have a much wanted pregnancy and whose problem has been diagnosed either because of a previous experience or as the result of screening. The decision to terminate the pregnancy is usually reached only after much thought and anguish. The consequence of termination is, therefore, very much like the spontaneous loss of a more advanced pregnancy, that is to say, of a grief reaction. Their psycho-social recovery may be assisted by granting them the dignity of a naming and burial. Most late terminations of pregnancy involve the induction of labour and a prolonged process of giving birth. This can be a distressing and traumatic experience, and psychological recovery will be improved by sensitive and compassionate handling by the doctor and nursing staff.

Psychological aspects in early pregnancy, of miscarriage and of termination

- Problems in early pregnancy have a psychiatric dimension
- Early miscarriage is associated with grief reactions
- Therapeutic termination does not cause increased psychiatric morbidity
- Late termination = 30% incidence of depression

Hysterectomy

Before surgery, the level of psychiatric morbidity is high. Approximately half of all patients undergoing hysterectomy meet the criteria for mental illness, the majority having mild depression and anxiety. Postoperatively, the level of psychiatric morbidity is halved at 6–8 months. Most who are depressed or anxious following surgery are ill before surgery or have a previous history of such illness. The number of women who become ill for the first time following hysterectomy is probably no higher than one would expect in the general female population. The overall view is that hysterectomy does not lead to an increase in psychiatric morbidity nor to other adverse sequelae. For the majority of women, their sexual function is either unchanged or improved after hysterectomy. The outcome of marital satisfaction and social function shows similar findings.

Factors related to poor outcome

It was once thought that an absence of physical pathology at postoperative histology was a predictor of poor psycho-social outcome. There is no evidence that this belief is true. The best predictor of postoperative satisfaction and good outcome is the amount of distress and disability caused by the dysfunctional uterine bleeding before operation, rather than the objective amount of blood loss or the presence of uterine pathology. A previous psychiatric history increases the risk of a psychiatric episode following surgery. It is likely that women whose anticipated fertility was abbreviated by hysterectomy will face particular emotional problems following operation and may well need extra support and counselling.

Patients awaiting hysterectomy will benefit from a clear explanation of their condition and the procedures that are likely to be faced. They will all benefit from reassurance that their sexual function need not be affected and that most of them will experience an improvement in their general emotional and physical health. However, it is not uncommon for women in the first 2–3 weeks after hysterectomy to feel tired, lethargic, emotionally turbulent and over-sensitive and occasionally weepy. Both patients and their carers need to be assured about this occurrence and its essentially benign nature.

Sterilization

Like hysterectomy, sterilization in women has acquired a reputation of leading to psychiatric problems and a deterioration in sexual function. Modern studies do not confirm this reputation. Apart from the fact that modern studies tend to use prospective standardized methodologies, the population being sterilized in the 1990s is very different to that of 30 years ago. The most dramatic change has been in the frequency of its use. It has become an increasingly frequent and commonplace choice of contraception in all parts of the world for women who have completed their families. There was a 12-fold increase in the rate of female sterilization between 1960 and 1975, and it continues to increase. There have been similar increases in other countries. Previously, sterilization was performed predominantly on older women in poor gynaecological health, with large numbers of children and in conditions of social adversity. It was on medical recommendation and frequently carried out shortly after childbirth, abortion or some other gynaecological procedure. Nowadays, sterilization is a widely accepted form of contraception used by women of all ages and social classes. They are, therefore, more representative of the population as a whole. Forty per cent of couples in the UK over the age of 35 years are now sterilized. Sterilization usually takes place at the request of the woman as an interval procedure unrelated to either childbirth or abortion. Women being sterilized have fewer children and are in better general health than previously.

There have also been major changes in surgical technique. Sterilization now usually uses micro-laparoscopic surgery, and is theoretically potentially reversible; in previous years it involved laparotomy. The general view is that, pre-operatively, patients awaiting sterilization throughout the world differ little in their psychiatric and socio-demographic characteristics from the general population, and postoperatively there is no evidence of adverse psychological sequelae. This is true not only of Western Europe but also of most other countries in the world. The majority of patients report an improvement in their sexual and marital relationships and physical and emotional wellbeing following sterilization.

Risk factors for adverse outcome

The rate of psychiatric disorder following sterilization is, in general, no higher than that in the general female population. However, for women who are sterilized immediately following childbirth, there is an increased risk of suffering from postnatal depression. A previous psychiatric history and ambivalence or uncertainty about sterilization is also a risk for psychiatric disorder. Postpartum status, previous psychiatric history, ambivalence and marital discord are also risk factors in deterioration of psychosexual functioning and regret. Some authors have also suggested that in cultures where femininity is strongly associated with fertility and where there is guilt and shame about contraception, great care should be exercised to ensure that patients are properly prepared for sterilization. Regret, often measured by a request for reversal of sterilization, appears to be most strongly predicted by marital breakdown and subsequent remarriage.

Infertility and assisted reproduction technologies

Infertility is a common problem. The exact prevalence of people who wish to conceive but cannot is difficult to quantify. Nonetheless, a reasonable estimate of the incidence of infertility is 120 couples per 1000 of the population, which means that at least one couple in eight will need specialist help some time in their lives to conceive, usually following a period of infertility of 2 years or more. Infertility and its treatment is widely accepted as being distressing, and assisted reproduction as being particularly stressful.

It is important to understand the commonplace and ordinary emotional reactions and experiences of these patients so that they may be forewarned, their experiences validated and appropriate reassurance given. It is a commonly held belief amongst the lay public that psychological factors contribute to infertility and interfere with its treatment. This may provide a rich source of guilt and anxiety to the patient. It is important for the professional involved in their care to have a critical understanding of the likely contribution of psychological and psychiatric factors in aetiology and treatment. They should be able to identify vulnerable patients who require special attention and be aware of common psychiatric disorders when they occur. It is also important to be able to predict those at particular risk of developing problems following successful treatment, that is to say, postnatal psychiatric disorder.

Psychosocial factors in the aetiology of infertility

Despite the widely held view that worry, stress, lifestyle and 'trying too hard' are all contributory causes of infertility, there is little to suggest that psycho-social factors play a major part in the aetiology of infertility. Compared to a wide variety

of controls, patients under investigation for infertility or on assisted reproduction programmes do not differ significantly. They are, however, more affluent, married longer and tend to have more stable marriages and personalities. The overwhelming impression is that they are a psychologically healthy and highly motivated group of people.

However, in individual cases, psychiatric disorders may contribute towards infertility. These are *eating disorders*, both anorexia and bulimia nervosa, *alcohol abuse* in both men and women, *sexual problems*, *drug abuse* and certain *psychotropic drugs*, particularly neuroleptics. If at assessment these problems are identified, psychiatric assessment should be sought.

Common 'syndromes' of psychological experience

These are consistently described in female patients, and include the following:

1. *Infertility becomes part of the female identity* – Irrespective of age, social background, career and lifestyle, infertility rapidly becomes incorporated into the identity of the woman, with an associated sense of failure, isolation and being different to other women.
2. *Preoccupation of priority* – Infertility and striving to conceive quickly become the most important issues in the woman's life and her main topics of thought and endeavour. Most women describe the process of trying to conceive as dominating their mental and social life, and other achievements become of less importance.
3. *'Monthly mourning'* – Each month, ovulation is anticipated, and there is mounting excitement for the following 2 weeks. Menstruation is associated with the feelings of profound disappointment and loss, only for the cycle to be repeated.
4. *Selective abstraction and vigilant focusing* – Women become preoccupied with physical changes signalling ovulation and conception or its absence, and the world seems full of pregnant women, as does the media.
5. *Social changes, isolation and avoidance* – It is common for women to change their social life to avoid contact with friends and relatives who are pregnant or who have small babies in order to avoid embarrassing comments about fertility.
6. *De-libidinization of sex* – Sexual activity is often confined to ovulation, and loses its spontaneity.
7. *Work, secrecy and shame* – Most couples tell very few people, even amongst their immediate

family, of their infertility problem, often because of embarrassment and guilt. The investigations are often very time-consuming for women, and can be humiliating and embarrassing and difficult to explain to employers (e.g. artificial insemination, postcoital testing, etc.). For this reason, many people give up their jobs, believing that the stress of working may hamper their success.

8. *Phases of despair* – The emotional reaction to infertility investigations often follow a series of peaks and troughs of optimism and focused activity alternating with phases of humiliation, hopelessness and distress. It is common when infertility investigations and treatments have been going on for some time to also go through phases of ambivalence, and for this state of mind to be concealed from both her partner and gynaecologist.

Effects on the marital relationship

Although at the onset of the investigation and treatment, couples are united in their commitment and desire to have a family, their coping styles, although normal for their own sex, are different from each other's, as is the priority that the process has in their lives. This difference between male and female coping styles and priorities tends to widen as time goes by and with the number of unsuccessful treatments. This widening gap between male and female coping styles and attitudes is essentially normal, but can nonetheless be a source of great distress. It should be remembered that often these couples have been together for a long time and have valued their intimacy. They may find, therefore, the sense of alienation from each other particularly hard to bear. It is important that those involved in their care should be aware of this potential and that men and women may require different types of psychological help to ameliorate their distress. The main differences between men and women are that men tend to show more suppression of emotions than women, and this process increases with the passage of time. They are more likely than women to use activity and problem solving as a way of coping with their distress and are more likely to feel that they are in control of what is happening to them. Women, on the other hand, are more likely to feel guilty and responsible for their problems, are more likely to engage in medical risk taking than men and have a greater desire to talk and confide their problems in others. Men are more distressed by the effect on their sexual life, and women by the loss of sense of intimacy.

Psychiatric disorder

At the onset of the investigation and treatment, the overall rates of anxiety and depression in both men and women are the same as the standardized norms from the sex. However, as the treatment proceeds, differences emerge. Women are more likely to develop clinical depression than men: the rates of depressive illness in women are higher than in the general female population and become more likely as the treatment cycles progress. The prevalence of depressive illness in an in vitro fertilization programme is approximately 25%. Men, however, experience more clinical anxiety than women. The rate of clinical anxiety does not increase as the treatment progresses but is substantially higher than in the general male population. The prevalence of clinical anxiety in men on an in vitro fertilization programme is 38%.

Adjustment to motherhood

There is a surprising lack of follow-up studies to both successful and unsuccessful treatment, and no studies of the rates of psychiatric disorder following childbirth in this population. However, there is good reason to believe that the rates of psychiatric disorder following childbirth might be elevated because of the constellation of known risk factors for postnatal depression in this group of women. In addition, women who become pregnant as a result of assisted reproduction, particularly in vitro fertilization, may have emotional adjustment problems following childbirth. They are more likely to have multiple births and more likely to have high expectations of themselves and their coping abilities. The ordinary vicissitudes of motherhood may be particularly distressing to a group of women who regarded themselves as fortunate to have a child.

Psychological aspects of infertility

- Infertile patients are, in general, a psychologically healthy population
- There is no justification for in-depth routine psychiatric screening but there are specific conditions that justify psychiatric referral
- Men and women differ in their attitudes to infertility and their reactions to the treatment process.
- It is important to anticipate and validate common experiences.
- Men are vulnerable to developing anxiety states, and women to developing depressive illness during treatment
- Women are probably at increased risk of developing major postnatal depression following successful treatment

---

33 Medico-legal aspects of obstetrics and gynaecology

The processes of human reproduction present major political and social problems in all countries. Although the issues addressed in this chapter relate particularly to the UK, they are generally reflected in most societies in Europe, North America and Asia.

CONSENT

When a woman agrees to a surgical procedure, it is important that the implications both in terms of benefit and risk are explained to her before embarking on the procedure. Indeed, it is a fundamental law of medical and legal practice that a doctor must obtain consent from the patient for any particular medical or surgical treatment and that without appropriate consent a procedure may constitute an act of assault or trespass to the person.

Secondly, the patient must receive sufficient knowledge of any proposed treatment to make a valid choice of whether or not to consent. The consent form provides evidence that consent has been given to a particular procedure, but it only has meaning if it is evident that the patient could indeed understand the nature and implications of any particular procedure.

In explaining the nature of a procedure to any woman, it is important to explain the purpose of the operation and the potential complications. Given that there may be a range of complications to any particular operation, how far is it necessary to go to explain all the potential complications to the woman given that it may induce disproportionate anxiety to explain a series of very remote risks?

In general terms, a risk in excess of a 1% chance should be explained to the patient, although this is a guideline rather than an absolute figure.

A common example which addresses the issues of inferred consent is the information given to patients before sterilization about potential failure. During the 1980s a substantial number of legal actions were based on the alleged failure to inform patients that there was a significant risk of failure and that pregnancy could follow any sterilization procedure. The patient would generally allege that no advice was given about the risk of failure and subsequent pregnancy and that had such advice been given, either the woman would not have had the operation or she would have continued to use contraception. In fact, it is both highly unlikely and highly illogical to continue using contraception after a sterilization procedure. Over the last 15 years, it has become common practice to include reference to the risk of failure and subsequent pregnancy in the substance of the consent form.

The failure of a sterilization procedure in either a male or female subject may be due to a method failure where, in the case of a female, the clip is applied to the wrong structure or cut through the Fallopian tube and therefore results in persistent tubal function and pregnancy – usually within 6 months of the sterilization procedure. The second cause of failure, applying to both the male and female, is recanalization of the tubes – a process that may occur some years after the procedure. This is an unavoidable risk of the sterilization procedure. Despite a consent form that acknowledges the risk of failure, errors in technique are generally indefensible.

It is important that consent is obtained by a member of staff who is medically qualified and who signs the consent form with the patient after explaining both the nature of the procedure and the potential complications. It is also important to ensure that the details concerning the patient's name and those concerning the operation are correct. For example, it is not sufficient to write 'sterilization' as the operation when the procedure may be laparoscopic clip sterilization, as the different methods of sterilization carry different implications.

The consent form must always be available and must be checked in theatre before any operation is commenced.

Consent

- Consent must be informed
- Purpose of the procedure
- Potential complications
- Consent forms must specify the operation
- Consent forms must be signed by the doctor jointly with the patient

---

LITIGATION IN OBSTETRICS AND GYNAECOLOGY

The last 10 years has seen an explosion in malpractice claims against the medical profession, particularly in obstetrics and gynaecology. When a patient decides to make a claim against her doctor, she will approach her solicitor. If the solicitor considers there is justification, he or she will advance the action by issuing a summons and seek access to the relevant case note records and then lodges an application for a hearing. If the case is to proceed, it will be heard in the High Court by masters of the Queen's Bench Division. Cases may also be heard in the County Court if the costs are below a certain figure. In the UK, cases are heard before a judge and not before a jury. There may be a long time lapse – both between the issuing of a summons and its hearing and between setting a case down for trial and the actual date of the trial. Medical litigation is expensive, and it is not, therefore, surprising that most plaintiffs in the UK are supported by Legal Aid. The Statement of Claim outlines the nature of the case, and it is up to the defendant to respond and to refute the allegations. The legally aided litigant has considerable advantages, as the Legal Aid fund meets all costs and therefore there is no sanction for failure. Advice is taken from experts on both sides, and documents and expert reports are exchanged before the trial. The trial is an adversarial process, and the onus is on the plaintiff to prove that the staff failed to provide a reasonable level of care with the result that the patient suffered unnecessary injury.

During the course of any trial, the major evidence tends to be drawn from the case notes. As a Resident Medical Officer, it is important to remember that case notes will be examined in great detail and constitute a legal document. It is, therefore, important to record facts properly, and the following guidelines should be followed:

1. Entries into case notes must be clear, concise and factual
2. All entries should be brief and free from personal comment
3. Entries should always be initialled and dated
4. No attempt should be made to alter entries in case records without countersigning the alteration.

If a letter is received from a solicitor asking for information with a view to initiating legal action, it is important to:

1. Notify one's medical defence organization
2. Notify the complaints officer in the Trust and the solicitors who represent the Trust.

Litigation commonly ensues where there are complications following a procedure or where a child is born that is brain damaged or dead. The majority of gynaecologists/obstetricians will be the object of a litigious claim during their professional careers, but the risks can be minimized by:

1. Careful adherence to the principle of not undertaking procedures for which one is inadequately supervised or trained
2. By careful and considerate provision of information to the patient before any surgical procedure, information concerning the procedure and any subsequent postoperative complications
3. Prompt action if there are abnormal findings in any tests that require intervention, e.g. an abnormal heart rate recording during labour demands a decision which may be to take no action, to perform a fetal scalp blood sample to look for fetal acidosis or to deliver the infant by Caesarean section – what is not acceptable is to ignore the recording and take no action, or fail to make a decision which is recorded in the case notes.

Minimizing the risks of litigation

- Keep accurate, factual records
- Sign and date all entries in case notes
- Keep patients well informed about their condition
- Make decisions on abnormal test results

DISCLOSURE

The doctor normally has an ethical obligation to keep secret all those details of a personal nature that may be revealed during consultation and treatment. The duty is not, however, absolute, as confidentiality may be breached under certain special circumstances. It must be remembered that unauthorized disclosure of information about a patient without that patient's consent is not a criminal offence, but it does expose a doctor to disciplinary procedures by the General Medical Council. Disclosure may involve matters of public interest, particularly where the patient may provide a risk of damage or violence to the public or her immediate relatives.

AIDS and HIV infection are not notifiable by Statute, although the General Medical Council in the UK advises that doctors 'should make every effort to persuade a patient of the need for their General Practitioners and sexual partners to be informed of a positive diagnosis'.

There are some acts of disclosure which are compulsory by law, and these include:

1. Notification of births and deaths
2. Notification of a termination of pregnancy
3. Notification of a treatment cycle in in vitro fertilization
4. Notification of artificial insemination by donor.

THE ABORTION ACT 1967

The Abortion Act 1967 radically changed the nature and availability of medical termination of pregnancy in the UK, and had the effect of both legalizing and liberalizing abortion.

Under the present law, termination of pregnancy may be performed under the following four conditions:

1. That the pregnancy has not exceeded its 24th week and that the continuance of the pregnancy would involve greater risk than if the pregnancy were terminated, of injury to the physical or mental health of the pregnant woman or any existing children of her family
2. That the termination is necessary to prevent grave permanent injury to the physical or mental health of the pregnant woman
3. That the continuance of the pregnancy would involve risk to the life of the pregnant woman greater than if the pregnancy were terminated
4. That there is a substantial risk that if the child were born it would suffer from physical or mental abnormalities as to be seriously handicapped.

Under the conditions of the Act, the decision to terminate a pregnancy must be agreed by two practitioners unless the practitioner 'is of the opinion formed in good faith, that the termination is immediately necessary to save the life or to prevent grave permanent injury to the physical or mental health of the pregnant woman'.

Termination of pregnancy must be carried out in a hospital vested in the Secretary of State for the purposes of his functions under the National Health Services Act 1977. In other words, premises must be licensed for the purpose of termination of pregnancy.

Notification is also a statutory requirement, firstly of the intention to perform an abortion and secondly of the actual termination and any complications during or after the event. It is, perhaps, difficult to understand why so much emphasis is still laid on notification where the Act itself is very liberal and in the context of a legal framework that does not require notification of sterilization – a procedure that has far greater implications for social planning.

THE HUMAN FERTILISATION AND EMBRYOLOGY ACT

This Act was first introduced in 1990, and provides the Statutory Authority that regulates all matters relating to assisted reproduction. The Act is long and complex, but should be read by all personnel involved in these procedures. The Act is administered by the Human Fertilisation and Embryology Authority, which consists of:

1. A Chairman and Deputy Chairman
2. Such numbers of other members as the Secretary of State appoints.

This Authority has the following duties:

1. To keep under review information about embryos and any subsequent development of embryos and about the provision of treatment services and activities governed by this Act, and advise the Secretary of State, if he asks it to do so, about these matters
2. Publicise the services provided to the public by the Authority or provided in pursuance of licences
3. Provide, to such extent as it considers appropriate, advice and information for persons to whom licences apply or who are receiving treatment services or providing gametes or embryos for use for the purposes of activities governed by this Act, or may wish to do so
4. Perform such other functions as may be specified in the regulations.

Overall, the Human Fertilisation and Embryology Authority has the power to licence and supervise centres providing assisted reproduction and to decide which particular procedures shall be acceptable within the terms of reference of the Act. It also has wide-ranging powers under the Clinical Law including, under Warrant, the rights to enter premises 'using such force as is reasonably necessary' to take possession which may be required as evidence of breech of the law and to take steps necessary to preserve such evidence.

BIBLIOGRAPHY

Chamberlain G V P (ed) 1992 How to avoid medico-legal problems in obstetrics and gynaecology, 2nd edn. RCOG, London

Clements R V 1994 Safe practice in obstetrics and gynaecology. A medico-legal handbook. Churchill Livingstone, Edinburgh

Index

Essential Obstetrics and Gynaecology

Benjamin Black

Barts & The London

To my family

For Churchill Livingstone:

Publisher: Timothy Horne
Project Editor: Janice Urquhart
Copy Editor: Rich Cutler
Indexer: Helen McKillop
Project Controller: Nancy Arnott
Design Direction: Erik Bigland